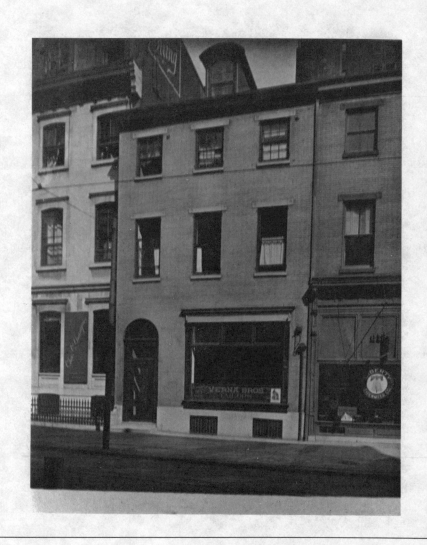

913 Walnut Street
1891

An Informal History
of

W. B. SAUNDERS
COMPANY

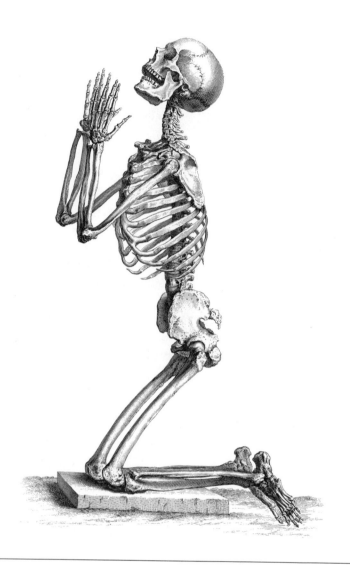

This is an illustration from the great
Cheselden OSTEOGRAPHIA (1733),
republished by Saunders in 1968 with foolhardy courage
and splendid elegance.
It depicts an editor who has wasted away in prayerful waiting
for manuscript from a dilatory author.
But others say it is an author who has pined away while
attending proof from his procrastinative publisher.

An Informal History
of
W. B. SAUNDERS
COMPANY

On the Occasion of
Its Hundredth Anniversary

by John L. Dusseau
Retired Vice President and Editor

1988
W. B. SAUNDERS COMPANY
Harcourt Brace Jovanovich Inc.
Philadelphia, London, Toronto, Montreal, Tokyo, Sydney

W. B. SAUNDERS COMPANY
Harcourt Brace Jovanovich, Inc.

West Washington Square
Philadelphia, PA 19105

Library of Congress Cataloging-in-Publication Data

Dusseau, John L.

An informal history of the W. B. Saunders Company on the
occasion of its hundredth anniversary/by John L. Dusseau.

p. cm.

ISBN 0–7216–2801–X

1. W. B. Saunders Company—History.   2. Medical
publishing—Pennsylvania—Philadelphia—History.
3. Publishers and publishing—Pennsylvania—Philadelphia—
History.   4. —Philadelphia (Pa.) Imprints—
History.   I. Title.

Z473.W2D87   1988

070.5'09748'11—dc19   87–35444
                                                        CIP

THE W. B. SAUNDERS COMPANY: An Informal History   ISBN 0–7216–2801–X

*This book is dedicated
to all who wrote for
and worked for Saunders.
They were not always right
in either action or judgment,
but they strove to be.*

PREFACE

Anniversaries are the occasion not only for celebration but for the pleasure of nostalgic remembrance of things past—no doubt a form of ancestor worship—evident in the formal histories of several distinguished publishing houses. Generally, these commemorate particular slight events and particular small triumphs. This is not the objective of this history. It hopes, rather, to set out the principles of publishing as perceived and carried out by Saunders. Observation, rather than recording, is its purpose. Very few picnics, new buildings, relocations, ceremonial dinners, fires and awards will appear here. Instead, authors and their work and the long, tortuous path to publication will be the object of scrutiny. It is also hoped that this book may cast a small ray of light into the jostle of ideas and the flow of thought that have made contemporary medicine an instrument of hope.

When Orlando, the centuries-spanning hero-heroine of Virginia Woolf's fantasy, stands on a balcony overlooking Johnson's London, she observes: "All was light, order and serenity." But then a small cloud appears over St. Paul's. It gradually diffuses, grows black and soon covers the city. "All was dark; all was doubt; all was confusion. The eighteenth century was over; the nineteenth century had begun." At the time of Saunders seventy-fifth anniversary, it was possible to look back upon order and serenity; but already a small cloud had appeared over publishing, once the pursuit of right words but becoming the pursuit of right numbers—a goal marked by a tasteless but revealing term, "the bottom line."

But all is not dark, doubt and confusion. There are still today many publishing houses trying to achieve excellence in their books and intelligent handling of authors and their precious ware. Saunders is one of these houses, and the design of this history is to recall the elements of the past that continue to be necessary lodestones of the present.

J.L.D.

APPRECIATION

So many people have assisted in the preparation of this book that I am forced to the distasteful expedient of simply listing their names. But of these many, four have been unusually generous in the gift of time and thought. They are Paul Beeson, Al Meier, Bob Rowan and Lew Reines. Each has read all or large chunks of the manuscript and offered astute commentary on it. If the published book abounds in the customary clichés of publishing, this is due to tone deafness in its author, not to imperception in its critics.

I have reached the age where was becomes nearer than is, so I am especially grateful to Al Meier—and believe readers will be too—for his writing the section of the book on the ambiguous present; and Bob Rowan has written a splendid brief chapter on marketing—an activity whose maneuvers I admire but whose principles are veiled from me. In my own writing I have drawn upon many published accounts and have unobtrusively cited them in appropriate places. If credit is not always paid, I shall take comfort in an observation by Lang Parsons—most honest and forthright of authors—that to steal from one source is plagiarism, to steal from many research.

The list that follows fails by its very abruptness to express the deep sense of obligation I feel to each of these persons:

Susan Alon	John J. Hanley
Margaret Bloom	A. McGehee Harvey
George W. Brauckman	Carl Katila
Eugene Braunwald	Claire Brackman Keane
Francesco Cordasco	Ronald W. Lamont-Havers
Donna Ciccotelli	John N. Loeb
Judy D. Cottrell	Nancy Gray Luxon
Richard A. Davis	Marian McDermott
Helen Dietz	Judith Miller
James Eckman	Polly Morrice
Don W. Fawcett	Waldo E. Nelson
Sara A. Finnegan	Lynn Perkins
Jack Goellner	Robert G. Petersdorf
Arthur C. Guyton	Stanley L. Robbins
Ferenc Gyorgyey	David E. Rogers
Hazel Hacker	Sharon Romm

David C. Sabiston, Jr.   Irma Sway
Dorothy Saunders   Theodore vanden Beemt
John T. Scott   Evelyn Weiman
Lloyd H. Smith, Jr.   James B. Wyngaarden

Like other books of reminiscence, this one may well have had more readers in preparation than it will in publication. Four who read it with understanding care and helpful suggestion are Lorraine Kilmer, its skilled designer; Carolyn Naylor, its mother-hen production supervisor; Elizabeth J. Taylor, its indulgent editor; and my wife Sheila, its faithful partisan.

I can no other answer make but thanks,
And thanks.

Twelfth Night

J. L. D.

x

CONTENTS

PART I PERSPECTIVE

1 *The Argument* 3

2 *Author and Publisher* 7

3 *Writer and Editor* 11

PART II PUBLISHING

4 *Origins* 17

5 *John B. Murphy, Theodore Roosevelt and the Saunders Company* 27

6 *Artist and Book* 41

7 *The Todd-Sanford Clinical Diagnosis by Laboratory Methods: The Story of a Specialty* 47

8 *Admiral Rozhestvensky Charts the Course of a Textbook: The Maximow-Bloom-Fawcett Histology* 51

9 *The Cecil Textbook of Medicine: Its Six Editors* 59

10 *The Christopher Textbook of Surgery and Book Writing in Chicago* 83

11 *Rochester, Minneapolis and Boston: Serendipity* 89

12 *Hopkins and Saunders: A School and an Artist* 101

13 *Nelson's Textbook of Pediatrics: The Green Bible* 109

14 *Conn Current Therapy: Saunders at Work* 113

15 *The Kinsey Report: A House Divided* 123

16 *Friedberg and Braunwald: The Heart of the Matter* 141

17 *Robbins and Guyton: Two Authors and Their Ways* 145

18 *Nursing Education: An Encyclopedia/Dictionary of Nursing and Its Genesis* 151

19 *The Selling of Saunders Books* 157
    by Robert B. Rowan

20 *Beyond Philadelphia* 167

PART III   PROGRESS AND PICTURES 173

PART IV   THE PRESENT

21 *A Decade of Change* 243
    by Albert E. Meier

POSTLOGUE 261

INDEX OF NAMES 263

PART I
PERSPECTIVE

Because it deals with the vital interests of individuals and societies—with life and death, and with so much that matters in between—medicine has long had an unusually complex and intimate relationship to cultural and social developments at large. Medical history involves social and economic as well as biologic content and presents one of the central themes in human experience. After all, what is more basic in the life of any people than life itself?

Richard H. Shryock

1

The Argument

A hundred years, even of survival, is a respectable length of time; and much of what we think of as modern progress emerged in the past ten decades. In the last quarter of this century the world of publishing has changed almost as much as the world itself.

The fact of change suggests that we think about where we have been and where we are, that we consider the nature of the book—what it is and what it may become. The technical or teaching book is an ancient and useful device for the storage and retrieval of information that has certain distinct advantages over more mechanical means. Above all, it can readily be consulted, either for isolated pieces of information or for a contemplative review of ideas. The book, too, has a certain luxury of presentation. A reference text in physiology may use information from physics and chemistry not as a formal expression of those disciplines but as subtle adaptation to the concept of function. A book can also afford to give a reserved answer, whereas the machine must deal in certainties; and nothing is more fatal to science or medicine than absolute certainty. Finally, the book can be read with pleasure. Gibbon's *Decline and Fall of the Roman Empire* is a ponderous work of erudition, but it is also one of the great delights of the English language. Felicity of expression too makes medical ideas memorable and compelling. How vividly the simplest words may stir the mind. Even to say the phrase "Addison's disease" is to summon up a vision of the long story of exploration of diseases of the ductless glands and of disturbances of chemical equilibrium and of how Addison's great monograph on the subject was regarded in its day as a trivial medical curiosity.

At about the time Saunders was getting started, the incomparable Sarah Bernhardt was playing Cleopatra on the London stage to sellout audiences. In her final scene she stabbed to death the slave who brought her news of Mark Antony's defeat at Actium. She stormed, raved, wrecked the scenery in her frenzy and, finally, as the curtain fell, dropped to the stage in a shuddering, wailing, convulsive heap. Tumultuous applause always greeted this performance and once, as it died down, a British matron was heard to say to her neighbor, "How different, how *very* different, from the home life of our own dear Queen Victoria."

How very different the brave new world of publishing threatens to be. Behind the attraction of electronic storage, retrieval and communication of knowledge is the curious notion that knowledge has somehow outstripped man's capacity to assimilate it. That man can create what he cannot understand seems at best a dubious proposition. But, more important, there is at the heart of this naive belief in the might of the machine not only the powerful force of laziness but subconscious belief in magic. Men will always seek some button to press to obtain wisdom, some mumbo jumbo to achieve salvation. The magic we must work is neither in mystic numbers nor in machines, only in the capacity to think hard and well.

The intellect can truly function only amidst a welter of data, a profusion of conflicting concepts and the manifold persuasions of beautifully marshaled and sometimes unconsciously skewed documentation. Richness of thought is our only resource that can be mined for so long as man endures. Those who call for its hedging and hoarding undervalue its power. How often the complaint is heard that too much is published. That it all must be digested, abstracted, assimilated, coded for usefulness. No charge could be farther from the truth.

The attempt to overedit, overselect, oversimplify and overabstract the product of the mind and to underuse the mind itself must result in a destructive statism of science. Surely, much that is published is drivel, but to drive out the eccentric and the strange and the seemingly unacceptable may be to drive out genius. Lewis Thomas, the Biology Watcher, advises us on this point:

> The real surprises, which set us back on our heels when they occur, will always be the mutants. We have already had a few of these, sweeping across the field of human thought periodically, like comets. They have slightly different receptors for the information cascading in from other minds, and slightly different machinery for processing it, so that what comes out to rejoin the flow is novel, and filled with new sorts of meaning. . . . What we need is more crowding, more unrestrained and obsessive communication, more open channels, even more noise, and a bit more luck.

The information-storing machine can be the instrument of only established doctrine: but fashions of the mind and spirit and even the shapes of truth do change. In the seventeenth century the Chancellor of Cambridge, Dr. John Lightfoot, culminated years of meticulous study in his announcement that "heaven and earth, center and circumference, were created all together, in the same instant, and this work took place and man was created by the Trinity on October 23, 4004 B.C., at nine o'clock in the morning." Lightfoot could not have known that on the very morning before the hour he so precisely specified, a highly cultivated people, and one well equipped to savor the achievements of science, crowded the great cities of Egypt, all unaware that their world had not yet been created.

In one vision of a changed future, books of course will not disappear; but they will take on a character quaint and ornamental. The library will be a cunning contrivance of tangled tape and circumambient circuitry. In this technological rat's nest will be an antiquarian alcove containing a few ancient

4

examples of the bookmaking art and perhaps even a stuffed editor reminiscent of Jeremy Bentham, who can still be seen seated behind his desk in a closet of the University of London. And the learned journal? It too will depart. The physician and the biomedical scientist will subscribe not to a journal but to a push-button answering service. And the answering service will give back the abstracted views of the contemporary Chancellor of Cambridge, Dr. John Lightfoot.

The new era will mean that the voice of the author and the voice of the editor will be stilled. In their place will be a placid corps of MBA's—all nicely gotten up, intelligent, industrious and profoundly ignorant of the nature and purposes of books. The life of the mind will have become the life of the machine. But this is a vision that may not be realized, and the book may survive as depository of information and source of knowledge.

2

Author and Publisher

All these editorial blokes, I understand, get pretty careworn after they've been on the job for a while.
                                                    Wodehouse: *Very Good, Jeeves*

What distinguished the formative years of the Saunders Company was faith in the writer and confidence in the editor, the latter not always easy to maintain but fortified by the commanding presence and perceptive understanding of Ryland Greene and by the powerful examples of Maxwell Perkins, Bennett Cerf, Harold Ross and Alfred and Blanche Knopf. This is not to say that intelligent management and effective marketing did not play significant roles in the success of Saunders, but underlying them was the realization that splendid books can be neither found nor written by astute managers.

The late Adlai Stevenson used to delight in the Talmudic legend that in man's history the heavens themselves are held in place by the virtue and shining integrity of twelve just men. They are totally unaware of this function and go about their daily work, their humble tasks—as teachers, workers, farmers (never, alas, editors)—and meanwhile the rooftree of creation is supported by them alone.

The publisher may not always appreciate that the heavenly effort of publication is supported by the author, who all unknowingly keeps in motion the celestial dynamics of book creation and provides the very sun under which publisher and bookseller alike flourish.

If this be oversight, there is reason for it. As L. Quincy Mumford has observed, the creation of a book is a tripartite affair. The author, whose ideas move in inky symbols across the page, says: The book is mine. The artist, who gives vivid life to the author's words and combines them in patterns of new insight, says: This is my book. The publisher, who weaves together the work of author and artist into a meaningful fabric of beautiful and understandable simplicity, says, too: This work is mine. But in the instance of the *scientific* book, the publisher is but performing his professional duty and but earning his livelihood in the work he does. The author in his writing is alone in not performing a professional task. His profession is that

7

of physician or biologist or mathematician; his writing is work like that of the twelve just men who support the firmament—an extra function.

There is no alternative to an editor's dangerous avowal of faith in the author—faith that, by Scriptural definition, is the sum of things hoped for and the evidence of things unseen. Any authors reading here will know only too well how often the editor's faith rests indeed on the evidence of things unseen. Things seen have not always been regarded as essential to truth. In the ninth century the Bishop of Ravenna prepared a great history of the Church, and had this to say in his preface:

> Where I have not found any history of these bishops and have not been able, by conversation with aged men or inspection of the monuments or from any other authentic sources, to obtain information concerning them, in such a case, in order that there might not be a break in the series, I have composed the life myself, with the help of God and the prayers of the brethren.

When Saunders was coming of age, the image of the physician was indissolubly connected with a stone home on a corner lot. On the driveway before its two-car garage stood a Buick automobile. These are symbols of solidity and stability. It was in those days quite safe to sustain some kind of medical emergency past 4:30 in the afternoon. The physician was a central figure of community life. He presided at birth, presided at the miracle of healing and presided at death.

For many complex and good reasons that image has changed. The mind of medicine has moved from the patient's bedside to the laboratory bench. This move has meant a thousand-fold increase in medicine's effectiveness, but it has also meant a new kind of impersonal medicine.

But, of course, the physician is no less a person than ever he was. One of the great pleasures of publishing medical books is to see in the creative process of writing the intense individuality of the physician-writer. A great deal of the best writing is still done on the kitchen table at midnight. Such writing is done without computers and without a team of experts. The author is equipment and team all in one. This is because his motivation is the lonely but compelling one of creation.

If the impulse to write is a whim, it is a whim of iron. One thinks back upon that rhapsodic romantic, Dante Gabriel Rossetti, who upon the suicide of his beautiful young wife impulsively tossed into her grave as an act of desperate penance the only manuscripts of much of his recent writing. Later he had her dug up and published the poems.

The book then, comes from within, within the writer's mind, within the reader's mind. If it is a fine book, we may say of it that it is the outward and visible sign of inward and spiritual reality—a reality that is at once dedication and hope.

Above all, the author must be industrious. He must have that capacity for sustained, incredible work that all have seen and at which all must marvel. His industry must spring from a sense of devotion, but this must be a balanced zeal, not an unreasoning fanaticism. In fine, the author's sense of dedication must be a scientific avowal, not a self-confirmed appointment. It must consider facts, but be aware of the relative nature of truth.

The author, too, must see himself and his work as going on timelessly and as overriding all ordinary and human difficulties. There are enough people to attend to the usual concerns of the world. Someone must attend to writing and someone else to the delicate sensibilities, the confusing unreality and the rare endowment of the author.

In his fine survey of William H. Welch's influence on modern medicine, Donald Fleming thus reviews the history of the teaching book. Hellenistic Alexandria saw the birth of what we now recognize as the textbook in science. It came into being as a recognition of the fact that the advance of science requires the forming of a consensus of expert opinion, a consensus intended not to repress innovation but to create general acceptance of the current status of knowledge as a springboard for further advance. It is this notion of the necessary expert consensus and of the equal necessity for its authoritative formulation that gave rise to the textbook in the broadest meaning of that term.

Thereafter, the pursuit of the scientific consensus never ceased, and with the understanding of its necessity arose the notion of the almost sacred character of the book: the book that represents the best of which the author is capable, the considered account of contemporary knowledge. The book then, as it concerns the reader, the writer, the editor, is the record and explanation of scientific knowledge by an expert mind, acknowledged to be an authority, hence an author.

What then is put down—accurately, precisely and wisely—as the truth springing from acute observation of specific circumstances will itself never change and will always have value. It is only the circumstances that will change and so create not a larger truth but a different truth.

And yet there is danger, too, in the very notion of the scientific consensus. It can become authoritarianism; editors, referees, site visitors and grantors of funds can become commissars of science, together standing like an embattled Maginot Line against every imaginable or unimaginable change in the scientific status or advance in human thought.

There is no rule that says arrogance cannot be combined with genius in the acknowledged authorities of science. One has only to think of the tragic figure of Ignaz Semmelweis, who not only found the means to prevent childbed fever but also recognized it as septicemia. There can be little question that his madness and death were mediated by the charges of charlatanism leveled against him by the orthodox Viennese obstetricians of his day.

Not only may new truth arise, but circumstances and fashions of the mind change too. As George Bernard Shaw has observed, the mystic, calculating the number of angels that can be accommodated on the point of a needle, is now Sir Almroth Wright, computing the number of streptococci contained in a specific volume of serum. Somehow, sevens and angels are out of fashion, while billions and streptococci are all the rage. This is not to say that either calculation is ridiculous, or that either is not, within its own frame of reference, a legitimate search for truth. Both sets of ideas stretch credulity; both rest for their acceptance on the authority of a writer. Very few of those who believe these data have seen either the angels or the streptococci. The achievement of truth rests on the scientist; its expression rests upon the writer. Ideally, they are the same man.

The scientific consensus is a necessity—but like all necessities it not only may, it sometimes must, be discarded and shattered. What editor would not wish to have the wisdom, courage and foresight to have published Harvey, Vesalius, Newton or Morgagni, whose lives were given to the destruction of the established consensus? The message they give us is not that we should reason together but that we should reason separately. Lord Rutherford put it nicely: "Every good laboratory consists of first-rate men working in great harmony to ensure the progress of science; but down the hall is an unsociable, wrong-headed fellow working on unprofitable lines, and in his hands lies the hope of discovery."

The dream of the editor is not the vision of beautiful copy or the product of bland orthodoxy. It is, rather, the dream of the great book—the timeless and classic contribution. There are always enough capable compilers—there are never enough great writers either in fiction or in science. Small as is the supply of truth, it has never been exceeded by demand.

Perhaps it is possible to exaggerate the delicate sensibility of the author. Joseph Wechsberg provides a mild corrective: "The intimate memoirs of sensitive writers convey the impression that they were extremely vulnerable—susceptible to cold stares and cold drafts—human mimosae. In point of fact, most writers are hard crabs underneath their soft shells. They have to be tough and resilient to function at all."

However impressive and elegant are sound scholarship, richness of erudition and originality of thought, they are not a wholly satisfactory substitute for the ability to swim in rough waters. In life, in medicine, in science, even in publishing there are plenty of situations in which the waters are indeed rough; and often the editor must exercise a calming and moderating influence. He should have too the happy knack of fostering the productive capacity of authors and of enhancing the exercise of their creative powers. Perhaps this is a role played less through participation than through protection; but in any event the happiest moment of the publisher's life is the first glimpse of a truly superb published work in whose realization he may consider himself to have played a small part.

3

Writer and Editor

There is with us not only a mythic attachment to the word but nothing less than assignment of sublimity to the *right* word. "A thing said walks in immortality if it has been said well." The writer is the inspired maker of words, and the editor is their keeper.

The first requirement for teaching, learning and communication by scientists and professional persons is the existence of an agreed-upon vocabulary of terms. The first and vital step in understanding any discipline is mastery of its language. The editor plays a part, albeit modest, in enforcing a necessary stability of language. Although an editor may have authority, he may not pretend to dictate. The language of science, or any language for that matter, has not descended to us in a state of uniformity and perfection. Johnson put this ambivalence bluntly in the preface to his *Dictionary of the English Language*: "I am not yet so lost in lexicography as to forget that *words are the daughters of earth, and that things are the sons of heaven*. Language is only the instrument of science, and words are but the signs of ideas. I wish, however, that the instrument might be less apt to decay and that signs might be permanent, like the things which they denote."

Language has always been subject not only to growth and decay but to vagaries of taste and to whimsicality. "When I use a word," Humpty Dumpty said in a rather scornful tone, "it means just what I choose it to mean—neither more nor less." "The question is," said Alice, "whether you can make words mean so many different things." "The question is," said Humpty Dumpty, "which is to be master—that's all."

Humpty is telling us that the great secret of good speech and fine writing is *command* of language—something neither readily taught nor easily learned but which forges images forever engraved on the mind. "I dress the wound," said Ambroise Paré; "God heals it." "Wounds," said John Hunter, "have a tendency to heal."

Early in his career a young Saunders editor was commissioned to visit a distinguished French publishing house to discuss what seemed an unsound situation. The French publisher was still trying to bring out a translation of the fifteenth edition of the *Howell-Fulton Textbook of Physiology*, although in the meantime two later editions had been published. The purpose of the visit was simply to persuade abandonment of 15 and taking up of 17. Faltering French was sufficient to convey this message; and the Gallic managing director thoughtfully considered it and its attendant cost. He cleared his throat preparatory to decision. "We shall continue," he said, "with the fifteenth edition; for physiology—it does not change." He was, of course, right—physiology does not indeed change—only our understanding of it, of its vocabulary, so to speak.

Precise words are a hallmark of the novels of Ivy Compton-Burnett. Sometime after her death, beneath the sofa cushions on which she had awaited death, was found the manuscript of her final unrevised novel, *The Last and the First*. In it when the put-upon young Heriots and Grimstones meet for tea, a minor Heriot says, "We have been looking forward to the day." A Grimstone replies, "We would have done so, but the faculty has faded through lack of use."

Unlike the Grimstones, an editor spends his working editorial life in constant high expectation. Scarcely a week goes by when he does not hope to publish a work of distinction and value. This is both the challenge and reward of publishing. If the editor cannot feel enthusiasm for his authors and their writing, who then will? An editor should take great personal pride in his list of books and in the innovative ideas of his authors, for not everyone will appreciate fresh approaches to old material. Consider the lengthy review of the first edition of Gray's *Anatomy: Descriptive and Surgical*. Its beginning strikes but the opening chords in a crashing crescendo:

> It is a serious thing to review a book like this of Mr. Gray's. One sits down to the task with the oppressive feeling of sadness which comes over a man when he has seen a wrong done, when he finds the occasion of such wrong has been unnecessarily sought for, and that the ill deed is after all ill done. It is grievous not so much to do what is fitting under such circumstances, as to come in contact with such a necessity; especially when it compels us to turn reproachfully upon one whose first essay deserved and received our commendation.
>
> Mr. Gray has published a book that was not wanted. It is low and unscientific in tone; and it has been compiled, for the most part, in a manner inconsistent with the professions of honesty which we find in the preface. Mr. Gray has worked without fairly appreciating the intellectual condition and requirements of the present race of Medical students. A more unphilosophical amalgam of crude anatomical details and crude Surgery we never met with. Mr. Gray rests contented with such unalloyed descriptions of parts that must be crammed for examination, or that may be cut in operations, as would be welcomed by a college of Barber surgeons. Where was the need for this? Elementary books we must have; but let them be the first rounds of a scaling ladder, not the useless ledges of a treadmill. [*Medical Times & Gazette* (March 5, 1859). First two paragraphs only—mercifully somewhat shortened.]

A publishing house is a few people and a body of ideas. The few people that count are those who manage its product, and the ideas that count are those that bring freshness and imagination to books. Editorial creativity and excitement will endure so long as editors may speak and act in the name of excellence and usefulness in writing—rather than in the name of strategy, as if strategy were some disembodied capacity to sell any product, whether shoddy or superb.

That great architect and builder, Mies van der Rohe, once said, "God is in the details." And so it is with publishing. Corporate exhortations to make more money no doubt serve some purpose; but they have no relationship to effective publishing, whose heart is careful attention to detail. What makes the good book better and gives every book a look and feeling appropriate to its character and purposes is the firm handling of a multitude of details. Editorial work does not consist of taking manuscripts out of envelopes and giving them to someone else to worry over.

One frequently hears from some aspiring author that he has important things to say but doesn't know how to say them. This is essential nonsense. Incomprehensible and disorderly writing arises not from inability to write but from the simple circumstance that the writer has nothing to say. Such work cannot be patched up, for the process of writing is identical with the process of thought. If the latter is vapid and disorganized, so will be the former. This is why first-rate physicians and scientists are unfailingly good writers. Clarity begins at home.

Everyone knows what an editor should be: He should be capable of imagination and of independent judgment. He should not be uncritically excited by every prospect that comes his way; he should know how to evaluate teaching effectiveness and writing skill. Editorial aggressiveness and editorial sheen are part of good performance; but underlying the push and patina must be solid intellectual perception—above all, perception of the worth of fine writing, of sound science, and of honest endeavor.

In the increasingly sophisticated and disillusioned life of Western man, there still persist about the elegantly written and eloquently spoken word those autochthonous elements of wonder and pleasure deriving from our primal sense of the numinous in all things. In the finest writing one has a feeling of infusion by a spirit creative and perceptive—a spirit significant to the structure of life and pervading the whole domain of culture and intellect.

The Saunders Company has always been aware that the care of words is an awesome care. In the 1940s it hired Lloyd G. Potter away from the Mayo Clinic to become Associate Editor and later Vice President and Editor. One of his immediate acts was to create the first true Editorial Department of any American medical publishing house—a department charged not with the procurement of manuscripts but with their expert refinement toward clarity, accuracy and intelligibility. The polishing of diamonds and of words is costly, but a necessity in the pursuit of excellence. Saunders authors too learned from gentle redaction. Soon several were able to distinguish between foreword and forward; but there persisted dear to the heart of a favorite author the phrase "Low and behold." Lord Beaverbrook did not fully understand the process. "You know," he said, "we have a system. I speak at this end and there is a machine at the other end and it comes out as a leading article." Only a Britannic peer could waive the rules of writing. Whatever the artful ingenuity of Beaverbrook's machine, it cannot capture the beauty that is eloquence of the mind.

Of course, rules are meant to be broken, else the sun would still be revolving around the earth. E. B. White was a soft-spoken iconoclast who distrusted the rules of writing, especially that prohibiting a terminal preposition. He delighted in the story of the father going upstairs to read to his little son but accidentally bringing along the wrong book. "What," the boy asks, "did you bring the book that I don't want to be read to out of up for?" But then few are the sentences ending in five prepositions, but few too are those whose style and invention make sensible rules senseless.

The experience of editing can also be a humbling one. When Saunders brought out Jean Hamburger's elegant two-volume *Nephrology*, its translation was done by Anthony Walsh, a scholarly urologist of fine-honed Irish temperament, who worked away at his formidable task with dutiful zeal and fine-tuned prose. However, as with many big books, the nearer it got to publication, the farther behind schedule it fell. At last Walsh sent in the final batch of manuscript; but the editor noticed on looking through it that four manuscript pages were unaccountably missing. Obeying an ancient adage, he seized time by the forelock and translated the missing pages himself. The book was published to pleasant success and critical praise, Gus Dammin, Pathologist-in-Chief at the Peter Bent Brigham Hospital, paying it a nice Boston tribute. "Its textual citations and its references," he said, "recognize judiciously the work done at Harvard." The editor, then, visited Tony Walsh in Dublin with a sense of pride in shared accomplishment. "Yes," said Walsh, "it was a good experience all the way except for one curious episode. As I neared the end of galley reading I ran across one passage of such inexact translation and inept style that I thought I must have dozed off in writing it. Then I noticed that its four pages of manuscript were not done on my typewriter. How in the world," he asked, "could such a thing happen?"

"I cannot," said his listener, "imagine how it could happen."

In the worlds of science and writing, equanimity is not always easily come by. In a curious memoir, Mrs. Osler—perhaps whimsically, perhaps wistfully—said of the great physician-writer: "It was all very well of William to preach Aequanimitas, but I noticed that when there was trouble at home he invariably had important engagements elsewhere and left me to cultivate the quiet mind—if I could."

PART II

PUBLISHING

Morgagni's life was uneventful, that of a man of science who lives remote from the world of affairs. His hours were filled with conscientious teaching, indefatigable labours in the dissecting-room, consultations, and an extensive correspondence with his professional colleagues. There did not yet exist an abundance of periodicals eager to publish the most trifling observations, to make the most seemingly inconspicuous ideas widely known. In the eighteenth century, an investigator who believed himself to have discovered something new began its dissemination by communicating with his colleagues, subjecting his observations to their criticisms. A letter of the kind, swelled to the size of a monograph, was read aloud in a friendly circle, was passed from hand to hand, gave rise to discussion and to control-experiments. There was no thought of publication until matters had ripened. The letters exchanged by the scholars of those days are stimulating reading. They give us a lively impression of the workshops of research. People disclose their personality much more freely in letters than in printed publications. If we know the history and biography of learned men of the eighteenth century better than those of their fellows belonging to earlier epochs, this is because of the innumerable letters which have been preserved in manuscript, and some of them in print.

Henry E. Sigerist

4

Origins

The history of almost all scientific publishing houses is comparatively ancient and genuinely honorable. That of the Saunders Company shares this pleasant character. The house was founded on March 4, 1888, and hence is sufficiently old to feel the force of a past tradition of gentlemanliness in publishing in which an amateur's love of books played a greater role than an accountant's regard for favorable balance sheets.

The founder of the business was Walter Burns Saunders, one of several children of an impoverished cleric. He and a brother had heeded the sage advice of the times and gone West and unaccountably managed to salvage a bale of cotton from the storm-swollen Mississippi River. With his half of the proceeds from this windfall young Walter Burns went into the second-hand book business.

It soon dawned on the youthful bookseller that selling individual copies of individual books wasn't as profitable as selling thousands of copies of the same book. He decided to become a publisher of medical books. A charming story has it that his wife Louise—with a fine disregard for practical realities— used her own modest savings to stake him to his first publishing venture.

The physical beginnings of the house were small—scarcely 1,000 square feet of floor space at 33 South 10th Street, Philadelphia. This location was selected because of its nearness to Jefferson Medical College and Hospital. Later moves brought the location virtually across the street from Jefferson, from which the publisher got its early authors.

Why did Walter Saunders go into medical publishing? Fundamentally, of course, as a business venture; but behind his decision was sound knowledge acquired from the used books he handled and sometimes read. The late nineteenth century witnessed great advances in medicine with the promise of other forward strides in the offing. Bernard's elucidation of the mechanisms of blood supply; Ludwig's invention of the kymograph; Virchow's conception of the function of white blood corpuscles; Hertz's demonstration of electromagnetic waves—the basis of today's radio, radar and television— all of these and many others were making medical history, and the medical

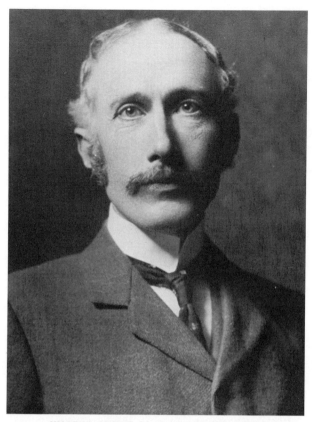

WALTER BURNS SAUNDERS (1859–1905)

He founded a company of like-minded men and women who believed in books, in the people who write them and in the people who read them.

profession was seeking definitive knowledge of them and their uses in preventive and curative medicine. Saunders recognized this urgency and did something about it. He laid down three principles for his venture, but they are the commonplace ones of all publishers. A difference may have been that he not only enunciated them, he paid them some heed. Here are the guideposts he set himself:

1. Authors must be leaders and authorities actually doing the things about which they wrote.

2. Prompt service must be afforded in getting books to customers.

3. Books must be produced to meet the highest standards of the book craftsman's art.

It is interesting evidence of Saunders' belief in these principles that he had scarcely begun publishing when he bought a printing press, so that books bearing his imprint might be well and handsomely produced. It was a repossessed machine of some years, and the tiny premises could not properly accommodate it so that its flatbed had to shuttle in and out of an open window as it printed. Presumably the "pressroom" closed in the coldest weather.

In November of 1892, W. D. Watson was hired by Saunders as an errand boy after some haggling over his demand for a salary of $2.00 a week (he was getting $1.76 at the law office of John Marshall Gest). He stayed for 60 years, becoming Executive Vice President and both familiarizing and concerning himself with every operation of the company. He liked to get in early each morning and zip quickly through piles of mail, thereby informing himself of practically everything. He was a busybody but a salutary one; his shrewdness as a manager kept the house on its steady course when Walter B. Saunders died suddenly in 1905 and it continually restrained unwise enthusiasms. Publishers, ever since the invention of movable type, have been known to harbor idle dreams.

Young Walter Saunders found soon enough that wanting to be a publisher was not quite the same thing as becoming one. The early days were bleak ones, and the handsome but elderly press had to be hocked in order to buy the paper on which to print books. His initial try was Hobart Amory Hare's *Quiz Compend of Physiology*—a question-and-answer book priced at $1.00. This was the first title of a series of twenty-four. These Quiz Compends sold well over 250,000 copies before they were discontinued because—and here

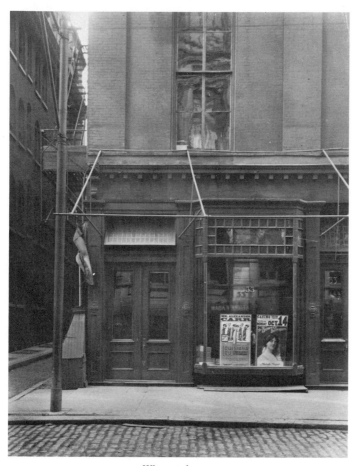

Where it began.

again their publisher showed his sagacity—they had become inadequate to include the advancing knowledge of a rapidly developing science of medicine. This famous "Blue Series," as they were called (bound in blue cloth with silver stamping), played an important part in establishing the Saunders name, particularly among medical students.

Another series, more pretentious in size and character, was begun. It was known as the Saunders Manual Series. The books in the series were written by leading physicians of the day—names that even now are spoken with profound respect. J. Chalmers DaCosta's *Surgery*, DeSchweinitz's *Diseases of the Eye* and other definitive texts appeared in this series.

In 1892 the Saunders Company published the first of the American Textbook Series. This was the *American Textbook of Surgery**—a collaborative work edited by two of the greatest surgeons of their day, if not of all time. They were W. W. Keen of Jefferson Medical College and J. William White of the University of Pennsylvania. This book sold 40,000 copies, a truly tremendous sale in those days. This first volume in the series was followed in 1894 by a two-volume work on the *Practice of Medicine* edited by William Pepper of the University of Pennsylvania, one of the outstanding teachers and clinical investigators in America at that time.

About the same time it became evident that the house not only was successful but—like all publishing houses, even today's—was understaffed and physically cramped for space. It moved to 925 Walnut Street. This was a four-story and basement building, the garret of which was the room occupied by the famous physician Chevalier Jackson, Sr., during his student days at Jefferson.

In this period printers of medical books in Germany were getting exceptional results with lithography. Saunders went to Europe to look into the matter and came back with a contract under which the Lehmann *Hand Atlases* were to be translated and published in English over the Saunders imprint. There were twenty of these *Hand Atlases*, all magnificently illustrated with the finest examples of German lithography. They covered the entire field of medicine and were immediately successful.

From this time on, leading medical teachers and authors looked to Saunders for their publishing. The names of John H. Musser, John B. Murphy, Isaac A. Abt, Nicholas Senn, J. Collins Warren, William H. Howell, Charles L. Scudder, Henry W. Stelwagon, Carl Huber, Howard A. Kelly, Thomas S. Cullen, Berkeley Moynihan, and a score of others rapidly appeared on the title pages of Saunders books.

What emerges from this sketchy picture is the courage with which the founder of the publishing house tackled vast programs. Translation, for example, of the ponderous multivolumed Nothnagel *System of Medicine* must

---

*This was to be followed by Keen's monumental eight-volume *Surgery*. In it Keen revealed for the first time the carefully kept secret of the surgery he performed on President Cleveland for cancer of the mandible. Definitive reference works of many volumes were to become a hallmark of the Saunders Company.

have been a venture requiring a rich store of fortitude, patience and money, and it was only the first two that Walter Burns Saunders could then command.

He had by now had sufficient experience in his chosen field to perceive that one of the nicer aspects of scientific publishing is that successful textbooks have a way of going on almost indefinitely. This conclusion was fortified by bringing Ryland W. Greene into the house as Editor.

Walter Burns Saunders died in 1905 and was succeeded in presidency of the company by his widow, Louise Baugh Saunders. Mrs. Saunders had neither office space nor specific managerial responsibilities, although in her capacity as owner she had the authority and power to participate in the company's affairs; but she suffered from almost complete deafness and communication with her was largely in writing. She did attend speech school and there met Dwight Hotchkiss, whom she invited into the Saunders Company, where he was to serve for forty years as Editor of the *Medical* and the *Surgical Clinics of North America* (see also page 201). Mrs. Saunders continued as titular president until 1936, when she was succeeded by her son Lawrence. In the thirty years of her successful stewardship she is said to have now and then opposed the suggestions of Executive Vice President W. D. Watson; but it is difficult to guess at the nature of these issues when the voices of discussion and dissent are stilled. She did place absolute confidence in the editorial judgment of Ryland Greene, the man her husband had brought into the business and his equal in courage and single-minded energy.

The great medical textbooks, many of which are still pillars of the present house, were begun by Ryland Greene. Among these was the Maximow and Bloom *Textbook of Histology*. Its First Edition was a resounding failure, partly because the world of medical science then did not understand tissue study as Alexander Maximow did. To publish an unsuccessful, expensive textbook may be more a mark of folly than of courage but to undertake a Second Edition of the same work can be reckoned the decision of only a rare combination of bravery, stubborn belief and shrewd perception, for from the very outset of what must have seemed a dubious Second Edition, Maximow and Bloom went on to become one of the most highly respected and widely used textbooks ever published in the field of bioscience, its influence and reputation extending throughout the world.

Greene made an important contribution to the Saunders Company not only as editor but also as author. He was the single-handed anonymous author of the *American Illustrated Medical Dictionary*. For the first edition and many editions thereafter authorship was credited to W. A. Newman Dorland, M.D.,* for Greene did not have the necessary doctorate in medicine. It now celebrates its eighty-eighth year in its Twenty-Seventh Edition, now known as Dorland's Illustrated Medical Dictionary and composed by computer from an entry file converted to magnetic tape. It is the largest-selling medical book

---

*It is certain that Dorland had nothing to do with preparation of the dictionary manuscript, but it is believed that he read with some care a complete set of galley proof of the first edition. He was then a member of the Committee on Nomenclature of the American Medical Association and had a natural interest in medical lexicography.

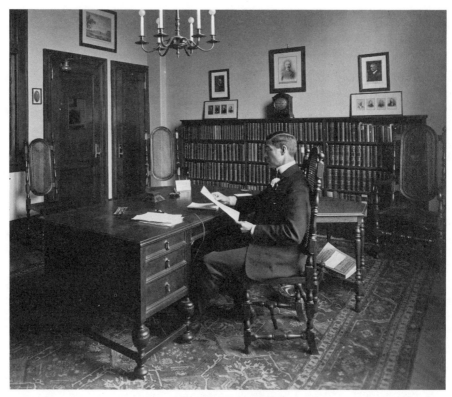

RYLAND W. GREENE

Perhaps the greatest scientific editor of all time, Ryland Greene left the Saunders Company a rich heritage of well-established successful textbooks. He ruled his domain and indeed the whole Saunders Company with an iron hand; but toward his authors he was unfailingly courteous and generous, for he knew from the experience of writing *Dorland's Medical Dictionary* that the way of authorship is a long and arduous one of many untoward turnings.

ever published. But the making of dictionaries is fraught with peril. In the interest of economy of space a later Saunders editor ruled that portraits should be deleted from the book—an order carried out so thoroughly that general paresis is no longer illustrated in the *Dictionary*.

In a roundabout way Ryland Greene also made a significant contribution to Lea & Febiger, an older and highly respected publisher, likewise situated on Washington Square, whose founder also promptly bought a press with the four hundred dollars the Marquis de LaFayette advanced in order that culture might take printed form in the newborn United States of America. In 1925 Saunders had published the first edition of William Boyd's *Surgical Pathology*—the beginning of a long and friendly relationship with a mildly iconoclastic, perpetually cigarette-smoking, and more-than-occasionally-martini-drinking Scotsman transported to Canada by allure of new and untried ways. He was actually trained in psychology but somehow persuaded the people at Winnipeg that he was a pathologist. When he first began work, he was dependent for his studies in anatomic pathology on cadavers imported, like himself, from the British Isles. They came preserved in malmsey, but, as he used to say with a sigh, "spoiled for drinking, you know." Neither cigarettes nor martinis nor constant work were to spoil his long life of thinking, teaching and writing or his complete enjoyment of it. Indeed, he inclined to believe that many seemingly wholesome medical admonitions spring more from puritanical bias than from solid research or human understanding.

One of the things Boyd richly enjoyed was the immediate success of his *Surgical Pathology*, and soon thereafter he completed his *Textbook of Pathology* and quite naturally brought it to Saunders, thereby posing a problem to Greene, for Saunders already published the great MacCallum textbook and had then a firm policy of not competing with its own authors. He therefore took Boyd by the hand—in the other the author anxiously clutched his manuscript—and walked him across the square to the offices of Lea & Febiger, who thus became the publisher of one of the most widely used, elegantly written and deeply cherished medical books ever written. It is said Van Antwerp Lea, dour senior partner of the house, was wont to say: "In five minutes the Saunders editor did more for Lea & Febiger than our own editor did in twenty-five years."

If one may subvert chronology and digress a little, it is possible to imagine that this episode had its unpleasant effect at Saunders, for the MacCallum was never again revised. Arnold Rich, distinguished Hopkins pathologist, took it on and realized after three years of work that he had succeeded in making countless revisions of MacCallum's first chapter but could not bring himself to that decisiveness of statement so necessary to textbook writing. Teaching may inquire; but it cannot be an endless debate.

Great editor though he was, Ryland Greene was no more infallible than the next fellow. He once wrote to his editorial associate, Wayne Marshall, a note that still exists. It says, "Do not call on Dr. Goodman." Who will ever know what occasioned this abrupt command; but what a fatal abstinence it was, allowing the first solid stone in the foundation of the Macmillan medical division and also eventually involving Saunders in the publication of five separate textbooks of pharmacology, all of them relative failures compared to that glorious sun of enlightened pharmacodynamics—Goodman and Gilman.

One of Ryland Greene's last projects—typical of Saunders authors and editors—was the Bockus *Gastroenterology*. It came from Philadelphia; and this is in itself remarkable, for editors, like professors on sabbatical leave, often seek in Timbuktu the diamonds that might be found in their own back yards. No one in Newark attends postgraduate seminars in Jersey City. Its contract called for a book of five hundred printed pages. To what must have been Greene's satisfaction its first edition was published in three volumes of more than a thousand pages each, and at present it appears in seven volumes—a Saunders book in the solid tradition of length devoted to rich clinical experience and astute observation. The American stage could offer no finer histrionic spectacle than that of Harry Bockus on the podium peering anxiously at the handwritten questions handed up to the rostrum during his lecture. In fact, he always had in his coat pocket a dozen or so questions he had already written out against the circumstance that either no or hazardous queries might be forthcoming. "The physician," he used to say, "should be prepared." And he was.

He was not quite so prepared for the later appearance on the Saunders list of the Sleisenger and Fordtran *Gastrointestinal Disease*—also a work of some magnitude but essentially different from the Bockus, for it does indeed explore and build upon the scientific foundations of gastroenterology, whereas the Bockus rests on the discipline and the skill of seeing and doing. One of the necessary imperatives of medicine is to present truth from its different points of view and to express the separate findings that arise from those differing viewpoints.

On August 11, 1949, Ryland W. Greene died while at work on revision on the *American Illustrated Medical Dictionary*—a task from which neither old age nor illness deterred him. Perhaps an incident in the publication of Thomas Cullen's classic work, *Embryology, Anatomy, and Diseases of the Umbilicus*, will act as summary of his spirit of publishing. It is taken from Judith Robinson's biography, *Tom Cullen of Baltimore:*

> Early in May of 1916 Mary Greene Cullen was dying. Tom's new book, whose progress she had followed from week to week with proud and confident affection, was finished. Final corrections made, the printed sheets had gone to the bindery. Only the index page proofs had still to be corrected and the title page and dedication to be set when Mary Cullen's elder son received the last of all the messages that brought him to her side. It came too late to let him leave Baltimore that day.

> Tom Cullen called Philadelphia and, though it was Sunday, got through to R. W. Greene, Vice President and Editor of W. B. Saunders Company, his publishers. He asked help. If it could be done, he had to have a copy of the new book before the express left Baltimore for Toronto Monday afternoon.

> He had it. Early next morning, in Saunders Philadelphia plant, a printer and a binder were at work. Title page and dedication were hand set and run off on a proof press. The printed sheets and illustrations for a single volume were assembled with blank outer sheets, trimmed and bound in their covers. Then index, title page and dedication were pasted to the empty end pages. Saunders editorial vice-president brought the completed volume to Baltimore. Mary Cullen's last gift from her boy Tom was ready in time.

Walter Saunders was not a believer in journals, but in 1912 the Company began publication of the *Surgical Clinics of John B. Murphy*—the progenitor of the *Surgical Clinics of North America* and the *Medical Clinics of North America*. These two bimonthlies, issued in alternate months, have circulations that are in excess of many of today's leading medical journals. Over ensuing years this pattern of book-journals built around invited articles on specific topics has been pursued and amplified, so that there are now thirty-four publications of this kind bearing the Saunders imprint.

The present success and standing of the Saunders Company can be traced directly to sound and shrewd beginnings. Important innovations such as entrance into college publishing and into nursing, dental medicine and veterinary medicine are simply extensions of experience and familiar ideas. Independent publishing by W. B. Saunders, Ltd., of London, establishment of a Canadian distribution center, sustained attention to distribution and translation of Saunders books throughout the world—these are but building upon established patterns. Even the publication of books of such wide-ranging diversity as the Conn *Current Therapy* and the Kinsey-Pomeroy-Martin-Gebhard volumes on sexual behavior followed an in-built tradition of daring and innovation. Slide sets, tape series, motion films, programmed texts, microfiche cards, filmstrip presentations, Linofilm typesetting, computer-controlled composition and electronic publishing would all have been unfamiliar to Walter Burns Saunders, but he would have found them neither strange nor inappropriate to his purposes.

In 1936 Lawrence Saunders, son of Walter Burns Saunders, was elected President of the publishing house his father had founded. His wife Dorothy was also much interested in the world of publishing, traveled with her

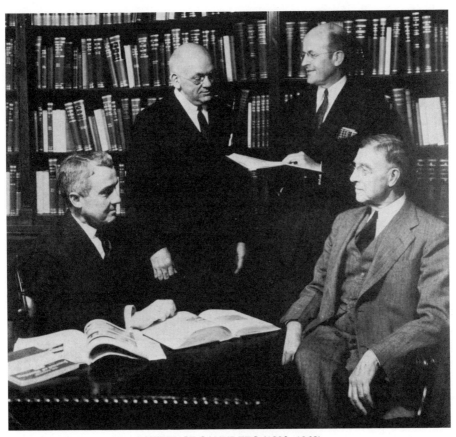

LAWRENCE SAUNDERS (1890–1968)

A son who carried on the tradition of integrity in publishing established by his father. Like many other publishers, he thought profit a pleasant thing, but he thought publishing good books a still better thing. He is shown here seated at his desk with the other officers of 1938: W. D. Watson, LeRoy Smith, and R. W. Greene.

husband on his many business calls abroad and served with sensible intelligence as a member of the company's Board of Directors for twelve consecutive years. Lawrence continued established traditions and strengthened ties of friendship with the American Medical Association, the American College of Surgeons, the Mayo Clinic, the Lahey Clinic, Johns Hopkins University Medical School, the National Academy of Sciences and the National Research Council. For all of these the Saunders Company at one time or another acted in the role of semiofficial book publisher or publishing consultant. Among the many significant volumes arising from these friendly associations were the *NRC War Manuals*—brief instructive studies of the special problems of wartime medicine from authorities of the greatest eminence. A fine example of them was the Pillsbury-Sulzberger-Livingood *Manual of Dermatology*—abundantly and beautifully illustrated, bound in sturdy cloth, and priced at $2.50, for Lawrence Saunders believed his company should earn no profit from these manuals when so many others were called upon to make a much greater sacrifice in a just cause.

In 1964 in honor of his golden anniversary with the Company, it established in his name a Fellowship in Medical Art at Johns Hopkins University School of Medicine, for the quality of medical art was one of his enduring interests. (See also Chapter 9.) His concern for excellence in the making of books lives on in the fellowship and in the publishing house that bears his father's name. Lawrence Saunders died on August 22, 1968, after a lifetime of service not simply to the welfare of the company but to the highest ideals of publishing. In that same year W. B. Saunders Company was acquired by CBS Inc., thus terminating eighty years of independent management and ownership of the company by the Saunders family. The acquisition might be said too to mark the esteem and respect that a small publishing house had earned for itself by a father-son adherence to sound principles and high ideals. It might also mark the circumstance that William Paley, then Chief Executive Officer of CBS Inc., was ever one to recognize a good thing when he saw it. He had long ago forsaken a small but flourishing cigar business to bet on a mysterious tube said to be able to transmit pictures.

5

John B. Murphy, Theodore Roosevelt and The Saunders Company*

John B. Murphy was one of America's wisest and most effective surgical teachers; but his fiery temperament and belligerent egomania clouded during his lifetime and obscure even today the fact that he also made significant contributions to the progress of healing disease and repairing trauma through surgery.

In 1849 at St. Mary's, a tiny log church in Appleton, Wisconsin, a circuit-riding priest united in marriage Michael Murphy and Anne Grimes, immigrants brought to America by Ireland's potato famine. The couple went home to the sixty acres of rich farmland Michael had cleared in back-breaking labor and to the spacious log cabin he had built for his bride. On December 21, 1857, their sixth and last child was born, John Benjamin Murphy, from birth a restless child who would become a restive, defiant man unable to brook opposition or suffer fools gladly. His mother, intensely ambitious and better educated than most Irish immigrant women, saw clearly that in America education was necessary not only to success but to solid accomplishment as well. She shared her son's early interest in medicine and realized that something more than a cursory apprenticeship was the lodestar of achievement, encouraging him to work his way through Rush Medical College and an internship at Cook County Hospital. He then practiced surgery with Dr. E. W. Lee but was attracted by the magnet of Vienna, at that time the world's leading medical center. He studied there for two years and returned to Chicago in the spring of 1884 to embark on a distinguished and sometimes embattled surgical career. In worldly matters he displayed an obdurate pigheadedness and grasping zeal, but he was never reluctant to change medical views that did not conform to his own experimental findings.

In the late nineteenth century few surgeons appreciated that operation without septic complications would vastly extend the scope of surgery; but

---

*The facts of Murphy's life are drawn from Loyal Davis's invaluable biography *J. B. Murphy* (Putnam, 1939).

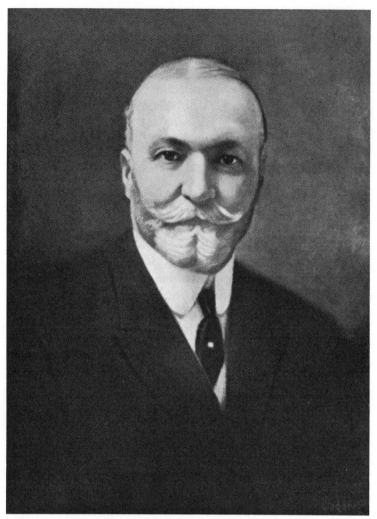

John B. Murphy: Stormy Petrel of American Surgery.

Murphy did, and the best-known of his surgical contributions—the Murphy button—revolutionized gastrointestinal surgery by making possible anastomosis and approximation of portions of the intestine without sutures. Murphy told of his experience with the button in a lengthy article in the *Medical Record* in 1892 (Vol. 42:665) and described boldly what he had accomplished: "To lessen the risk to the life of the patient, I have devised a mechanical means to dispense with the need of sutures, the necessity of invagination, the possibility of non-apposition, the sloughing through of disks, the digestion of the catgut, the almost insurmountable difficulties of technique of operation, the prolonged and fatal exposure of the abdominal contents and the protracted anaesthesia."

In 1896 he introduced end-to-end suture of blood vessels by means of invagination, the intima being brought into apposition with the adventitia. Before then others had transplanted pieces of artery or vein by means of magnesium rings; but all these attempts had failed because of septic complications. Murphy described in the *Medical Record* (Vol. 51:73) his successful result with uniting a femoral artery severed by a gunshot wound, concluding with satisfaction his account of the first recorded repair of a divided human blood vessel: "A pulsation could be felt in the dorsalis pedis on October 11th, four days after the operation. There were no oedema of the leg and no pain. The circulation was good continuously from the time of operation. The wound suppurated; drainage was inserted, but at no time did the patient's temperature exceed 100.8°F. December 8, 1896, the circulation is perfect, the wound has healed with the exception of a small superficial ulcer, one-third of an inch in diameter. The patient has not had an unpleasant symptom since the operation. January 4th, patient is walking about the ward of the hospital, has no oedema and no disturbance of the circulation."

But the concept of working with open blood vessels was too daring to be accepted in Murphy's day. Extensive reconstructive vascular surgery was still a half century distant. Similarly, Murphy had remarkable results with bone grafts, which usually do not succeed unless the tissue used is autogenous. This too was work that was neglected until its later pursuit by Fred H. Albee of New York.

Secure in his position as Chicago's most eminent surgeon and in his felicitous marriage to a devoted, beautiful wife, Murphy nevertheless remained a defensive anxious person excessively fond of himself, of the limelight, of money, and of his own convictions. He had, too, an almost destructive capacity to embroil himself in disputes in which his very vehemence tended to defeat what may indeed have been valid positions. But his surgical skill was never open to question; and at a time when many surgeons, trained before effective anesthetics were available, operated with merciful but careless haste, Murphy was cautious and meticulous. Berkeley Moynihan wrote with sincerity and appreciation of his expert surgery: "He believed in safe and thorough work rather than in specious and hazardous brilliance; all was honest and simple—no false move, no part incomplete, no chance of disaster."

In 1912, when Murphy was at the height of his dazzling career, another bigger-than-life figure overly fond of the limelight appeared in nearby Milwaukee—Colonel Theodore Roosevelt, as he was then almost always called—to seek a third presidency of the United States as nominee of the Progressive Party. On his way to the Milwaukee rally, the former President was shot and wounded in the chest by a madman named Schrank, who was saved from lynching by the crowd through the candidate's intervention. Roosevelt's own life was probably saved by the thick manuscript for his address tightly wadded into his coat pocket. Never one to miss a golden opportunity, the heroic Colonel announced that he would go on with his address. He thrilled his vast audience as he apologized for his faltering speech ("I'll do the best I can, but there's a bullet in my body") and as blood visibly oozed through his shirt front. His hearers roared their admiration and that night in Milwaukee he could have been elected President of the World. Nevertheless, he would fail of his bid, just as Murphy would fail of election of the American Surgical Society.

It was arranged that the wounded Bull Moose would go by train to Chicago and there be met and attended by four surgeons—Arthur Dean Bevan, L. L. McArthur, A. J. Ochsner, and Murphy. Under circumstances that have never been satisfactorily explained and amidst confusing communication, Murphy boarded the train at the Clybourn Street Station before it reached Chicago and spirited Roosevelt away to Mercy Hospital under his care alone. His critics cried that he should be tried for kidnapping a President of the United States. In any event, his patient received excellent care, and Murphy wisely resisted some pressure from well-wishers to remove the bullet. Indeed, Roosevelt may have actually ordered that he be placed under Murphy's sole care—as a politician he knew he needed working-class Catholic support and he liked the name Mercy Hospital—but it was an odd circumstance that Murphy never notified McArthur and Ochsner of Roosevelt's whereabouts, nor did he ever discuss the change of plans with them, although he did call on Bevan as a consultant. High-handed he was.

X-ray studies showed the bullet to be embedded in Roosevelt's right fourth rib; and roentgenograms—much less common then than today—were widely reproduced in newspapers with arrows pointing to the bullet and appropriate plaudits to Murphy, who now issued his second bulletin on the famous case. It was a model of formal, cautious statement, but it contained an altogether irrelevant sentence that came to haunt its author. "We find him [Roosevelt] in magnificent physical condition due to his regular exercise and habitual abstinence from tobacco and alcohol." The patient himself may have suggested this out-of-the-way passage; for he knew, but Murphy did not, that he was about to sue for slander a small-town newpaper that had accused him of alcoholic overindulgence. At the trial much was made of Murphy's sentence; but under oath he had to admit that he had no real knowledge of Roosevelt's exemplary abstemiousness. The ambitious politician and the ambitious surgeon were much alike—they disdained caution, but they also disdained people and even facts that stood in their way.

Murphy's famous clinics attracted students and surgeons from all over the world, and he performed his surgery before them with dramatic explanations and wide-ranging excursions. His notes became *The Murphy Clinics*, published by Saunders and the forerunner of *The Surgical Clinics of North America*. Murphy was an effective but scarcely polished speaker who wrote, Loyal Davis said, "as though he were trying to scratch himself out of a steel cage." He dimly suspected this deficiency and spent years hunting for an editor who would refine his style without ever changing whatever he spoke or wrote. He was astonished that he could never find anyone who could perform this redactorial legerdemain.

Murphy had a way of building suspense in discussing a case. His arguments would warm imperceptibly, a coherent chain of questions narrowing until slowly a sense of excitement, of impending revelation, arose. All the discussion and argument led to something everyone sitting on those benches fairly ached to learn. As the end approached, as the time for climax neared, a question barked at his audience would hang unanswered in the silence. In a clangorous, almost menacing voice, his face strained, his arm outstretched in dramatic gesture, Murphy would hurl the question at one after another, until at last the answer appeared. And then, after a final brief summary, the clinical journey was over, its end well worth its anguish, its course colorful and compelling.

Then he would operate. Throughout the operation he would talk for the hospital record and for his *Clinics* notes. He wasted no time as he talked, operating all the while and expressing aloud the purpose of each operative step. "Let the record show" became a familiar expression in his clinic. When the operation was done, he would draw his stool near the front row of seats, cross his legs, rest his elbows on his knees with his gloved hands clasped together, and talk of surgery in general, of the specific case at hand, or even of his errors. He had at last caught up with his ambitions, but he still had to prove to everyone that he was master and that no one could outfox or put him down. Like Dickens in his American readings, he stood at the center of a storm of his own making.

And, indeed, the course of the *Murphy Clinics* was a stormy one. Daily telegrams and letters flew from Chicago to Philadelphia with recriminations, unreasonable demands, threats to withdraw the *Clinics* from publication and repeated dismissals from his office of the young and brilliant artist Tom Jones, the devoted secretary and recorder Miss Margaret Maloney and his harried editor Dr. S. Solomon. All of these people were under contract to and paid by Saunders, so that Murphy could scarcely fire them; but he did so regularly with outraged denunciations of their incompetence and disloyalty and with tears freely flowing from the accused. Nevertheless, the staff somehow hung on and the *Clinics* somewhat continued. But a culmination in trauma and fury was reached on October 27th, 1914, extending for a week of fiery communication. The following wires and letters tell its story.

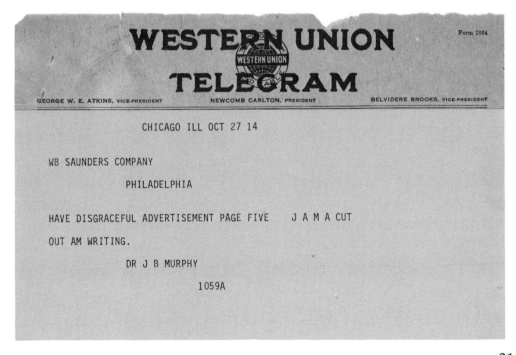

WESTERN UNION TELEGRAM

Form 1864

GEORGE W. E. ATKINS, VICE-PRESIDENT   NEWCOMB CARLTON, PRESIDENT   BELVIDERE BROOKS, VICE-PRESIDENT

CHICAGO ILL OCT 27 14

WB SAUNDERS COMPANY

PHILADELPHIA

HAVE DISGRACEFUL ADVERTISEMENT PAGE FIVE   J A M A CUT

OUT AM WRITING.

DR J B MURPHY

1059A

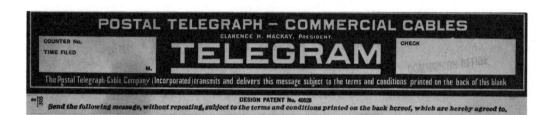

October 27, 1914

Dr. J. B. Murphy

    2526 Calumet Ave.,

        Chicago, Illinois

TELEGRAM   RECEIVED   ADVERTISEMENT   PAGE   FIVE   IN   JOURNAL

HAS   BEEN   REMOVED.

                        W. B. Saunders Company

DR. JOHN B. MURPHY
2526 CALUMET AVENUE
CHICAGO

October 27, 1914.

W. B. Saunders Company,
  W. Washington Square,
    Philadelphia, Pa.

Gentlemen:

About a year and a half ago I had a distinct understanding with you that you were to run no advertisement in any
journal that had not been OK.d and passed by me. On looking over
the Oct. 24 issue of the Journal A. M. A., I find on page 5 of the
advertising department an outrageous advertisement of the Clinics.

I certainly feel that I should bring suit against you
for liable for publishing such an article concerning any work which
I am doing. You cannot use my Clinics in such a crude and
boastful manner as you have in this advertisement, and I want the
advertisement taken out at once. And I want substituted in its
place in this journal an apology to the readers for having published such an article. You have the material for the last number of the
Clinics that you will get from me, unless this is corrected and
corrected instantly, and so that I may know that the apology is
what I want please submit it to me before sending it to the Journal
A. M. A. The Clinics are not second hand goods and they cannot be
advertised in that way. You have violated your contract and I shall
hold you responsible for this violation.

Respectfully yours,

Rec'd
10/29/14

33

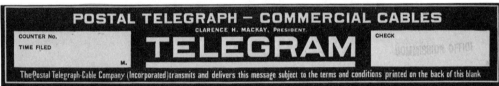

October 29, 1914

Dr. J. B. Murphy,
2526 Calumet Ave.,
Chicago, Ills.

     Will publish full page apology in Journal.
Mailing you copy today.

        W. B. Saunders Company.

34

October 29th, 1914.

Dr. John B. Murphy,
    2526 Calumet Avenue,
       Chicago, Illinois.

My dear Doctor Murphy:

       Personally replying to your letter of October twenty-seventh, I am greatly distressed at the annoyance that has been caused you by the advertisement in the "Journal of the American Medical Association" of October twenty-fourth. I have given instructions to our advertising manager to do everything possible to make a satisfactory apology. I have told him to make this apology emphatic by devoting to it an entire page in the Journal. He is submitting to you copy for this apology, which I trust will make such reparation as is possible under the circumstances.

       You are entirely correct as to the understanding that advertisements were to be submitted to you. I find that this was done for a time after you made this request, but that owing to the fact that such a large number of advertisements on the "Clinics" were being published constantly, it did not seem advisable to keep bothering you with the small details. I see, however, that this was a mistake, and hereafter proof of every announcement will be sent to you. I hope in this way any further annoyance may be avoided with regard to the advertisements of the "Clinics."

       Very truly yours,

R.W.GREENE

October 29, 1914

Dr. John B. Murphy,

2526 Calumet Ave.,

Chicago, Ills.

Dear Sir:-

    We are just in receipt of your letter of the 27th and are
enclosing a copy of the full page apology we propose to publish
in the Journal of the A.M.A., November 14th. This is the earliest
date on which we have an available full page and it would seem to
us to be advisable to publish this apology as a full page advertisement rather than as a portion of another announcement.

    If our apology is satisfactory, will you please be good enough
to O.K. the copy and return it to us; or, else to inform us that it
meets with your approval.

                              Yours very truly,

                              W. B. Saunders Company,

                              Per

October 31, 1914

W. B. Saunders Co.,
    W. Washington Sq.,
        Philadelphia, Pa.

Gentlemen:

        Enclosed is the copy of the apology you sent me
corrected as I wish it to appear.   You say this will be a full
page advertisement and published in the issue of November 14th.   I
want you to make it a half page advertisement and have it appear
in the November 7th issue, in the space where the advertisement was
to appear. The space belongs to you, and I see no reason why it
cannot appear then. If it is not published until the 14th, that
will give the profession so much more time to talk about the announcement, and it should be stopped at the very earliest moment.

                Respectfully yours,

                                    RBMurphy

I shall expect the — proof of the various advertisements. I am not too busy to look them over. JBM.

37

Nov. 2, 1914.

Dr. John B. Murphy,

2526 Calumet Avenue,

Chicago, Ill.

Dear Sir:

I have your letter of October 31st. enclosing
the copy of the apology corrected by you. We will, of course,
publish it just as you have indicated.

It was impossible for us to get this in the November
7th issue, as this number went to press last Wednesday. Immediately on receipt of your first telegram, we arranged to
omit the advertisement to which you took exception, from the
Journal and replace it with other material. The journal goes
to press ten days ahead of publication date.

Very truly yours,

W. B. Saunders Company,

per

R W GREENE

Thereafter, things certainly grew no calmer—how could they—but the incidence of explosions slowed. This was no doubt due to a certain judicious forbearance on the part of Ryland Greene, the Saunders editor, for he never mentioned that no proof of the offending advertisement had been submitted because it was in fact written by that master of self-glorifying superlatives, John B. Murphy, the often petulant petrel.

ADVERTISING DEPARTMENT

Murphy's Clinics

An Apology

On page 5 of our 13 page advertisement in THE JOURNAL for October 24th, there appeared an announcement of Dr. Murphy's Clinics.

Dr. Murphy takes great exception to the manner in which this announcement was presented. He feels that the statements there made are too boastful and not in good taste.

We gladly meet Dr. Murphy's demand that we publish an apology to him and to the medical profession.

W. B. SAUNDERS COMPANY

The full-page advertisement from the *Journal of the American Medical Association*, November 14, 1914.

And here is the offending part of the long-ago ad. Its unabashed superlatives seem innocuous enough compared to today's more subtly misleading representations. But perhaps even then "a certain clinical history means a *definite lesion*. Not usually, but *always*" seemed more positive than facts might warrant.

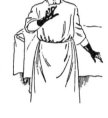
His *Murphy Clinics* continue today as the influential *Surgical Clinics of North America*. Their originator died on August 11, 1916, while vacationing on Mackinac Island—an illustrious figure who had the gift of scientific imagination but over whom there still hovers a shadow of enigma and ambivalence.

6

Artist and Book

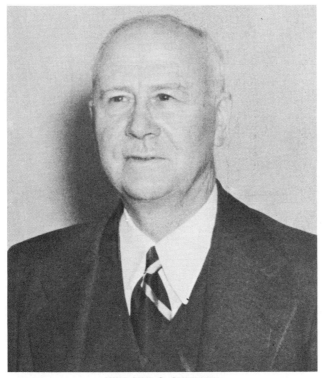

WILLARD C. SHEPARD

Usually called Shep but sometimes Jeff—in obvious reference to his long association with the gangling Tom Jones. The face in this picture has a look of wispiness—perhaps even of vagueness. But appearances can be deceiving. Behind that fey facade lie iron determination, vast fortitude and the intellectual capacity to make visual a truth or concept arising from the wilderness of detail that is modern bioscience.

Walter Burns Saunders was intensely aware of the value of original artwork, sharing Mumford's view that the artist gives vivid life to the author's words. Indeed, advertisements for the *International Textbook of Surgery* contain the phrase "with new brilliant artwork expertly executed in Mr. Saunders' personal art studios." Whether the word "personal" here is exact may be questioned; but advertisers have long taken undue liberties with words ("Our store will hereafter be closed on Wednesday afternoons for your greater convenience").

Then as now, authors, editors, production managers and cost accountants all deplored the dilatory, costly, but essential work of the artist. In 1924 Saunders had begun publication of the eight-volume, elegantly illustrated *Bickham Operative Surgery*—a work that proved to be of immense value and influence but that also utterly exhausted Bickham's physical and financial capacities. What a despairing but familiar cry from the heart this is:

New York, June 24, 1923
Apt. 1--440 Riverside Drive

Dear Mr. Greene,
          The time of exhausted resources that I felt certain was approaching--and which was the entire basis of my several stressed letters upon this subject, in the recent past--seems now so near at hand, that I am writing--am simply compelled to write--to ask (based upon your recent letters of kind offer), to ask you what is the maximum monthly amount we could arrange for me to draw against my future Royalties, beginning with next month, July, and extending over twelve months, if needed.
          I have always asked that the Firm would defer taking the 1/2 Royalty to repay themselve for my part of the picture-expenses, during the first year of the revenue from the Book (1924)--so as to give me time to get upon my feet again.
          I shall not ask for a continuation of a monthly advancement on the Royalties for one month longer than actually needed for meeting imperative expenses--but I would have to have some definite knowledge in advance, as to what I could systematically depend upon, in order to know how to plan. Naturally, I would want--and it would be to my advantage--as quickly as possible, when once on my feet, to discontinue the monthly amounts--and to pay back my part of the Pictures--so as to feel that, thenceforth, the Royalties would be untramelled--and that I was not running upon a debt basis--but upon a revenue basis.
          I exceedingly regret being placed as I am--and having to make any such request--and the more so, because we both know that I would not have been brought to the necessity of being placed where I am, had not the publication been delayed the nearly two full years it will have been, beyond all calculations--according to which all the books would be now issued and on the market and the resulting revenue assured to us both. It is only because what was to have been naturally expected, though our mutual planning, has not transpired, that things have reached their present predicament--in consequence of which I am literally driven, with hurt feelings and humiliation, and through no personal fault of my own, to ask the Firm to make the most ample provision within their power, to aid me meet my financial difficulties.

Very sincerely,

Warren S. Bickham

Lawrence Saunders, too, saw that authors of profusely illustrated, multi-volume works simply could no longer manage on their own. He therefore created in 1946 the Saunders Art Department with a gifted director and an annual working fellowship in medical art. His choice of a director could not have been wiser.

W. C. Shepard was born in Canadice, New York, in 1896. He came from what were once called "humble beginnings" but that might well be called rich beginnings—a family understanding the necessity for hard work but equally appreciative of the work of the mind, a family experiencing not deprivation but the frequent difficulty of making ends meet that were pretty far apart.

In pleasant rural surroundings Shep lived a happy and placid childhood, but early in boyhood he took the counsel of Horatio Alger and became an expert telegrapher. This skill stood him in good stead during the long years of his training as artist, often interrupted in order to accumulate enough money to keep going. From it he also picked up a kind of ten-word terseness of speech that, like the telegram, could sometimes be disconcertingly pointed.

Having followed the advice of one famous author, he now heeded that of another and went West. Telegraphy took him as stationmaster to the southernmost bastion of the Southern Pacific Railroad where he once forget-fully neglected to put on his shoes when rushing out to greet the biweekly Cannonball and was promptly bit in the ankle by a rattler. A true woodsman, he at once slashed the sting points with his pocketknife and was at that age able to reach his ankle by mouth in order to suck out blood and venom. He was put aboard the baggage car and spent a fretful night of fevered tossing on mail sacks in the not-unlikely expectation of death.

Unfortunately, the train was headed not for Los Angeles (site of the Southern Pacific Hospital) but for Yuma, and quite some time elapsed before he got any medical attention. After six weeks in the hospital and pronouncement of recovery, he was discharged with a bill not only for medical care but for train fare first to Yuma, then back to Los Angeles. Stationmasters are not treated quite so cavalierly these days, but then there aren't many stations either.

The telegraphic trade took him to what was a vast, almost uninhabited desert, the Imperial Valley. The wires were not exactly kept humming in that lonely outpost, and Shep took to making sketches of the strange, beautiful and limitless plains.

There entered upon this desolate scene an anonymous prospector who either was or fancied himself to be a connoisseur of art. In either event, he had the wit to see the young telegrapher was a true artist. Upon his recommendation Shep moved on to the Chicago Art Institute, where he studied by day, worked as a telegrapher by night and occupied his free time in sketching.

On the bulletin board of the Art Institute there one day appeared a letter from an unknown fellow named Max Broedel, saying in effect that there was a genuine need in America for anatomical-surgical artists and that he was prepared to train them at Johns Hopkins University, where it was said to be easier to become a professor than a student.

Below the tappetty-tap-tap surface of every Horatio Alger telegrapher lies a concealed adventurer. Shep went to Baltimore not really moved by Max's letter but by the timeless urge of wanderlust. He studed with Broedel for three years, becoming the master's preeminent pupil; and he richly enjoyed the experience, perhaps because he and Max were cast from the same artistic but not the same characterologic mold.

At last he had reached the end of the beginning, and in 1915 he left the white marble stoops of Baltimore for the green hills of Berkeley as Staff Artist at the University of California. There he worked with the great Herbert Evans, who did an unforgivable thing. He told the young Broedel student that his interest was in having on hand a capable surgical artist, but then rigorously devoted the artist's talents to painstaking microscopic drawings. If there's one thing Shep hated more than deception it was making histologic drawings. He at once quit and left for Chicago, where he worked with the equally distinguished Arthur Bevan, whose lionish roars concealed a timid mouse.

There are two versions of the reasons for this hasty departure. Evans always maintained that microscopic vs. surgical drawing was a smokescreen debate and that the real issue was Shep's acquaintanceship made on August 15, 1915, with Alice C. Shaw, who had come to Berkeley to attend a wedding and stayed to take a Master's Degree. Along about the time of Shep's departure, another attractive wedding had summoned Alice to Chicago, and Evans always believed that Shep's real motive in leaving for Chicago was to persuade her to attend a wedding of her own.

As with many artists, there was about Shep a mild otherworldliness, which was complemented and corrected by Alice's decided this-worldliness. If Shep arranged many a fruitful union between artist and author, Alice facilitated unions between wary bachelors and consolable widows.

Just after Shep's arrival in Chicago, he had a second profoundly important encounter—that with Tom Jones. Tom—equal in skill, taller in stature, more outspoken in sentiment—made with Shep as fine a creative union as Alice made with him a perfect connubial union. Tom was then at the University of Illinois and had already begun work with the irascible John B. Murphy. Although they were a little separated in space, Tom and Shep were close in spirit and in motive.

The two artist friends worked together on many projects of far-ranging and diverse nature; but their talents were most effectively pooled in the Jones and Shepard *Manual of Surgical Anatomy*—one of the first medical books to appear in both maxi and mini sizes and one from which borrowing of figures (both acknowledged and unacknowledged) has become more extensive than that from any other single medical source.

Wide as the influence of the *Manual* was, it may not have been as great as that of the Homans *Textbook of Surgery* (Charles C Thomas), for which Shep single-handedly did all its superb line drawings. They were recognized upon their appearance and are still reckoned today to be absolute models of clear, simple, instructive schemes of surgical principles and surgical procedures. They have never been equaled in medical literature in their effectiveness.

In 1946, when men of similar age might be contemplating the distant pleasure of retirement, Shep contemplated instead an entirely new career. He came to the Saunders Company as its Art Director, the first such post established in any medical publishing house the world over. He came upon the recommendation of Tom Jones and the invitation of Lawrence Saunders.

It soon became evident what Shep would do. He would introduce a new order of quality into books. He would guide and instruct many a young artist who would feel only the kindness of his touch, scarcely conscious of its directive force. Shep may not have always known where the artwork was but he always knew what it was and what it was supposed to do.

Not long after Shep's arrival preparation of the Bickham-Callander-Shackelford *Surgery of the Alimentary Tract* got under way and was carried out under the sole authorship of Shackelford. As it neared completion, he submitted a Preface containing these words: "A uniquely kind and valuable artist is Mr. Willard C. Shepard of the Saunders art department with whom I worked intimately. He has the patience of Job, the anatomical knowledge of a modern Leonardo and an artistic ability second to none. It was amazing how he corrected anatomical inaccuracies and how quickly he sketched a likeness of what I was trying to express in words. To him I owe an especial debt of gratitude."

At that time the Saunders Company had an absolutely rigid policy specifying that all its own people were anonymous. The Preface was changed to express instead a general acknowledgment of the capability and helpfulness of the Saunders staff. Proof of the revised expression of gratitude went out.

There followed a rather explosive letter from that usually nonexplosive and kindly gentleman, Richard Shackelford. He said that the Saunders staff was indeed capable and helpful and was generally conceded to be so. But that was not what he wanted to say. What he wanted to point out was the extraordinarily imaginative, skillful and courteous help he had had from *one* particular person of the Saunders staff. With a whistling sound of sad resignation the balloon of rigidity suddenly split, releasing the pent-up hot air of policy. Thereafter the prefaces to Saunders books were allowed to mention the specific help of real people and thereafter too Shep's name led all the rest.

7

The Todd-Sanford Clinical Diagnosis by Laboratory Methods: The Story of a Specialty

Dr. James C. Todd, youthful Associate Professor of Pathology in the Medical Department at the University of Denver and pathologist to four of the city's busy hospitals, still found time to publish in 1906 and 1907 a series of articles entitled "Laboratory Diagnosis for the Practitioner." These were brought together as a small privately published book (*A Syllabus of Lectures upon Clinical Diagnosis*), the basis for *A Manual of Clinical Diagnosis* published by Saunders in 1908—how rapidly things moved in those days!—a book that in its long vigorous life has exerted a great influence on clinical pathology itself and become a standard teaching text.

In the first decade of the twentieth century clinical pathology could scarcely be called a recognized specialty. General practitioners and internists employed what is now considered clinical pathology as a part of physical diagnosis. Bacteriology, chemistry and physics had just barely begun to be applied to medical diagnosis in the living patient; but advancing knowledge and demanding skills would soon make it impossible to regard laboratory medicine as a simple adjunct to physical diagnosis. The early clinical pathologist was a physician who began using new methods of precision that enabled him to see more and penetrate further than was possible with the five senses. The *Syllabus* provides a rather modest picture of the emerging discipline: "A kitchen table, with a few shelves for bottles, screened off in a corner of the office will suffice for a laboratory." And here is the ancestor of the modern blood cell calculator: "Some workers divide a slide box into compartments by slides, one for each variety of leukocytes, and drop a coffee bean into the appropriate compartment when a cell is classified." Only two types of leukemia were recognized, myelogenous and lymphatic. No clinical importance was attached to the platelets.

Four years later a second, enlarged edition appeared with the new title *Clinical Diagnosis: A Manual of Laboratory Methods*. Important additions included Benedict's test for sugar in the urine, blood culture in typhoid fever, the Wassermann test for syphilis, new chapters on bacteriologic methods and use of vaccines, and photomicrographs taken by the author. These were all harbingers of things to come; but a few incidental notes can hardly be called prescient: "The hematocrit cannot be recommended for accuracy, although it seems to be gaining in favor"; and of pernicious anemia: "It is frequently impossible to diagnose this disease from the blood examination."

Thereafter the book grew steadily in scope, size and authority; but Todd had long suffered from serious illness and had written all editions of his book while bedridden. The fifth edition, published in 1925, was to be the last he would do alone. In it acute infectious mononucleosis was mentioned for the first time and the index outline of laboratory findings in important diseases appeared; it long remained a valuable feature of the book. Arthur H. Sanford, of the Mayo Clinic, joined Todd as coauthor of the sixth edition and continued as its sole author for five editions thereafter.

For the sixth edition Saunders offered what was a reasonable continuation of the existing contract with Todd, specifying a graduated scale of royalty return to Sanford; but because of his long-continued ill health Todd was anxious to secure a fair share of royalty for his wife, and Sanford was understandably concerned that in the event of his death his wife too should have a satisfactory return from the book. They therefore hired a lawyer to review the submitted agreement of publication; but few authors realize that lawyers cannot earn a living by outright approval of offered contracts. The lawyer drew up an extraordinarily complex agreement that foresaw every possible contingency except the end of the world and the circumstances that were actually to occur. Dr. Todd died in January of 1928, and his wife was to outlive him by more than forty years, and Mrs. Sanford too was to long outlive her husband. The fact that each of them had a substantial royalty share was to make sensible royalty provisions for new authorship almost impossible in the event of Sanford's disability or death.

Meantime the book itself, now *Clinical Diagnosis by Laboratory Methods*, continued to grow in size and influence. Its eighth edition, published in 1935, provided for the first time a separate sixty-page chapter on Clinical Chemistry, and its Preface forthrightly said that "clinical pathology has become a recognized specialty of medical practice."

After publication of the eleventh edition (1948), it became increasingly clear that the book's future might be jeopardized by its existing royalty commitments. Dr. William MacFarland (associate medical editor at Saunders) was dispatched to discuss with Sanford arrangements for future editions—the meeting to take place in Chicago during sessions of the American Society of Clinical Pathologists at the Drake Hotel. It was one of those occasions on which a practical end is sought; but MacFarland, for all his education in science and knowledge of books, was not precisely a practical sort. His encounter recalls an adventure of the mullah Nasrudin—an Oriental Everyman given to Franklinesque pronouncements—who was once hired by a pedagogue to ferry him across a very wide river. As soon as they were afloat, the scholar asked if it was going to be rough.

"Don't ask me nothing about it," said Nasrudin.

"Have you ever studied grammar?"

"No," said the ferryman.

"In that case, half your life has been lost."

Soon a terrifying storm blew up, and the crazy cockleshell of a boat began to fill with water. Nasrudin leaned over toward his companion.

"Have your ever learned to swim?" he asked.

"No," said the pedant.

"In that case, schoolmaster, *all* your life is lost, for we are sinking."

The meeting was at breakfast. For two and a half hours editor and guest discussed the book, its strengths, its weaknesses and its commanding position as a reference text. Finally, Mac summoned up courage to ask about future authorship. "Dr. Sanford," he said, "have you given any thought to possible coauthorship for the next edition and to a plan for royalty division?"

"Young man," came the reply, "I have enjoyed greatly our discussion of what is undoubtedly the finest teaching text available in clinical pathology. But I am not Dr. Sanford; I am Dr. William Collins of New Orleans."

Sanford, who had been stewing and fuming for three hours in the hotel lobby, was by then in no mood to discuss either his possible demise or division of his royalty return. However impressive are our ideas and however strategic our plans, they are not a wholly satisfactory substitute for the ability to swim in rough waters; and in publishing there are plenty of situations in which the imperative need is merely to keep afloat.

Benjamin B. Wells joined Sanford in preparation of the twelfth edition, published in 1953. It was possibly the least changed of the many editions of the book; and it was clear after Sanford's death in 1959 that Wells could not carry on the book alone, although he was a man of wide medical learning and vast experience. But his experience was too diversified for sharp focus on the specific area of clinical pathology. Having studied medicine and also earned a doctorate in chemistry, he was certified in internal medicine and in pathology and he had done important work with Kendall at the Mayo Clinic. He had served too in various schools as chairman of medicine, as chairman of pathology and as dean. He had written for Saunders an excellent book on *Interpretation of Laboratory Tests* and had been briefly the Saunders medical editor. He was also an accomplished musician and a man of wide-ranging other interests—in short, a protean figure able to do well anything to which he turned his attention, but attention whose span was brief.

Upon Sanford's death it was justly said of him and of Todd that together they had witnessed the dramatic growth of a new specialty and had helped spread its wings and bring it to full-fledged maturity. This was also a critical point for the future of *Clinical Diagnosis by Laboratory Methods,* and again the Saunders Company was wonderfully fortunate.

Israel Davidsohn, Director of Pathology at the Chicago Medical School, Chief of the Department of Experimental Pathology at Mount Sinai Hospital Medical Center and dean of American clinical pathologists, accepted coauthorship with Ben Wells of Edition 13. This was for Davidsohn a true labor of love and dedication to the idea of the value of a standard reference text in his specialty, for he was no longer a young man needing either fame or publication, and he may have suspected that Wells was by now sufficiently far removed from clinical pathology to make an altogether appropriate coauthor. For the first time the book would become a collaborative effort, and this too may have signalized that clinical pathology had come of age— a discipline so exacting in its skills, so sophisticated in its techniques, and so sweeping in its scope that it could no longer be fully encompassed by one mind.

Writing books and editing multi-authored books are entirely different intellectual tasks, and Israel Davidsohn proved ideally suited to the latter. His Old World charm and Viennese courtesy partly concealed an extraordinarily penetrating and critical mind. No slipshod contribution to the book could escape his sharp evaluation; and the thirteenth proved to be the most successful of all its editions.

For that edition a young and then scarcely known clinical chemist, Norbert W. Tietz, contributed a detailed and eloquent chapter on Clinical Chemistry; and this in turn led to his doing a superb *Fundamentals of Clinical Chemistry*, in which he displayed a Davidsohnian dedication to perfection that at once dismayed and inspired his contributing writers; and, a decade later, he would write his splendid *Clinical Guide to Laboratory Tests*, one of the most genuinely useful books in laboratory medicine ever published.

As time for preparation of Edition 14 of the Todd and Sanford neared, Ben Wells withdrew from authorship, and Davidsohn realized that he must have help with the task ahead not only because of its immensity but to insure continuity of authorship and objective. John Bernard Henry, at that time Professor of Pathology and Director of Clinical Pathology, State University of New York, Upstate Medical Center, had, like James Todd before him, prepared an excellent series of laboratory manuals for his own students, and these were well known to Davidsohn and Saunders. He accepted the invitation to join Davidsohn, and Edition 15 or the Todd-Sanford became larger and more widely accepted than ever.

John Henry must be, by any count, one of the busiest men on the American medical scene. Nevertheless, he has been able some way to find time, despite his post as Dean of the School of Medicine of Georgetown University, to create with single-minded devotion thorough revisions of the Todd and Sanford. Now in its seventeenth edition, once again under a title change— *Clinical Diagnosis and Management by Laboratory Methods*—it is still the authoritative expression of the whole range of clinical pathology and is, by the miracle of hard work and judicious compression, briefer than its two preceding editions. Even in his new post as President of the State University of New York, Upstate Medical Center, John Henry finds those resources of mind and energy indispensable to the right doing of a splendid book—a man little like that Oxford don of whom it was said that the time he could spare from the adornment of his person he devoted to the neglect of his duties.

Admiral Rozhestvensky Charts the Course of a Textbook: The Maximow-Bloom-Fawcett Histology

8

Of all history's wars, the one most predictable and senseless, the one accompanied by the most glorious acts of heroism and the most awesome acts of folly, was the Russo-Japanese War. It was to become the story of a Russian fleet of forty-two aged, badly equipped and ill-manned men-of-war under the command of an irascible, courageous aristocrat, Admiral Zinovi Petrovitch Rozhestvensky, who placed duty to his country and to his emperor above all else and who would lead his fleet on an incredible eighteen-thousand-mile odyssey sabotaged by perfidy of his subordinates and corruption of his superiors and beset by the hostility and mockery of the world—culminating in the eventual destruction of his fleet and his force in a battle the most decisive since Trafalgar.

The Sino-Japanese War had, to everyone's astonishment, ended in complete victory for Japan and its possession of Port Arthur, the most northerly ice-free port on the Asiatic mainland; but by 1897 it was in Russian hands because of pressure from Germany and France—a betrayal and humiliation the Japanese could not forget. In 1904 Admiral Togo with his powerful and highly trained fleet recaptured Port Arthur for Japan in an attack astonishingly similar to the later onslaught on Pearl Harbor. The Russian Second Pacific Squadron, under the command of Admiral Rozhestvensky, was readied to avenge this defeat and retake Port Arthur. In theory its firepower was tremendous; but Russian shipbuilding was a leisurely, inefficient process oiled only by bribery, and many of the Russian behemoths were top-heavy and slow. Further, the fleet was eighteen thousand miles away from its target; and coal was to be the problem that might end the whole perilous venture, for most of the long journey would be through unfriendly waters where no bases would be available. The armada, depending on its speed, would consume between 500,000 and 600,000 tons of coal. The Russians too were handicapped by absolute conviction that Japan was an upstart nation of puny people unfit for war or imperial ambition.

After a series of heart-breaking difficulties, mutinies, insubordinations, breakdowns and mad directions from St. Petersburg, Admiral Rozhestvensky miraculously brought his fleet intact to within a hundred and fifty miles of the islands of Japan. By chance the day was the anniversary of the Czar and Czarina's coronation. The chaplain in full canonicals led the toast: "On this, the great anniversary of the sacred coronation of their Majesties, may God help us to serve with them our beloved country. To the health of the Emperor! The Empress! To Russia!"

Before the brimming glasses could be drained, the call to action stations sounded through the fleet. The great battle of Tsu-Shema (Donkey's Ears) was about to begin. In planning its strategy the Russians had a secret weapon at their command. A high-ranking Japanese naval officer was in their pay and giving to the Russian military precise details of Admiral Togo's battle plan. Almost on the eve of battle Russian intelligence officers were beginning to wonder whether they were actually harboring a counterspy; but just at that moment the officer and all of his family were executed for treason, and the Russians knew that their man had indeed been a traitor to his country. What they did not know—perhaps even could not imagine—was that the officer had volunteered this sacrifice to persuade the Russians of the truth of his revelations. Admiral Togo's immediate attack and its swift and hazardous maneuvers came as a total surprise. The Russian Second Pacific Squadron was utterly destroyed; more than five thousand men were killed; and over 200,000 tons of warships either sunk or captured. To escape further slaughter, the few remaining vessels surrendered and a handful of survivors, including the badly wounded Rozhestvensky, returned to a Russia afire with discontent and the spirit of revolt.

Another survivor of the devastating disaster was Admiral Nikanov, the father of a son Fedor by a ballerina of the Russian Imperial Ballet. Perhaps it may be conjectured that the charming ballerina saw little future in the military. In any event, she turned her attention to science and married Alexander Maximow, Russia's greatest bioscientist, whose classic monograph on *Inflammation* antedates in its findings the later work of many investigators and is still admired today as a pioneering study of great foresight and exactness. When the revolution came, Maximow, his wife and young Fedor Nikanov bribed their way through border guards with laboratory alcohol and escaped over frozen Lake Ladoga to Finland. They eventually arrived in America just as the new socialist regime was being denounced here for what was presumed to have been the execution or death in imprisonment of Russia's most eminent scientist. Maximow took up his study of tissue culture at the University of Chicago and soon began work on his *Textbook of Histology*, but was able to complete less than half of its manuscript before his death in December, 1928.

Here Margaret Bloom, wife of the late William Bloom and worker with him in histologic researches, takes up the story of how her young husband, an anatomist with a recent doctorate in medicine from Johns Hopkins University, came to be the coauthor of the *Textbook of Histology*.

> At the time Maximow died Bill had been working in his laboratory for several years as a Research Fellow in Anatomy and had had the opportunity to read those chapters of the Histology which had been completed, as well as rough

drafts of others. The state of the manuscript at the time of Maximow's death and the subsequent completion of the book are described accurately and in detail in the preface to the first edition (1930). Maximow had also made many original drawings to illustrate the text and had secured permission to reproduce others which had appeared in various scientific publications.

After Maximow's death Bill was asked to remain at the University of Chicago to continue the work of the tissue culture laboratory which Maximow had directed. When Bill's fellowship expired, he was appointed to an assistant professorship in the Department of Anatomy. Professor Bensley and the other senior members of the department felt that the textbook should be completed and persuaded Bill to undertake what for a young scientist was a monumental task. As for what the book meant to Bill, his feelings were mixed, both during the period of preparing the first edition and throughout the years of revisions. He was well aware of the broadening of his scientific outlook as he sought to acquaint himself with as much of the vast amount of histological literature as possible. But he begrudged the time spent on the book, as this left less time for the research projects which were always his primary interest.

Maximow was imposing in appearance, with the dignity and formal manners typical of European professors of his generation. His military bearing was probably acquired during his student years at the Imperial Military Academy of Medicine in St. Petersburg. He was proficient in a number of languages. His command of English was excellent and he conversed and lectured as fluently in English and German as in his native Russian. While at the University of Chicago, he observed a rigid routine from which he rarely deviated. His teaching was scheduled for the early morning. The remainder of the day he spent in the laboratory, except for an hour's walk in midafternoon. On days when there was no teaching, experiments were often begun early in the day and continued through into the evening.

Despite the intensity with which he worked, Maximow could relax when he was vacationing. During the summer of 1928 he gave a series of lectures at a number of universities in Germany. After his scheduled tour, he went to Italy, to Madonna di Campiglio, one of his favorite vacation spots in the Dolomites. There Bill and I joined him for a week. In his earlier years Maximow had been an enthusiastic mountain climber. By 1928 hiking at this altitude was too strenuous for him, but he was able to enjoy the magnificent scenery as he rode on a mule along the steep trail to the foot of one of the glaciers. He took pleasure in pointing out to us the various wild flowers along the way, identifying each by its botanical name.

When Bill was a first-year medical student at the Johns Hopkins University in the fall of 1919, the first lecture in the Histology course, given by Professor Florence Sabin, described the investigations of a very great Russian scientist, A. A. Maximow, who was reported to have died in the Russian revolution of 1917. Some years later, when Bill was Associate Pathologist at Michael Reese Hospital in Chicago, he learned that Maximow had escaped from Russia and had joined the faculty of the University of Chicago. Professor R. R. Bensley, Chairman of the Department of Anatomy, was among those who had received letters from Maximow, expressing his desire to come to the United States and obtain a position at an American university. Bensley was delighted with the possibility of acquiring Maximow for his department. Negotiations followed and, after many months, Maximow arrived in Chicago with his wife and sister, and his wife's son.

Bill first heard Maximow lecture at a meeting of the Chicago Pathological Society and soon afterwards had the opportunity of meeting him at the University and showing him microscopic preparations of some of his research material. From the time of this first brief meeting, Bill was determined to work with Maximow. Later, when Maximow agreed to take Bill into his laboratory,

Professor Bensley warned Bill that he would find Dr. Maximow a most stimulating professor but an unbelievably hard taskmaster. Bill learned that both statements were true, but that Maximow drove himself harder than any of the people in the laboratory.

I met Madame Maximow only three or four times. On these social occasions she was gracious and friendly, but I never knew her well. She had been a ballerina in Russia and taught ballet for a while during the years she lived in Chicago. As you know, Madame Maximow had a son named Nikanov, but I was not aware that his father was an admiral.

Margaret Bloom refers in her account to the Preface to the First Edition of the Textbook. Here are pertinent parts of it:

At the time of his death, Professor Maximow was writing a Text-book of Histology. This was to be based as far as possible, both as to text and figures, on human material, and the functional aspects of the structures described were to be emphasized. For this work he had collected much new material and had made many new illustrations. He had completed the sections on the male and female generative organs, the urinary tract, the organs of special sense, and epithelium. In rough manuscript he left the sections on the blood and connective tissue, the gastro-intestinal tract, the blood vascular and lymphatic systems, the spleen, the integument, and the mammary gland.

None of the chapters on the Nervous Tissue were written by Professor Maximow in their present form. His papers included some notes and drawings which were helpful in a general way as indicative of the line of treatment contemplated. There was also available the Russian text of 1918 in which the nervous tissues are treated very fully. A complete translation of these Russian chapters and the notes and drawings were placed in the hands of Professor Maximow's colleague, Professor C. Judson Herrick, and these served as the basis upon which the present text was written. In reorganizing this material and bringing it up to date, the attempt was made to conform with Professor Maximow's method of treatment as far as practicable; but the twelve years since the Russian text was published have been very fruitful in this field and much of the discussion which was apposite at that time is now out of date. The section dealing with the physiology of the nerve fibers and part of that on the synapse have been taken from a more complete treatment of the correlation of structure and function of nervous tissues by Professor R. W. Gerard. These chapters, accordingly, are to be regarded not as a posthumous publication, but as an entirely new formulation of the theme, the responsibility for which rests chiefly with Professor Herrick.

I have written the sections on the biliary and respiratory systems, the pancreas, the endocrine glands (with the exception of the suprarenals) and the introductory chapter. In all of these sections I have conformed, in general, with Professor Maximow's ideas on these subjects. In addition, I have thoroughly revised the sections on cartilage, bone and muscle, which were based on translations of parts of his Principles of Histology (Russian), and his rough manuscript of the blood vascular and lymphatic systems, the spleen, integument, mammary gland, gastro-intestinal tract, the blood, connective tissue, and the blood-forming and destroying tissues.

Much of Professor Maximow's manuscript was left in Russian. For their careful translations of this and of portions of his Principles of Histology (in Russian) I am indebted to Doctors G. Hassin, O. T. Hess, and E. Piette.

William Bloom

Chicago, Illinois
September, 1930

The youthful assistant professor of anatomy had taken on a very large burden; but Madame Maximow—as is perhaps customary with graceful ballerinas—was not one to concern herself with the burdens of others. In fact, her first proposal was that Bloom be allowed to complete and carry on the textbook purely for the honor accruing to him from association with the work of her illustrious husband. Madame Maximow lived to be an irascible nonagenerian, who once in a while came over from Paris to complain to Saunders about her paltry royalty return. In all those years she always referred to Bloom, by now a distinguished scientist of the first order, as "Professor Maximow's little assistant." The paltry return was by no means minuscule, for Madame Maximow had driven a hard bargain, insisting that the lion's share of royalty go to the lioness. For once, Ryland Greene did not protect the legitimate interests of the man who was to do most of the work.

It is true that the first edition of the textbook was a comparative failure; but the second and all editions thereafter have been resounding successes, and "paltry" is scarcely the term to use in describing their royalty return, As with many splendid reference texts, the *Histology*, by the impressive weight of its authority, achieved a wide use outside the strict domain of the classroom. All bioscientists find they need its authoritative description, illustration and analysis of microscopic structure, and conscientious teachers have always recognized that the text that invests the skeleton of facts with the flesh of thought is a stimulus and challenge to the minds of students.

William Bloom was a proud man grown confident in his scientific judgments and his mastery of classical histology; but by the early 1960's he concluded that care of the world's most respected text in histology was becoming too much for him and that he was unable himself to bring to it the rich elucidation of ultrastructure that electron microscopy could provide. Also, established concepts in hematology and lymphology to which he had contributed were being challenged by new immunologic findings and radiolabeled tracer studies. He took a cautious view of these new developments and perhaps felt he was not the person either to evaluate or to incorporate them in his book.

Author and publisher quickly agreed that the ideal collaborator was Don W. Fawcett, the youthful Professor of Anatomy at Harvard and one of the two or three great pioneers and perfectionists in the use of the electron microscope. Fawcett was probably attracted to this formidable task by reasons much like those that had motivated the young assistant professor Bloom to its doing. The textbook itself was firmly based on the researches of many leading figures of microanatomy in its most fruitful descriptive period around the turn of the century. It afforded, too, the opportunity to accelerate the incorporation into descriptive morphology of the exciting new information made possible by a powerful new device—a stream of electrons controlled by magnetic fields. Finally, it also offered a compelling reason for the specialist to become a broadly informed generalist—precisely what an effective teacher must be. And what a fine thing his acceptance has been for the *Textbook of Histology*.

From the Eighth Edition on, the care of the book has been his. In reviewing for *Science* the Fifth Edition of the Weiss *Histology: Cell and Tissue Biology*, R. P. Gould said this: "Fawcett and Bloom (the tenth edition of the original Maximow and Bloom) appeared in 1975 and was the work of Don Fawcett. It is a splendid book, well written, accurate and beautifully illustrated; it shows all the hallmarks of its author's approach to the subject, being scholarly, meticulous, balanced, and revealing Fawcett's marvelous appreciation of the visual appeal of the subject. It is perhaps not surprising that at least five of the contributors to Weiss's volume were at some time working in the Department of Anatomy at Harvard when Fawcett was chairman there."

Fawcett also found time to write and later revise for Saunders his magnificently illustrated atlas, *The Cell*, which, like the *Histology*, has found use outside its own sphere, especially among those studying or working in genetics and comparative biology. It is interesting that the German translation of the First Edition of *The Cell* was apparently too early in its definitive character for its audience, for initially it failed to sell at all. It was only after it had been available for five years that it suddenly sprang into widespread use, both as a reference tool and as a teaching text in cytology and microscopy.

The beard does not make the philosopher—nor the anatomist. But for Don Fawcett it is singularly appropriate—elegant, precise, formal, perhaps even slightly forbidding, it recalls Elizabethan noblemen or nineteenth-century Russian professors. Its austere look conceals a heart and mind of passionate cares and concerns—care lest medical students and medical educators be deluded into belief that there is some easy magical way to understanding medical science; concern lest the growing overpopulation of the underdeveloped world create desperate hunger and starvation in millions; apprehension that the rapacity bred of need and hunger destroy the few survivors of some of the world's most beautiful animals.

Fawcett is a superb observer and photographer of the birds and animals of East Africa, especially of the great cats—so inscrutable, so wise in their ways, so responsive to nature in all its forms. Their coats in patterns of wonderful symmetry suggest the esthetic beauty of fine structure; and perhaps to Fawcett both suggest an artist's design in all the manifestations of life. A Saunders editor once suggested to him that an atlas of his pictures (*Dr. Fawcett's Animals*) would have enormous appeal; but other matters now occupy his mind, for in 1980 he forsook Boston for Nairobi to take up work in the International Laboratory for Research on Animal Diseases. Here is his account of a decision that must have seemed strange to many of his friends and colleagues:

> Dorothy and I have embarked upon a new adventure intended to make our later years more enjoyable. The life of a professor of some reputation in the U.S.A. is now an endless series of committee meetings, grant applications, progress reports; service as a reviewer of papers for familiar journals and others one has never heard of; writing letters of recommendation for scores of former associates who are being considered for promotion or chairmanships; distinguished scientist lectures, etc. The professor comes to know the airports of the

world like a forceps or pipette in his own laboratory. There is little time for reading or writing and no time to think except in the bathtub which still forms an effective moat against the continual outside bombardment of one's consciousness. So we have recently left it all behind for a more peaceful life in Kenya.

The laboratory is in Kabete about 10 miles west of Nairobi, 90 miles south of the equator at an elevation of 5500 feet—situated on a hill with a fine view of the Ngong hills so fondly described by Karen Blixen, who for some obscure reason chose the unattractive pseudonym Isak Dinesen. We will live in a little 2 bedroom house on the site. ILRAD is supported by the Food and Agriculture Organization of the U.N. and a consortium of foundations and its mission is to do something to combat the two principal cattle diseases that kill 60 to 80,000 cattle a year and make millions of square miles in East and Central Africa unsuitable for animal husbandry. One disease is caused by a trypanosome and has the tsetse fly as its vector; the other is caused by a theileria (an organism similar to that of malaria) which is transmitted by the cattle tick *Rhipicephalus appendiculatus*. The laboratory is beautifully equipped and I am in charge of the Electron Microscope Unit. It will be an interesting experiment to see if I am too old to learn the literature of a field of biology almost entirely new to me. In any case, it will be a refreshing change and just possibly I may be able to do something useful for the developing countries of Africa. As a reproductive biologist I was not very successful in doing something about the population explosion—maybe as a parasitologist I can help feed the excess humans by keeping their cattle alive. Kenya now has a population doubling time of 16 years (32 for the world) and more than half the population is under 17 years of age.

This is for him an adventure in humanitarianism untried in its circumstances and unfamiliar in its challenge; but so is the writing of books that assist learning and rest on scholarship. The definitive reference text that goes beyond classroom needs supports Fawcett's heretical view that if students are well prepared, agile in mind and eager to learn, the differences in modalities of medical education will of themselves have no significance. It has been said that revamping the medical curriculum is like rearranging the lifeboats on the Titanic—it ignores the iceberg. So too Fawcett's recent work in parasitology enforces the view that a solid foundation in research defies narrow specialization and permits a broad spectrum of use.

It is a curious circumstance of medical history that when Fawcett began to work on East Coast fever, he discovered that the classic paper on the life cycle of the pathogenic parasite had been written by Cowdry and Ham in the early 1930s. Three North American anatomists, all authors of textbooks of histology, had been attracted to the study of the same obscure protozoan at different points in their long fruitful careers. Here is part of Arthur Ham's letter responding to one from Fawcett:

Dear Don,

It is really terribly important work that you are doing in Kenya. I heard somewhere recently that of all places Africa was falling behind in being able to produce the food they require and so I'd think it would be an enormous help if you could find some way to enable them to raise cattle successfully. Looking at Kenya superficially one would think they could raise enough food to feed an enormous population.

That the trypanosomes change their surface antigens every couple of weeks or so must be a real challenge to immunologists. However the way things are going these days they will probably find out something new and fundamental that will apply to immunology in general when they solve the problem, and it may account for some phenomena hitherto not understood in other areas.

Dr. Cowdry and I worked in the Veterinary laboratory at Kabete. Dr. and Mrs. Cowdry were provided with a house nearby. My wife and I lived in Nairobi and I recall I bought an old Studebaker car to drive back and forth from the Norfolk Hotel each day. I had to take a Kenya driving examination and the last part of it was to back through an acreage of stumps without hitting any.

I certainly appreciate your problems of getting into the proper mood to revise your textbook, for it seems to me the situation with regard to a histology text has become very complicated. The time allotted in medical schools for histology has become less while the content of its subject matter has grown. This seems to have led to a lot of students wanting books of the core type to enable them to more or less memorize such parts that will enable them to pass the type of examinations now given. Then there is always the question of how physiological a histology text should become. For my eighth edition I took on a younger co-author, Dave Cormack, from our department in Toronto, with the understanding that this was the last edition I would work on and that from now on it was up to him if there were to be any further revisions. I have since turned my attention to a secondary interest in economics.

Sincerely,

Arthur Ham

The "proper mood" in which to revise a reference text can only be one of toil and compromise, for even the most thorough of textbooks can never manage every detail that its author knows to be important in the synthesis of knowledge and the analysis of data.

Look around the world: contemplate the whole and every part of it: You will find it to be nothing but one great machine, subdivided into an infinite number of lesser machines, which again admit of subdivisions, to a degree beyond what human senses and faculties can trace and explain. All these various machines and even their most minute parts, are adjusted to each other with an accuracy which ravishes into admiration all men who have ever contemplated them.

Hume: *Dialogues*

9

The Cecil Textbook of Medicine: Its Six Editors

Of all great collaborative reference works it may be said that their value and usefulness rest on the experience and wisdom of their individual writers; and several of the separate contributions to the *Cecil Textbook of Medicine* have become in their own right small classic statements on various aspects of disease, read and reread, cherished and quoted—a unique example is Fuller Albright's "Introduction to Diseases of the Endocrine System," an essay that appeared little changed over many editions because it was essentially timeless in its observations and appraisals. But, in a larger sense, it is the editors of such works who give them unity and coherence, quality and perspective, who fashion from the disparate work of many a single whole responsive to the needs of teaching and of practice, reflecting the emphases and discoveries of contemporary medicine.

It will, therefore, be the intent here to try and capture something of the characters and capacities of the six fine editors who have made the *Textbook of Medicine* a standard reference source recognized and used throughout the world. Although not dichotomous by its nature, medicine embraces two fundamentally different points of view—the how and why—one concentrated on the practice or art of medicine, the other focused on its science or underpinning. The achievement of a proper balance and interaction between the two is one of the triumphs of good medical writing. It arises from the circumstance, for which physician, student and publisher must be grateful, that the finest minds of medicine have not hesitated to devote large parts of their busy lives to the making of books.

In the mid 1920s Russell L. Cecil had the wisdom to see that a single-authored textbook in medicine was no longer possible. For seven editions of his textbook he carefully sought out the best of physician-writers and created a work without parallel or competition. In those years it probably secured more than ninety percent of all medical textbook use in the English-speaking world and was translated into a dozen languages. Cecil relished its esteem and its usefulness and knew how to achieve both.

What his close associates felt of him shines through in the warm and sometimes indulgent anecdotes they recite about him, many of them about the days after World War I when he was the central figure of a small group of young physicians living together in New York, all of them destined for great distinction. They lived without great means in a boarding house on Sixty-second Street that young Cecil adroitly managed. The way Dave Barr used to tell it, Russ generally seemed to dine on lean, loin lamb chops while his put-upon boarders choked on gristle. And this may have been at least figuratively so, for Cecil both treasured and knew how to secure the good things of life. When he was in his mid-seventies he taught himself fluent command of Greek that he might enjoy Greek poetry without the interposition of awkward translation. He was an artist, too, of real talent who, unlike many artists, took great pleasure in his own work and the work of others. His prose and his painting and his personality had a Churchillian flavor.

There was another side of the many-faceted character of Cecil that some of his closest friends scarcely knew—he was a radical, if by "radical" we mean one who gets at the root of things. In 1937 there appeared a two-volume report of the American Foundation Studies in Government, entitled *American Medicine: Expert Testimony Out of Court.* The evidence brought together there indicated that many people lacked the medical care they needed; that there should be better integration of the services of general practitioners and specialists; and that group practice seemed to offer enough advantages to patients to warrant a more extensive trial. Evidence was also presented concerning the relative merits of state medicine and voluntary health insurance as means of assuring comprehensive medical care for all levels of the population.

Within a few months of the publication of *Expert Testimony,* a group of medical men headed by Russell L. Cecil formulated and made public a set of principles and proposals designed to improve medical education, medical research and medical care. Part of that document follows:

Principles

1. That the health of the people is a direct concern of the government.

2. That a national public health policy directed towards all groups of the population should be formulated.

3. That the problems of economic need and the problem of providing adequate medical care are not identical and may require different approaches for their solution.

Proposals

1. That the first necessary step toward the realization of the above principles is to minimize the risk of illness by prevention.

2. That an immediate problem is provision of adequate medical care for the medically indigent, the cost to be met from public funds.

3. That public funds should be made available for the support of medical education and for studies, investigations, and procedures for raising the standards of medical practice. If this is not done, the provision of adequate medical care may prove impossible.

4. That public funds should be available for medical research as essential for high standards of practice in both preventive and curative medicine.

5. That public funds should be made available to hospitals that render service to the medically indigent and for laboratory and diagnostic and consultative services.

The publication of the principles and proposals, which now seem sensible and even conservative, gave rise to bitter controversy within the medical profession. An editorial in the *JAMA* accused the signers of being traitors to their fellow physicians. The controversy and the reports that preceded it served to make the public aware of the fact that the AMA did not speak for all physicians and that there was a large group of distinguished medical educators, investigators and physicians who believed that American medicine was in need of improvement. Not many well-placed private practitioners of medicine would then sign a document giving rise to charges of betrayal from the powerful American Medical Association.

Cecil was from the South; but he was no post-bellum traditionalist. He was, rather, a completely modern man—urbane, witty and cosmopolitan—who astutely judged the worth of other men, but with a shrewdness tempered by compassion and an amused tolerance of human frailty. The comical antics of people, including himself, were his constant delight and he could tick off pretension in all its forms with salty humor and wry appreciation. Something of the South lingered in his courtesy and effusiveness. When he called on the phone—even if about trivial matters—he would cry out the given name of his hearer with a certain rising explosive ring that suggested a new world of exciting adventure was about to open up.

Occasionally he would reveal a persistence of the past in the old-fashioned values he cherished. In publishing there is a common practice, whenever a revision of a work is brought out, to destroy remaining copies of the previous edition. Custom or no, this was a practice that outraged Russ—not because it was happening to *his* book but because it could happen to any book. Deep within him stirred an old attitude from frontier days that a book—any book— was the precious product of man's intellectual creativity and not a thing to be willfully destroyed. His carefully preserved Virginia accent and especially his pince-nez also recalled the past. His rimless glasses danced on his indented nose in moments of mirth and pure delight and in moments of anger, but they never were dislodged from their perilous perch. They had, like their wearer, an old-fashioned stick-to-itiveness.

Cecil was recognized as America's leading authority on rheumatic disease and was a founder of the American Rheumatism Association, serving as its President in 1937–38; but he said of himself somewhat ruefully, "The rise and fall of focal infection was the rise and fall of Russell Cecil." The achievements of his scientific and professional life would have made his career distinguished and his name well known; but the book idea he initiated—and nurtured for over thirty years—made him the best-known American physician in the world, a position in which he took great pride.

And yet, despite his great intellectual endowment, his achievement and his human concern, there was about Cecil an odd sense of detachment toward his profession, his book and even himself, almost as if he were a spectator viewing judiciously his own enlarged life and career.

It was this very detachment that gave him the further wisdom to perceive that the scientific basis of medicine had so enlarged that his own background in science was no longer current or sufficient. Hence for the Eighth Edition he invited his friend Robert F. Loeb to join him as coauthor. This union of the abilities of a private physician and part-time professor of medicine with those of a full-time academic professor schooled in the biosciences was a happy one for the book and for its authors. Both men were dedicated to the idea of putting the key concepts of the scientist and the useful practices of the specialist into a form understandable and useful to the medical student and the physician. Under Loeb's editorship the book changed subtly, becoming less the repository of established doctrine and more the expression of advanced ongoing ideas in medicine.

Cecil and Loeb each had ample claims to distinction aside from the book, and each in the course of long careers had benefited many people; but it was their joint editorial venture that allowed them to exert a healing influence on many thousands of patients they never saw and a learning influence on many thousands of students and residents who could not experience at first hand their extraordinary ability as teachers. The two editors complemented each other—Cecil tending to worry more about the needs of physicians and Loeb about the needs of students. The latter concern made Loeb a tougher editor than Cecil, more interested in the impact of the book than in its strategy.

Robert F. Loeb was born in Chicago in 1895, the son of gifted parents. His mother, Anne Leonard, was the first woman to earn a doctorate in philology from the University of Zurich, then the language study center of the world. His father, Jacques Loeb, was a founding member of the Rockefeller Institute and of the Marine Biology Laboratory at Woods Hole—a physiologist who at the turn of the century brought the objectivity of chemistry and physics to the study of biology. Like his father, Robert Loeb insisted upon medical science as the basis for expert clinical practice and for the advance of medicine. Yet this belief never came between him and his humane concern for the ill patient and the overburdened student. This was the guiding light of his teaching, illumined by a capacity for detached and perceptive judgment that made him among the wisest of men. In 1947 he became Bard Professor of Medicine at Columbia University, carrying on and elaborating the great traditions of a famous chair.

Throughout his long and illustrious career he received scores of honors and honorary degrees; but perhaps he would have liked best of all the title "physician," for he was a master of the art of medicine. In his rounds, intense and completely immersed in the problems at hand, he created an electric atmosphere of concern and skill that compelled a response of confidence from the patient and an increment in reasoned understanding from students and residents.

In short, Bob Loeb was a scholar and an artistocrat—an aristocrat of the mind who cared little for fools and shoddy contrivance. He had the look and bearing of a Brahmin and this deceived some people, for he was at heart the kindest and gentlest of men who never forgot a resident's name or needed to consult a bedside chart to know the identity and illness of a patient. The most scientific of physicians, he knew that medicine is not only science but also art—the art of wooing nature—and that nature must be wooed not simply by correct measures by also by the ministrations of care, a tempting tray sometimes as effective as a drug in restoring health.

As a writer, he was disciplined and scrupulous. As an editor, he was shrewd and ruthless. A few of America's most eminent practitioners of medicine were to learn from him that their essays were trivial and foolish—entirely unsuitable to the most widely used textbook of medicine in the world. Never strait-laced or self-righteous, he was nevertheless a puritan who believed that life was an adventure in morality. Cecil once asked him what he could do about his intermittent claudication. He replied, only half-jokingly, "You can't do anything about it, Russ, for it is the voice of God telling you to have only one martini before lunch."

Humble yet proud, he shunned the limelight of formal lectures, the textbook being for him a means of dissemination of his steadfast principles and sometimes heretical ideas. In public and in private he did not hesitate to speak his mind, especially on matters that angered him—principally, sloppy thinking, lack of attention to significant details and publication of unjustified conclusions. Firm believer though he was in solid investigation as the rock upon which clinical medicine must be built, he could be coldly critical of ill-conceived, wasteful research. His essay on Clinical Investigation published in May of 1936 in *Science* (Vol. 83, No. 2185) ruffled a few feathers, as may be imagined from these paragraphs:

> There is no doubt that what we desire to save above all else is that backlog of solid and profitable research which has continued to advance medical science and which may be defined as a product of thoughtful and critical curiosity supported by ingenuity in experimentation. Whether or not the results are of immediate practical value is relatively unimportant, but that the stimulus to investigation should be a query either of fundamental or of practical significance is vital. Of two general approaches to research, experience has shown time and again through the ages that the outstanding advances in the realm of science have resulted from the efforts of individual investigators possessing the spark essential for creative work. To be sure, in this approach the full harvest of results may frequently be reaped only through the subsequent cooperation of others better versed in various technical aspects of the problems, but the fact remains that it is the individual investigator whose creative force furnishes the opening wedge. It is, consequently, this rare individual who above all is to be treasured and who deserves the support necessary to enable him to exercise his powers to the full.

> The largest group interested in clinical research is composed of individuals, many of whom are the clinical teachers responsible for the development of critique and a point of view among students of medicine. These investigators share in common one characteristic, namely, that of intellectual curiosity; they perceive the significance of fundamental observations and are frequently able to extend them, but their capacities for critical and thoughtful experimentation naturally cover a range so wide that the products of their scientific endeavors, while often good, are more frequently indifferent and occasionally very bad. Nevertheless, the progress of medical science is greatly enhanced by these gleaners. Consequently they, too, deserve encouragement and should continue to receive financial support. However, the time has come when the qualifications of the recruits for this class of investigators should be scrutinized

meticulously, because it is the futile efforts of the many lesser lights among these gleaners which lead to untold waste.

Another approach to clinical investigation has been developed in recent years and lies in sharp contrast to that already described. This is the *research project* which demonstrates in its point of view total ignorance of the means by which science has advanced. It attempts to force progress through regimentation of workers who lack the essential critical curiosity in the subject under investigation and it stifles the untrammeled play of imagination which often seizes upon a most significant by-product in the course of individual research. It is not the product of creative thought, but is usually initiated by energetic and misguided promoters inspired by the effectiveness of mass production in big business. It involves the wasteful expenditure of large sums of money. In other words, it assumes that scientific knowledge can be bought, and that dollars give birth to ideas. The research project in clinical medicine has proven consistently barren and has resulted in the disbursement of funds which, if applied to the endowment of individual investigators or university departments where creative thought is fostered, may reasonably be expected to further the progress of science. Hence I make my plea for the support of those individuals engaged in fruitful research, for the reapportionment of the limited funds available for clinical investigation and for their direction into recognized productive channels.

Loeb, who had made important contributions to the understanding of water and salt balance in health and disease, was fond of the story of an Irishman named O'Shaughnessy, who in 1831 made an inspired stab at truth. He recognized that a state of dehydration and shock was frequently the cause of death in cholera and correctly ascribed this deficiency to the diarrheal loss of water and salt, and also demonstrated a decrease in neutral and alkaline salts in the blood. He further recognized the salutary therapeutic effect of sodium chloride in the treatment of cholera and the value of injections of saline solution in diabetic coma. It was only fairly recently discovered that O'Shaughnessy was so dismayed at the charges of fraud and falsification leveled against him by the leaders of British science that he gave up medicine, changed his name, went to India, had a brilliant career there, in which, among other achievements, he established 3,000 miles of telegraphic communication, and was knighted for his pseudonymous accomplishments.

The story illustrated for Loeb that the medical establishment is not endowed with infallibility and that medicine should be a highly practical enterprise—illuminiated by science and guided by intelligence—but not too much different from establishing telegraph lines. Nor should it be a vainglorious venture but one dedicated to service and springing from soundness of heart and mind. No man in American medicine ever did more to make his vision of medicine a reality—a vision in which unity of spirit underlies diversity of means.

This portrait of Bob Loeb has been drawn in some detail, for the character it portrays—one of scholarship, scientific brilliance, humanistic concern and, yes, humility—is the hallmark of the four editors who were to succeed him. He and Cecil both retired from editorship of the textbook upon publication of its tenth edition, and Paul B. Beeson and Walsh McDermott took over the reins of a book well established and bearing the imprint of its previous editors. Like Cecil and Loeb, the new editors were united in their aim to provide in understandable prose authoritative clinical guidance and a reasoned scientific basis for the pursuit of medicine.

Paul Beeson was born in Livingston, Montana, but soon removed to Anchorage, where he underwent an Arctic survival course that was to prepare him for the cold English winters and but barely heated rooms of later years. He studied medicine at McGill University and after internship went into general practice in Ohio, where his father had started a group clinic, the experience giving the young doctor a sense of the importance of those elements that underlie intelligent care—the history and physical examination, an intuitive "feel" for the patient and an awareness of the physiologic rationale for drug use—elements that have stayed very much alive in him through a career distinguished for important research and large administrative responsibilities.

But for the long term general practice was not satisfying, and it was at the Rockefeller Institute where he fully developed his investigative skills. Eventually the siren call of Eugene Stead summoned him to Atlanta. When Stead left for larger challenges, Beeson succeeded him as Chairman of Medicine at Emory and there exercised his remarkable capacities as a clinician. In 1952 he left Emory to become Chairman of Medicine at Yale, where he put his stamp on the medical service as doctor and teacher. Never too busy to see a patient, he took great pains to show younger physicians the value of a sensitive patient-doctor relationship. But he always managed to find time for his laboratory and in the 1950s began his studies of pyelonephritis, culminating in a beautiful article in 1955 (*Yale Journal of Biology and Medicine,* Vol. 98:493) in which he laid to rest the idea of lymphatic and hematogenous pathways through which bacteria reached the kidney. Always mindful of both clinical experience and laboratory findings, he became convinced that the urethral catheter was an important source of urinary tract infection, and he demonstrated this in a simple but elegant experiment. Just as Bob Loeb twenty years before had upset the complacent equilibrium of research administrators, so too this finding upended a steadfast conviction of urologists, who hotly disputed his views. Nevertheless, he was to prevail, just as his findings in the pathogenesis of fever and in induction of the eosinophil response by bone marrow offered new ideas that were only gradually accepted.

One day in 1965 to almost everyone's astonishment Paul Beeson announced that he was leaving Yale to accept the Nuffield Professorship of Medicine at Oxford. There too he continued his investigative work with Hans Krebs. He also completely revised the Oxford introductory course for medical students, using the sciences of pathology, microbiology and pharmacology as bridges between preclinical study and clinical experience. For his accomplishment there he was made, just before his return to the United States, a Knight Commander of the British Empire; but he may have relished more his new American title: Distinguished Physician, United States Veterans Administration, University of Washington School of Medicine, where he rejoined his old friend Bob Petersdorf—also an able and devoted editor of a medical textbook.

Petersdorf had presented Paul with the Kober Medal in 1973 and had concluded his remarks by asking a question, to which he gave a nice answer.

> Why is the Association giving the Kober Medal to Beeson? Is it because of his investigative triumphs—it has been said that Beeson has more "firsts" than anyone else in infectious diseases. Is it because he is a good doctor, clinician and teacher who has been an inspiration to many young men? Is it because he has served as American academe's ambassador with courtesy, grace and friendliness? Or because he is the recipient of many honors? Is it because he has, as President of this Association, shown remarkable clairvoyance by warning us five years ago that we had better turn our attention to true clinical investigation? Or is it because he is a wise counsellor and warm friend who has helped countless young men attain their place in the academic world? All of these accomplishments are contributory, but in my view not any of them is the reason. Beeson deserves the Kober Medal because he has taught us, probably more than anyone else in academic medicine, how to live the academic adventure fully, how to live it with humility and humor, with style and graciousness, and to live it with an understanding and kindness for his patients, his students and his colleagues, in a spirit of giving to all of them more than he has received. In short, he has been the example of what the best in academic medicine is all about.

Throughout these years so busy with investigation, the practice of medicine and the burden of administration, Beeson still managed extraordinary service to the *Cecil Textbook of Medicine,* reviewing the sections for which he was responsible with scrupulous care and substantive suggestion. He is a perfectionist, and even a slight, trivial error in the published book (there were but two or three in all the years of his editorship) filled him with despair and dismay. In the midst of these concerns and commitments, especially his newly awakened interest in the plight of the aged and their inadequate medical care, Paul could even find time to read critically the not-inconsiderable writing of the Saunders editor, including substantial parts of this manuscript, and to offer valuable advice and just commentary enlivened by a salty wit.

Just as Cecil and Loeb complemented each other perfectly as editors, so too did Paul Beeson and Walsh McDermott. If Paul was inclined to worry too much, Walsh was inclined to hope for the best. If Paul was a shade overorganized, Walsh was a trifle underorganized, often exquisitely aware of the substance of a contributed piece but not so sure of its whereabouts. They were the fastest of friends and the best of collaborators.

In presenting him with the Kober Medal of the American Association of Physicians and later with the Founder's Medal of the Southern Society for Clinical Investigation, Bob Petersdorf—no mean rhetorician—tried twice to capture the spirit of Paul Beeson; but it does him no injustice to say that he failed, for Beeson is a man of seeming contradictions. Impatient with stupidity, he is patient with the long and tortuous path of research; fragile in appearance, he is indomitably strong in pursuit of the goals of perceptive medicine and a well-ordered society; gentle with friends, colleagues and the ill, he is abrupt and scornful with pretense and falseness; adaptable to environment and circumstance, he is unalterably opposed to dishonesty and says so; hopeful in his work, he yet feels that the work of achieving the good life for man has been scarcely begun and is now threatened by the senseless prospect of universal destruction. Perhaps he would say with Dwight Eisenhower, "Every gun that is made, every warship launched, every rocket fired signifies a theft from those who hunger and are not fed, those who are cold and not clothed." He would add "those who are ill and not cared for."

The doing of any great book brings with it mementos of triumph and of failure. Of these the one Paul Beeson most cherishes is a letter from the translator of the Chinese Cecil:

UNIVERSITY OF WASHINGTON
SEATTLE, WASHINGTON
U.S.A.

93 DU TIEN XIAN
JIUJIANG, JIANGXI
PEOPLE'S REPUBLIC OF CHINA

Feb. 18, 1983

Prof. Beeson
Prof. McDermott
Prof. Wyngaarden,

Dear Sirs,

May I, an ordinary Chinese physician, take the pleasure to inform you that your "Cecil Textbook of Medicine" has been translated by me into Chinese and will be published in 10 volumes within 3 years. Please pardon me for not being able to inform you beforehand. [The complete translation appeared in 13 volumes in 1984.]

Cecil's Textbook has a deep and wide influence in China as it has in the other parts of the world. Virtually all of our old clinicians received their medical education with the help of this Book. At the beginning of the fifties, as a medical student, I had heard a lot about Cecil and his famous textbook and longed to have a copy of it for reference. Since it was too dear for me, I went to our university library, but I was told that a number of students were waiting to borrow it and I had to wait patiently. Half a year later I eventually got the Book from the University library. With a most respectful and happy feeling I embraced it in my arms and returned to my dormitory. It was the 9th Edition of the Book, the most up-to-date edition available at the time. I immediately began reading it with "greedy" interest and was deeply impressed by its systematic, authoritative and strict description, accuracy and compactness. It seemed that I was travelling in a great magnificent and solemn palace. As the moon ascended outside my window, an odd idea suddenly rose before me: Why not try my best to translate the Book into Chinese?

Time went by very fast. After graduating from the University, I became a qualified physician. I don't believe in Fate, but fate did conduct me along a rough and uneven road. In 1957 owing to my suspicion of the "advanced" medicine of the USSR and my suggestion of learning from all advanced countries, not from the USSR alone, I was labelled as a "Bourgeois Rightist" and was sentenced to 12 years imprisonment and was put into prison where I served at a hospital. The accusation was that I didn't show profound respection for the poems by Mao and that I praised some medical authorities of the U.S. imperialists.

In 1972 one of my poor "counter-revolutionary" friends who had been released from prison sent me a copy of the 13th Edition of your Book. I was no longer a young student but a weatherbeaten, middle aged man. When I got the Book from my friend, however, I could hardly restrain my tears. Yes, I thought, it is the very time to begin my work—putting the Book into Chinese now!

It was, indeed, not only an odd idea, but also dangerous and ridiculous, for China at that time was carrying out a policy of excluding anything foreign, especially anything that came from the United States. A counter-revolutionary political convict, who has already been sentenced heavily, dared to think of doing such an unwise and impractical work during his imprisonment. But I was not at all impulsive in making the decision, for I firmly believed that a situation like this would not last long in China. No one in the world could be able to isolate and sequester our great nation and her economics, science and culture from the outside world endlessly. China would certainly return to the world and make her contributions to mankind. It was with this belief in mind that I determined to start my work—translating your Textbook into Chinese while in prison. I thought it was the only thing that I could do for my motherland in that time and in those very conditions. After spending innumerable nights and overcoming many inconceivable difficulties, I eventually finished my work in September, 1975. A month later, I was allowed out of prison. Having lost everything, including my wife and my only son, still I felt "wealthy" because I was back with my manuscript—a 3,400,000 Chinese word manuscript of Cecil's Textbook of Medicine (13th Ed.). I then returned to my tiny home town, Jiujiang, Jiangxi, where lived my poor, lonely and old mother who had, for years, sorrowfully waited for her only son's release and return.

Thanks to the 3rd plenary session of the CPC, the shame and mistreatment that I had put up with since 1957 were finally removed in 1980. The long-forgotten translation manuscript has at last the opportunity to serve the people. In the winter of 1980, thanks to the support of Professor Hwang Jiasi, director of the Chinese Academy of Medicine, who wrote a preface to the Chinese Edition, Inner Mongolia Publishing House decided to publish it and I happily began retranslating it according to its 15th Edition. Up till now I have finished about 3,100,000 words (some three quarters of the Book). The first volume of the Chinese Edition is now in print and will emerge this coming spring. It is predicted that the Chinese Edition will be heartily welcomed by our medical students and physicians. Everyone who is benefited by the Chinese Edition will of course be grateful to you, its original editors, and all its 277 contributors. Would you be kind enough to write some words for your Chinese Edition?

If there is a new edition in English, please inform me in time and I'll order it. Additions and omissions will be reflected accordingly in its Chinese Edition.

With best regards

Yours,

Wang Xiancai

Now the quiet voice of Paul Beeson tells something of the experience of being an editor for the two most influential and respected textbooks of medicine ever published in the English language. Perhaps its ardors pale in comparison with those of translating the *Textbook of Medicine* into Chinese; but they are real enough all the same:

In 1945, when I was in the Department of Medicine at Emory University, I received an invitation to write the chapter on typhoid fever for the Cecil Textbook of Medicine, and I was thrilled to have this recognition. Reviewers had said about previous editions that "the list of contributors reads like a Who's Who in American Medicine." The interesting thing about my invitation to contribute was that it came as a form letter, with a blank filled in for the title of the article I was to write. It was signed by a woman whose name I did not recognize, presumably Dr. Cecil's editorial assistant. I heard nothing from him directly. I did write about typhoid fever in the editions that appeared in 1947 and 1951.

In the latter half of the 1940's Tinsley Harrison of Alabama invited me to become a co-editor of a new textbook of medicine that would challenge Cecil. Its first edition appeared in 1950 under the title "Principles of Internal Medicine." Harrison's idea was that a medical textbook, rather than offering a catalog of diseases by organ systems should present subject matter in a way that simulates clinical practice. He planned that the first part of the book would deal with the interpretation of cardinal manifestations of disease, discussing such common signs and symptoms as edema and shortness of breath. He argued that a patient does not come in saying "I have hepatitis" or "I have angina pectoris;" rather he seeks a doctor's help because he is jaundiced or is having chest pain.

Harrison enlisted as other co-editors William Resnick, George Thorn, Maxwell Wintrobe, and Raymond Adams. The six of us had a number of week-long meetings, some of them in delightful places such as New Orleans or Jackson Hole, in which we planned the new "Harrison approach" and began to go over submitted materials. For me attendance at those meetings was an invaluable privilege—among the most informative and stimulating experiences of my professional life.

In 1952 I was invited to become chairman of the department of medicine at Yale and, of course, gladly accepted. This meant that I was going to be responsible for the direction of a much larger department, and I decided that I should give up the textbook work after participating in the first two editions of Harrison in order to devote all of my time to the affairs of the department at Yale.

After six years at Yale I was less daunted by the responsibilities of departmental chairmanship and felt that it would be advantageous for me and for the school to take a sabbatical leave. I did so in the academic year of 1958–59, working on a problem of the immunology of kidney infection at the Wright-Fleming Institute in London. This was an enormously valuable and refreshing year. Some months after my arrival in London I received a two-page letter from John Dusseau informing me that Drs. Cecil and Loeb would be giving up the editorship of the textbook after the 10th edition, and inviting me to join with Walsh McDermott as co-editor. This was an attractive offer from many standpoints. I was still awed by the reputation of the Cecil textbook and the thought of having my name on its spine was gratifying indeed. McDermott and I had by then become good friends. We had served on an NIH study section together and later, with Barry Wood, had formed a little society that met informally twice a year in New Haven, New York or Baltimore. The original purpose was simply to talk about the experimental work going on in our respective infectious disease divisions, with particular emphasis on work in progress rather than publishable results. This society grew spontaneously because even after younger colleagues had left our divisions, they always wanted to return and participate in these meetings. I was in no doubt whatever that I could work effectively and productively with McDermott. The Dusseau letter specified that I would be listed as first editor because it had been agreed between him and McDermott that the first name should be that of a chairman of a clinical department.

When I returned from the sabbatical in the summer of 1959, McDermott, Dusseau and I had a meeting to discuss the mechanics of editing the book and getting out the next edition in 1963. We did the 11th through the 15th editions, which appeared at four-year intervals during that time. We recognized the necessity to have some associate editors because of the rapid growth of specialization within the field of internal medicine, and in those five editions, we were fortunate to have the help of Fred Plum, Alexander Bearn, Philip Bondy, Carl Moore, Ralph Nachman, Marvin Sleisenger, Nicholas Christy, Phillip Marsden, John Murray, Roscoe Robinson, and Andrew Wallace. At the time of the publication of the 14th edition, although Walsh and I were at the conventional age of retirement from the textbook editorship, Saunders decided to ask us to serve for one more edition, the 15th, due in 1979. Jim Wyngaarden joined us as co-editor for that edition, and he and Holly Smith succeeded as editors for the subsequent editions of the textbook.

One of the events of the 20 years during which I was editor was my transfer from Yale to Oxford. I moved there in 1965 and returned—this time to the University of Washington, and from there I participated in the editing of the 15th edition.

By the 1960's the competition between Harrison and Cecil was neck and neck. Drs. Cecil and Loeb had acknowledged the attractiveness of the Harrison concept by inserting introductory chapters in each section of the book—certainly not substitutes for the large amount of space given to the cardinal manifestations in Harrison but presentations of the derangements of physiologic function in each organ system to be considered. Later on, because of the rapid progress in the basic sciences of genetics and immunology, we included entire chapters on these, dealing with them as basic disciplines without much reference to relevant specific diseases. We also had the problems of more extensive coverage of imaging techniques, ultrasound, angiography, and computed tomography. We, of course, were constantly on the lookout for descriptions of new diseases, new diagnostic techniques and new therapies, and also we had in mind the need to change authorship of various chapters as medical progress took place. There are disadvantages to the Harrison formula. The section of cardinal manifestations, so appreciated by junior medical students, is probably not as likely to be studied again by older users of the book, and it imposes a real handicap in terms of organization. Subjects are often dealt with in more than one part of the book. For example, one finds the principles of normal bilirubin metabolism in a chapter on jaundice, but the abnormalities of bilirubin metabolism may be dealt with in detail in another part of the book, a thousand pages later, under Diseases of the Liver. This is sometimes a nuisance, and it often requires some redundancy in coverage. By contrast the Cecil dogma has been to combine pathophysiology with the description of the disease. Cecil editors have felt that by minimizing duplication they gained more leeway for completeness and the encyclopedic features that have always characterized the work.

One of the main functions of the editors in a publication of this kind is to deal with the large number of contributors. Our first invitation usually went out at least a year in advance of the deadline for the manuscript, and a reminder letter was sent out about three months before the deadline. By and large, our experience was quite good in the matter of receiving manuscripts on time. This undoubtedly was due to the great reputation of the book at the time we took it over. Nevertheless, there are always crises and a few manuscripts did not come in on time. We quickly learned that in such cases there must be contact with the delinquent contributor by telephone, and occasionally we even had to rerun an article from the preceding edition with some anonymous updating by a good friend.

We did not follow a practice of rigid critiquing of the content of articles, because anyone invited to contribute had already appeared to be an established authority in the field. We realized that authorities can have differences of opinion, but we thought it appropriate to let each contributor present his own point of view. In perhaps four or five instances, over the 20-year period, something was submitted to us so disappointing in style and content that rejection was the only possible way out. As to details of the writing we felt no compunction about fairly extensive use of editorial pencils. Indeed, the use was needed surprisingly often. There were some crashing surprises when nationally respected people turned in very badly written pieces requiring extensive editorial repair. We asked ourselves who must have helped these people to compose their other articles!

When Walsh McDermott accepted coeditorship of the *Textbook of Medicine* with Beeson, he was Livingston Farrand Professor and Chairman of the Department of Public Health at the New York Hospital Cornell Medical Center. The title is significant because, of his many broad and compelling interests, the idea attracting his greatest attention was that of interaction—the interface between private and public good, private and public health. He saw that preventive and curative medicine are a continuum, not separate activities, and that advances in technology, the discoveries of science, the progress of medicine, the dissemination of fresh ideas affect populations as a whole. Successful adaptation to and utilization of the new may for the long term be more important than the act of discovery itself. He recognized, for instance, that the antiviral vaccines were made feasible only by the prior discovery of antimicrobials.

In a sense he saw the textbook as an instrument of adaptation. It would bring to the physician and student the meaning and implication of the new. It would not simply state, it would explain; it would tell not merely what to do but what to consider and what to expect. It would amplify the spread of knowledge within the framework of reason and the experience of the past. He once said of the textbook that the greatest compensation of its doing lies in "knowing that the volume goes to the remotest parts of the world—that somewhere, perhaps in an African jungle, some human being is getting correct treatment for his illness because a doctor or nurse has our book."

After graduation from Columbia University College of Physicians and Surgeons and a residency in internal medicine, McDermott served in various staff and faculty positions as an internist at Cornell University Medical Center; but he was never to lose sight of the role of basic research or of the effects of change produced by medical innovation.

During those years he played a pivotal role in deploying penicillin for civilian use, for the supply of penicillin during World War II was largely limited to military use, especially for the treatment of venereal disease, and was not available to the public for treatment of fatal diseases in which penicillin had been demonstrated to be a lifesaving agent. "I was with Dr. Joseph Moore," Walsh would say, "when a woman called in and said she had just talked to Dr. Chester Keefer and told him that if her husband could not get penicillin for his bacterial endocarditis, she was going to send him out to get syphilis, so he could be eligible for the drug from Dr. Moore's office." He also played a key pioneering role in the early demonstration and evaluation of streptomycin and of isoniazid in the treatment of tuberculosis, a disease he knew through firsthand acquaintanceship. As the antimicrobial specificity of antibiotics became increasingly apparent, he conducted many of the initial studies that clarified their pharmacologic action. But he was not content with the clinical trial of new drugs, because the process of adaptation was ever a significant consideration to him. He therefore studied the phenomenon of microbial persistence—why certain infections persisted after they had been bacteriologically cured; and this in turn led to important findings concerning the development of resistant strains of pathogenic microorganisms.

In 1966 and '67 Walsh served as Chairman of President Lyndon Johnson's Task Force on American Indians—a logical appointment because of his years of research on tuberculosis and other health-care problems among the Navajos of Arizona—work that documented the miraculous qualities of isoniazid. But these studies also demonstrated that technology is not all—health is by no means the inevitable result of health care. It is rather the result of a host of socioeconomic factors producing an environment in which medicine may or may not effect cures. Where there is malnutrition, inadequate housing, lack of proper sanitation, dependence on drugs or alcohol, destructive ways of life and the dreariness of closed doors of opportunity, medicine unaided can accomplish no lasting miracles.

This perception was part of his genius, for he saw the need for new local, national and international institutions to nurture scientific developments and apply them for man's benefit. He recognized that successful efforts would not occur randomly. New working arrangements would be needed to bring people together. The development of the health components of AID, the National Institutes of Health, the Health Research Council of New York, reoriented WHO health programs for developing nations, and the Institute of Medicine were, in part, his inventions. And, said Dave Rogers in his eloquent memorial, "the academic medical center and what it might do for mankind was his church."

The Saunders editor was aware of Walsh McDermott's countless commitments and responsibilities when discussion of his role in the textbook was first initiated. Walsh has already had more than one brush with death and he was, among his other sleight-of-hand performances, editing with consummate skill and no staff *The American Review of Respiratory Diseases*—a task he performed for twenty-five years without seeming effort. He accepted this new burden on his time and strength and never failed to give the book his best thought and work and to be at all times a counsellor and friend to the beleaguered Saunders editor, often called upon to review manuscripts almost totally inscrutable to him. In every great man—and Walsh McDermott was truly among the great—there is a secret wellspring of strength and perception of which he himself may be unaware but upon which he calls in time of need, and in Walsh's world medicine, his associates, students and books could always call upon his deep resources of strength.

He was the most outgoing and most generous of men, never unable to find time or ideas or support with which to help his friends, and they were beyond number. But there was also about him a strong sense of reserve. He spoke and wrote vividly and forcefully on a thousand topics. One can scarcely name a subject to which he could not bring the insight of fresh thought; but there were some subjects he did not dwell on—and one of these was himself. He was the master of reminiscence; but in his shrewd and often hilarious recollections of the past he himself figured only slightly. This was not due simply to a sense of modesty but rather to the sense of a man's belonging only to himself—not to the outside world.

He once wrote that a man may be judged by his sense of outrage; and outrage was a strong component of his own attitudes. He was the most benign of men; but he could not forgive meanness or cruelty or dishonesty, for he knew what a fearful toll these qualities exact on every life they touch. He loved humanity too greatly to condone inhumanity.

And he loved medicine and science too greatly to be blind to their faults and follies. He expected science to be painstaking and truthful and to improve the lot and understanding of man; but he did not expect it to perform miracles or to save the world. He knew that the world can be saved only by the ideals alive in man—ideals that spring not from the pursuit of truth but from a proper vision of life.

A part of his own vision was that the indwelling soul of man must be nourished and maintained in secret. He was a never-failing source of help, of astute criticism, of splendid performance—indeed, of constant inspiration. He made the publisher's task fun and his life exciting. His magic turned relationships into friendships. He gave himself freely to all who asked; but he did not often reveal himself. In all his relationships he preserved a delicate propriety.

In the *Journal of Medical Education* not long before his untimely death in 1981, McDermott summed up in his easy, engaging prose the aim of medical education. It is also the aim he sought constantly to realize in the *Textbook of Medicine:*

> Most of the time, when we need a physician, we don't need a very good one. The need for a high-quality physician usually comes only rarely, or perhaps never. But its coming is wholly unpredictable; it may come tonight for any one of us. And when it comes, if the moment is not properly seized, if a quality physician is not there, or if it not be appreciated in proper time that he or she should be there, the result can be disastrous. The catch is that the only person who can really tell you whether you need a middling-to-poor physician or a good physician, *is* a good physician. Thus, medical education as it concerns physicians must occupy itself with the development of graduates of high quality. This is not to say that we should not have various types of physicians' assistants, but they must be just that. The present discussion, therefore, is concerned with the education of physicians to a high level of quality—to be "good" physicians. The great vital principle of medical education and training of the highest quality lies not in impressive facilities or glittering diagnostic apparatus but in the deep-seated tradition of self-discipline.

A man for all seasons is a phrase of grandeur that can be applied precisely to Walsh McDermott. For him there was no foul weather in his friendships. For him no wintry clouds obscured the vision of what man might be. For him no miasma of despair or distrust impeded dedication to the noblest of professions.

As so many times before, good fortune (perhaps it should simply be called good luck) smiled on the Saunders Company, for with the Sixteenth Edition of the *Cecil Textbook* James B. Wyngaarden and Lloyd H. Smith, Jr. succeeded Beeson and McDermott as editors, affectionately and eloquently dedicating the book to their predecessors.

The two new editors are like their precursors in devotion to sound science, good medical care and effective communication. Indeed Wyngaarden's "Use and Interpretation of Laboratory Data" and the contributions of both editors to the sections on Human Genetics and Metabolic Diseases are among the book's brightest gems of distilled wisdom. But a change has come over medicine in which Wyngaarden and Smith have been active participants. In an introduction to the textbook ("Medicine as a Learned Profession") Smith quotes McDermott's definition, "Medicine is not a science but a learned profession, deeply rooted in a number of sciences and charged with the obligation to apply them for man's benefit." And Smith adds: "It is also a mutable body of knowledge, skills, and traditions applicable to the preservation of health, the cure of disease, and the amelioration of suffering. The boundaries of medicine blend into psychology, sociology, economics, and even cultural heritage. Disease may be encoded in the genome; disease may also be encoded by the deprivations of poverty and ignorance."

In this concept of the broad sweep of medicine, there is a key word—skills—for it is these that have grown enormously in complexity and effectiveness. The tools of research, of diagnosis and of life-support systems are wonderfully sophisticated instruments whose proper use alone requires profoundly expert understanding. The mere circumstance that hundreds of millions of isolated bits of information can be stored and retrieved mechanically opens up the possibility of use of statistically unlimited data in the analysis of disease and the synthesis of observation. It is a new world—one in which Russ Cecil and Bob Loeb and even Walsh McDermott might not have felt entirely at home.

While Walsh McDermott was still in medical school, President Herbert Hoover created a commission of scientists, intellectuals and community leaders, with a research staff of over five hundred expertly trained persons, to plot the course the United States should pursue through and beyond the 1950s. Nowhere in their massive thirteen-volume report on our future were even mentioned effective antimicrobials, or the birth-control pill, or DNA, or atomic energy, or computer technology, or space exploration. While everyone was looking west, the future dawned in the east in a brightness of discovery no one had even surmised.

In medicine improved technology has meant a new-found effectiveness; but it has inevitably also meant a certain impersonality, for the machine has a cool head and a cool heart. Perhaps today the electron microscope will serve as the symbol of the modern, scientifically trained physician. It provides a deeper vision. The intellectual concern of medicine has moved away from the bedside to the laboratory. No less humane than before, medicine is no longer intimate and comforting. Preventive measures in diphtheria are infinitely more useful but much less personal than the forgotten heartbroken vigil at diphtheria's bedside. At the center of this visibly changed world of medicine stand Jim Wyngaarden and Holly Smith—the former, when his editorship began, Frederic M. Hanes Professor and Chairman of the Duke University Medical Center and now Director of the National Institutes of Health; the latter Professor and Chairman of the Department of Medicine of the University of California at San Francisco.

Just as Eugene Stead had summoned Paul Beeson to Emory, so he brought Jim Wyngaarden to Duke, where Stead was busy transforming a collection of impressive Neo-Gothic buildings into an impressive modern medical school.

In 1985 Bill Kelley, Professor and Chairman of the Department of Medicine of the University of Michigan, presented to Wyngaarden the Robert H. Williams Award of the Association of Professors of Medicine. In presenting the award, Kelley quickly sketched in Wyngaarden's early life, for it is important to his later development. His father received his undergraduate education at Occidental College and at the University of Washington, going on to receive his doctorate in Semitic languages at the University of Pennsylvania. At the time of Jim's birth his father had joined the faculty of Calvin College in Grand Rapids as Professor of Old Testament Theology. He held this position for 37 years, teaching Hebrew, Old Testament History, and Theology until his retirement in 1961. Jim came then from a background in which scholarship and culture were prized, no commitment was undertaken lightly and the spirit, not the letter, of the law was a guiding principle. These are the characteristics that have marked his career and his life.

In 1944 young Wyngaarden matriculated at the University of Michigan Medical School, an institution the United States Navy had selected for him. Fortunately, the accelerated medical-school program had been abandoned at the end of World War II, and the restored four years of study not only proved refreshing and fruitful for him but also provided time and opportunity for research work that would have been impossible in the shortened program.

Upon his graduation from Michigan, first in his class and recipient of the first annual Borden Undergraduate Research Award in Medicine, he chose to pursue postgraduate training at the Massachusetts General Hospital and there, like other bright young men before and since his time, came under the exciting influence of Fuller Albright and Walter Bauer and also spent six months working in John Stanbury's laboratory. It happened that Stanbury spent much of that six months in Argentina on special assignment, and his young associate was able to work with more freedom and independence than might have been anticipated. The result was his first truly creative paper, "The Effect of Certain Anions upon the Accumulation of Iodide by the Thyroid Gland." Published in *Endocrinology* in 1952, the paper was a milestone in the developing study of thyroid pharmacology, demonstrating that perchlorate was ten times more potent than thiocyanate in discharging thyroid-collected iodide.

It was in later work with DeWitt Stetten of the National Institute of Arthritis and Metabolism that Jim first became interested in uric acid and purine metabolism—pursuits that would mark all his research, much of which was carried on at Duke University, where he accepted his first academic faculty appointment in 1956 as Associate Professor of Medicine. He had long recognized that overproduction of purines and uric acid was important in the pathogenesis of gout but that little was known about the regulation of purine metabolism. He began to look specifically at the control of the initial enzyme unique to purine biosynthesis and was able to demonstrate feedback inhibition by purine nucleotides. These findings constituted the most important scientific contributions of his career and were the basis for his election to membership in the National Academy of Sciences at an unusually early age.

In 1958 a plan he and John Stanbury had long discussed took final shape. They had considered for several years the idea of writing a book on inborn errors of metabolism and had quite naturally interested Don Fredrickson, who was later to become Director of the National Institutes of Health, in being one of its authors; but at the Young Turks' meeting in Atlantic City, whose boardwalk has seen the hatching of many a fine idea, they decided to do a contributed volume instead and together wrote out its table of contents and list of expert authors, many of whom were also strolling the boards. John Stanbury's brother worked for McGraw-Hill and put the authors in touch with Bill Keller, then the McGraw-Hill medical editor. Would that Stanbury's brother had worked for Saunders, for by the time the Saunders editor learned of the book Keller had already safely put it under contract.

In 1960 the McGraw-Hill Book Company published their largish volume— *The Metabolic Basis of Inherited Disease*—at once a pioneering effort and an extraordinary synthesis of ideas and findings, still undergoing analysis and maturation, related to the complex problem of how the structures of genes and their protein products in alteration affect function of the human body. It was published at a time when "inborn errors of metabolism" were being rediscovered and when new technologies, especially in molecular biology and immunology, were illuminating the genetic mechanisms of many diseases of obscure etiology. It was a daring work of advanced ideas and rich erudition. It could just as well have been called "The Heritable Basis of Metabolic Disease."

If not a precursor, there was an early parallel to it in medical significance— *Inborn Errors of Metabolism*, published in 1909 in England by Sir Archibald Garrod, who had noticed that patients with alkaptonuria excreted large quantities of homogentisic acid and that this abnormality had a familial pattern. He discussed his findings with William Bateson—an early figure in the great school of British geneticists—and together they concluded that explanation of the familial characteristic of the defect lay in its heritable nature as a recessive trait conforming to the rediscovered laws of Mendel. Garrod went on to postulate the theory that some diseases of lifelong duration are due to inactivity or absence of an enzyme governing a single metabolic step. His brief book set out the whole conceptual framework in which the nature of genetically determined disease was thereafter to be studied. He had established the basis for *The Metabolic Basis of Inherited Disease*, published half a century later, by demonstrating that a gene controls a chemical reaction through an enzyme acting as an intermediary.

The Saunders editor read Wyngaarden's chapters in the section on Disorders of Purine and Pyrimidine Metabolism in the Third Edition of what had become the most forward-looking reference source in contemporary medicine and decided that their author should join Beeson and McDermott as one of the editors of the Fifteenth Edition of the *Cecil Medicine,* for he is a man who stands at the cutting edge of medicine and looks at its advances from a perspective that extends from the past into the future. His own work, especially that on gout, done with Bill Kelley, has its roots in the work of Garrod and its intellectual culmination in the Kelley-Harris-Ruddy-Sledge *Textbook of Rheumatology,* whose two-volume Second Edition, published in 1981, sets a new standard and framework for the understanding of the rheumatic process.

The editor visited Wyngaarden at Duke University Medical Center in 1976 and there found a man of warm personality and steely determination to whom no demand of time or effort in pursuit of better medicine is too great and whose countenance of fools and foolishness is slight. It happened that he was just then completing construction of a new home, which he and the editor inspected. The physician's obvious appreciation of and pride in the intricate and careful structure of the house were a mark of his character— no detail was too small for his attention, no architectural concept too sophisticated for his understanding. One had the impression not only of a perfectionist but of a man who could tolerate nothing less than the highest excellence in his own work and that of his associates. It is a pleasure to quote part of his letter to the editor describing his experience with the textbook of medicine:

> Working with Saunders on the *Cecil Textbook of Medicine* has been one of the highlights of my life. From the beginning, working with you, Paul, and Walsh on the 15th introduced me to a new level of professionalism and competence in the publishing world. When you, Paul, and Walsh retired and Jack Hanley and Holly Smith came on, this high level of professional enjoyment and pleasure continued. Saunders has clearly been the finest medical publisher for many decades and I hope it can maintain its position. In the 17th edition I think we have a well-balanced and beautifully crafted book. We have introduced more illustrations without increasing the overall length, by urging each contributor to reduce his or her chapter by 10 or 15 percent. Not everyone could do it, but overall it worked quite well.

> I really enjoyed the one edition with Paul and Walsh and gained a new appreciation for Paul's quiet, steady, dedicated scholarship and Walsh's intelligence and controlled flamboyance. Working with Holly has also been a joy. As you know, we go back a long way, having been interns together at the Massachusetts General Hospital in 1948, and having had somewhat similar scientific interests although his were centered in pyrimidines and mine in purines. We served together on the President's Science Advisory Committee, on the Council of the Association of American Physicians, on the Medical Advisory Board of Howard Hughes Medical Research Institute, and now as co-editors of *Cecil.* Holly is a person of great and many talents and one of my best friends for over 35 years. Working together on *Cecil* keeps us in close contact, and I value this very much, having had to give up the Howard Hughes connection on coming to the NIH.

The innumerable honors and distinctions of Wyngaarden's career are not listed here, for they are but the confirming signs of achievement and of the trust the worlds of medicine and of learning place on those who safeguard truth and disseminate new knowledge.

In the nineteenth century an anonymous Viennese, asked by a foreigner to describe his government, coined the phrase *"Absolutismus gemildert durch Schlumperei"* (absolutism tempered by sloppiness). The Hapsburg empire and the traditional empire of medicine were not so dissimilar as one might offhandedly suppose. In both, Schlumperei sometimes had the saving grace of unseating highhanded certainty. Today mystical phrases like "integration of the basic sciences," "coordination of premedical and preclinical curricula," "comprehensive, holistic medicine," "computer-assisted learning," "study of the behavioral sciences and humanities" and "interdisciplinary team approach" are on every approved list of objectives and on every eminent tongue. But they may conceal an impulse toward mediocrity. In fact, they come perilously close to saying that medical education should be designed not for the gifted but for the dull average.

Jim Wyngaarden is a man to whom average is anathema. Just as Bob Loeb warned fifty years ago that the evolution of ideas is gradual, that the establishment of scientific truth cannot be purchased by large funding of small vision and that only the tireless, disciplined work of a creative mind can achieve greatly, so in his address as president of the American Association of Physicians Jim Wyngaarden warns anew that science is a demanding master that cannot allow mixed motives or divided attention:

> The reasons for the decline in research interests among young physicians are complex. A major one involves a re-evaluation of societal goals in the wake of Vietnam. This has led to greater emphasis on medical care of deprived segments of our society as a more pressing immediate need than basic biomedical research in the improvement of health and conquest of disease. Assessments of medical students' goals show a dramatic swing away from biomedical research beginning in the late 1960's. There is a feeling among some students that the technology of medicine has outrun its sociology. The primary care–family medicine themes have successfully played pied piper tunes.

> A second important factor is the instability of Federal support of biomedical research and training. Students, residents, and fellows observe young faculty uncertain of research support. There is a perception that the instability reflects a public value judgment. Young people tend to choose fields marked by high public approbation.

> A third factor is that of curriculum revision. One of the casualties of new medical curricula has been the excision of simulated research laboratory experiences that formerly characterized many of the basic science courses. The result is that many house officers now reach the end of residency training with no first-hand knowledge of the excitement of working in a laboratory. And in the absence of a military obligation far fewer are exposed to the sometimes decisive experience of an appointment to the National Institutes of Health. . . .

> In the last several years economic considerations have come to dominate career decisions. A high percentage of young physicians who in the past might have been willing to delay economic gratification and indulge a curiosity about the research life, now become victims of what one of my chief residents has called the 'resident-fellow-Porsche syndrome.' . . . What is needed is a period of time to discover the pleasures of measurement, of designing experiments, of executing them, and of analyzing results, of pursuing an idea that does not fit into conventional dogma, of testing one's creative imagination and experiencing the exhilaration of the experimental proof of a new hypothesis, however small the facet of the stone may be. The young physician cannot know whether this will prove to be consuming and gratifying unless the research life can be sampled for a year or more without incurring unwarranted economic or professional penalties.

Holly Smith, like Russell Cecil, was born in the South; and there is about his voice too that rising inflection of eagerness that evokes a response of expectation of great things to come or to be announced—one of the pleasures of our crowded lives. He is also that increasingly rare phenomenon in medicine—a scholar, a scientist, a full-time academician who is a superb physician. Rounds with him are like those with Bob Loeb—adventures in acuity and concern responsive to every nuance of the patient's illness and the student's learning needs, for the fine art of diagnosis is the art of unraveling implications.

When Smith was accorded the Robert H. Williams Award as Distinguished Chairman of Medicine, the University of California provided a news release setting out the principal points of his distinguished career. Its many pages list citations, honors, academic positions, and memberships in learned societies, including presidency of the Association of American Physicians, of the American Society for Clinical Investigation, of the Western Society for Clinical Research and of the Association of Professors of Medicine. These are the signs of accomplishment and have their parallel in the lives of many Saunders authors; but they also mark dedication to the advance of medicine and involvement in the ways through which that advance is initiated, supported and criticized.

In presenting the award, Marv Sleisenger pointed out that the careers of Holly Smith and Bob Williams have curious parallels. Both came from the deep South, both had brilliant records at Eastern medical schools (Williams at Hopkins, Smith at Harvard), both spent some years in Boston doing postgraduate work centered on endocrine and metabolic studies and both brought their careers to highest fulfillment in the West. Both too succeeded in attracting to their departments of medicine bright young investigators who would strengthen those departments. They used the persuasions of money, superb facilities, climate, scenic beauty, new challenges and even the excellence of restaurants to enlist the best. It is said that Williams never replied directly to questions about the number of days of sunshine in Seattle, but magnificent views of gloriously sunlit Mt. Rainier were part of his persuasive armamentarium.

Holly Smith entered Harvard Medical School in January of 1944, having never before been north of the District of Columbia. His brother Frank accompanied him on the train ride to Boston, for Frank was transferring to the third year at Harvard from the University of North Carolina Medical School. As a student Holly won the coveted Henry Christian Award and graduated *magna cum laude*. Internship and residency at Massachusetts General Hospital followed almost as a matter of course.

He then decided to extend his training in biochemistry as a background to serious medical research. Thereafter he studied purine and pyrimidine metabolism with DeWitt Stetten at the Public Health Research Institute of New York City and with Peter Reichard at the Karolinska Institute in Stockholm. Upon his return to Boston he turned his attention to the difficult field of enzyme assay and, with Hibbard Williams, discovered the enzyme defects of two distinct forms of primary hyperoxaluira. In these studies he came inevitably under the influence of Fuller Albright and Walter Bauer. Together they coordinated the emerging techniques of enzymology and molecular biology—the basis for long-continued distinguished work in the laboratories of the Massachusetts General Hospital.

In 1964, while on a sabbatical leave spent studying with Hans Krebs at Oxford, he was offered the Chairmanship of Medicine at the University of California, San Francisco. He may have been uncertain of the wisdom of such a move and decided to inform Dean Berry of the Harvard Medical School of his indecision. That great man was astonished that anyone should ever think of leaving Boston and may have provided the weight that tipped the balance, for he cried, "Why, Holly, we were *even thinking* of proposing you for an Associate Professorship!" (Italics Smith's.) Perhaps too Holly may have read Bernard De Voto in *The Saturday Review of Literature:* "New England is a finished place. Its destiny is that of Florence or Venice, not Milan. While the American empire careens toward its unpredicted end, it is the first American section to be finished. It is the first old civilization in America."

The San Francisco school had the reputation of being solid but provincial and unexciting, even though people like Julius Comroe, John Murray and J. Englebert Dunphy were on its faculty. But the imminent departure of the Stanford School of Medicine for greener Palo Alto gave the new chairman at San Francisco an opportunity to develop the services and strengthen teaching and research at the San Francisco General Hospital and the Veterans Administration Hospital. He had found his place.

Holly Smith, now Distinguished Service Professor of Medicine at San Francisco, serves also as a member of the Board of Overseers of Harvard University and as Chairman of the Scientific Advisory Committee of the Massachusetts General Hospital, some of whose old-guard members may still wonder why he left Harvard and may not even know that he transformed an unexciting school into one full of life and promise, staffed by talent, and urged on by that unrelenting drive that impelled its Chairman of Medicine from Boston to California to unsettle the West.

His would seem to be pretty full hands; but Holly not only brilliantly edits with Jim Wyngaarden the *Cecil Textbook of Medicine,* he also edits for Saunders a fascinating series of monographs on Major Problems in Internal Medicine and, with Sam Thier, an exciting textbook on *Pathophysiology of Disease.* He assisted too in the editorial development of Abe Braude's elegant *Medical Microbiology and Infectious Disease* and helps Jim Wyngaarden put together their *Review of General Internal Medicine.* In his spare moments he serves on the editorial boards of *The Journal of Clinical Investigation,* the *American Journal of Medicine* and the *Western Journal of Medicine.* The only visible sign of any approaching weariness is his recent decision to forego playing in the house-staff basketball games, "Each year," he says, "I'm a year older and they're the same age": but he's still the faculty tennis champ of UCSF and ready to take on all comers. Dean Berry, you muffed it.

For a quarter century the early *Cecil Textbook of Medicine* was without peer or real competition; and this was a very good thing for its publisher. But what every science-art needs is more conflict of ideas, more crowding of communication, more alternative approaches, so that it is a better thing for medicine itself and for students of medicine of all ages that there are now available five excellent textbooks of medicine. As of this writing they are:

Cecil Textbook of Medicine: Seventeenth edition. Edited by James B. Wyngaarden and Lloyd H. Smith, Jr. W. B. Saunders.
Harrison's Principles of Internal Medicine: Tenth edition. Edited by Robert G. Petersdorf, Raymond D. Adams, Eugene Braunwald, Kurt J. Isselbacher, Joseph B. Martin, and Jean D. Wilson, McGraw-Hill.
Internal Medicine: First edition. Edited by J. H. Stein. Little, Brown.
The Principles and Practice of Medicine: Twenty-first edition. Edited by A. McGehee Harvey, Richard J. Johns, Victor A. McKusick, Albert H. Owens, Jr., and Richard S. Ross. Appleton-Century-Crofts.
Scientific American Medicine: First edition. Edited by Edward Rubenstein and Daniel H. Federman. Scientific American.

The New England Journal of Medicine published a comparative review of these texts; and the reviewer, Dr. Robert M. Glickman, found that all were authoritative, carefully conceived, and fine in execution but that each had its individual excellences and individual differences. "It is comforting," he said, "to know that so many high-quality textbooks are available A textbook of medicine is one of the internist's most important possessions. It should be comfortable and feel right." There is, he concluded, no basis for judging one superior to the other. Only use will determine which most satisfactorily fills individual needs. "After that, probably more than one of these fine textbooks will earn a valued place on one's bookshelf."

There are also curious resemblances among them. All conclude that something like 2,000 closely packed pages are needed on which to present the full scope of contemporary medicine. All are multi-authored works; but two vary this approach: *The Principles and Practice of Medicine* is constructed to reflect the coherent views of a single institution—Hopkins—and the *Scientific American Medicine* to reflect the views of two institutions—Harvard and Stanford. Such confinement in choice of contributing writers may indeed result in a more cohesive presentation; but no school of medicine—even the very best—can afford the authority of writers chosen for their expertness from all over the world.

The *Scientific American Medicine* is the most expensive of the group and hence, perhaps, the least widely used; but its expense springs from its beautiful, open production, its fine drawings graphically visualizing intricate concepts and its monthly supplements updating selected sections of the whole. But it may be questioned whether the supplements are used as carefully as they should be, nor should it even be considered that they replace reading of the several splendid journals in bioscience and medicine.

Indeed, currency has become an American fetish, the English taking a more modest view of the moment. For this reason some of these textbooks, at an enormous cost to their editors, writers and publishers, are on a three-year revision schedule. One may question too whether this is necessary and whether it truly responds to need. Significant advances in medicine come slowly and require periods of analysis, confirmation and maturation before they can be said to be firmly established. All one need do is read the correspondence columns of the *New England Journal of Medicine* to discover that even the most thoughtful study—perhaps after years of preparation and even years in publication—may be disputed or refined by critical colleagues. In fact, some of the world's most powerful scientific discoveries have come about not by pursuit of the new but by need to uproot what seemed to be established ideas. Chester Keefer once said, "If physicians only knew thoroughly most of what was known ten years ago, they would be better doctors."

The work involved in the creation of these books can scarcely be imagined; but the world of academic medicine is sufficiently small so that it was possible for the editor of one publishing house to know, with varying degrees of acquaintanceship, almost all of the physician-scientists who gave an astonishing part of their lives to the five principal textbooks of medicine. He would say, with Dr. Glickman, "It is comforting to know" that dedication to learning and teaching is very much a part of the self-disciplined and selfless lives of our leaders of medicine.

10

The Christopher Textbook of Surgery and Book Writing in Chicago

In 1920 Loyal E. Davis, then Assistant Professor of Surgery at Northwestern University Medical School, suggested that he write for Saunders a brief book on *Neurologic Diagnosis*. This was completed and published in 1923—a nicely illustrated, straightforward account of presenting symptoms correlated with their anatomic, physiologic and pathologic bases. This may have been one of those books that fall midway between needs—insufficient for the neurologist, too much for the general practitioner or surgeon. It did not do well. But Ryland Greene, who could spot a comer at three hundred paces, was impressed with the youthful, vigorous Davis. Nevertheless, he declined to publish his next book—*Principles of Neurological Surgery*; and it, like Boyd's *Pathology*, went to a neighbor, Lea & Febiger. An in-house note from Greene comments that the *Principles* was not really needed. What was needed was a richly illustrated, definitive work in several volumes setting out both the scientific principles and technical details of neurosurgery—in short, a Saunders book.

This seemed to end forever the existing relationship between Davis and Saunders, for the young neurosurgeon was not one to forgive stupid errors, and he quite naturally saw Greene's decision as an egregious example of one of the worst of them. In fact, Davis refused thereafter to see any Saunders representative, even the local textbook man quite innocent and unaware of the act underlying the ban. It could scarcely then be foreseen that many years later Saunders would publish the last edition of the *Principles of Neurological Surgery* and also *Neurosurgical Contributions of Loyal Davis*, compiled by his son Richard Davis, also a neurosurgeon. The latter is an interesting volume, for it reproduces with commentary fifteen of the significant papers from more than two hundred that Davis had written, several with his mentors and colleagues Harvey Cushing, Allen Kanavel and Louis Pollock. These are accounts of meticulous surgical-anatomic studies, some of profound importance to neurosurgery. It is worthy of note that none of them was funded by a granting agency, either governmental or private, and that most of them were the product of an individual working in association with one or two colleagues. They antedate today's laboratory team efforts, grant applications, budgetary fussing and problems of space allocation.

While Lea & Febiger was publishing the *Principles*, another young Assistant Professor of Surgery at Northwestern, Frederick Christopher, also to become a prolific contributor to surgical literature, was single-handedly writing his *Minor Surgery*, published in 1929 by Saunders, with an appreciative foreword by Allen Kanavel. The book was an immediate success and was to go through six editions under Christopher's authorship, gradually growing with each edition—as all books do, presumably in response to expanding knowledge. It also enjoyed wide international esteem and use, and the sale of its Spanish translation was pleasantly large.

Encouraged by this experience and impressed by the value of the Cecil collaborative *Textbook of Medicine*, the still-youthful Christopher, now Associate Professor of Surgery, suggested to Greene his editorship of a multi-authored *Textbook of Surgery*. This was completed with contributions and valuable advice from Loyal Davis, now Professor of Surgery at Northwestern, and published in 1936. It, like the *Minor Surgery*, was an instant success and its Spanish and Italian translations enjoyed wide use. The *Textbook* became a standard teaching tool throughout America and most of the English-speaking world; and Christopher ably carried on its editorship through five editions.

At midcentury Christopher was ready to put the safekeeping of his books into other hands; and Alton Ochsner, Professor of Surgery at Tulane, and Michael E. DeBakey, Professor and Chairman of Surgery at Baylor University, took on this awesome task. Whether wisely or not, they elected to make the *Minor Surgery* a collaborative work; and some of its young contributing writers were to become America's leading surgeons, one of them, Denton Cooley, doing a nice chapter on removal of minor skin lesions. Although the book did quite well in its seventh and eighth editions, it had lost something of its cohesiveness and consistent point of view, so that the eighth became its last revision. Also, Ochsner and DeBakey were certainly two of the busiest surgeons on the American scene and found they simply did not have the necessary hours and energy to manage the *Textbook*. Too much time had already gone by, and Saunders was faced with the necessity to find at once a forceful, aggressive, distinguished editor who, by good chance, might have some familiarity with the book and its Northwestern traditions.

There was really only one choice—Loyal Davis (the E. had mysteriously disappeared along the way), now Chairman of Surgery at Northwestern, Editor of *Surgery, Gynecology and Obstetrics*, a power of tremendous force in American surgery and a tiger not on speaking terms with Saunders.

The young Saunders editor looked forward more with apprehension than hope to his visit with a figure said to be a reincarnated John B. Murphy, whose biography Davis had written with admiring care and published to acclaim. So much time had gone by since the last edition of the textbook that the editor had taken what he presumed to be the totally premature step of bringing with him a contract of publication already signed by Saunders. Despite his forebodings, he was kindly received by the leonine figure, listened to patiently and invited to dinner that very evening for further discussion.

Hastily canceling an already accepted dinner invitation from a long-standing and understanding author, the editor arrived a half-hour or so in advance and walked about in the chill air admiring the neighborhood. Not entirely accustomed to the elegant life, he found breathtaking the spectacle of Edith Davis, dressed in what seemed to him a coronation robe, majestically descending a regal staircase. Graciously extending her hand, Mrs. Davis said, "Would you mind hooking my gown? Loyal, you know, is so clumsy." Many a greenhorn resident must have been taken in by this pleasant ploy— but so was the editor. Carefully observing what instruments his host and hostess used during dinner, he managed to be reasonably alert and businesslike. Finally, Mrs. Davis asked, "Why are you being so coy, Loyal? Why don't you sign the paper the young man has so we can talk about something more entertaining?" And he did. Is it unimaginable that Davis may have said beforehand, "Edith, when we're about near the end of dinner, why don't you say, 'Loyal, why are you being so coy. . . ' "? Thus was the subtle triumph of reluctance and persuasion maintained.

The tiger-turned-tabby proved to be an altogether agreeable and splendid editor of the textbook who was perfectly aware that too much time had gone by since its last edition and knew what to do about it. Not one to pine away in patient waiting for late papers, as with the figure in our frontispiece, he waged a carefully planned campaign against the dilatory. Loyal Davis never did seem to have any trouble getting calls through evasive secretaries; and perhaps the image of an irate Editor of *Surgery, Gynecology and Obstetrics* gave wings to dawdlers. The Sixth Edition was planned, written, edited and published in record time and immediately recaptured its position as the leading text.

In response to an inquiry, Dr. Richard Davis has set out the reasons for his father's interest in carrying on a Northwestern book whose influence extended throughout the world:

> Dr. Loyal was 60 years old at the time he began this project, and had already won accolades as a clinical surgeon, laboratory investigator, teacher, editor of *Surgery, Gynecology & Obstetrics,* and Chairman of the Department of Surgery at Northwestern. Although someone unfamiliar with Dr. Loyal might have expected him, at this point, to rest on his laurels, he approached this self-assigned endeavor with his usual enthusiasm and interest.

> His reasons for accepting the assignment were many. Perhaps the most important motivation was his profound interest in medical education. He saw the textbook as his contribution to doctors of the future; it was his opportunity to teach surgery in the most logical and coherent manner possible. He also hoped that the textbook would gain exposure for Northwestern Medical School and his own Department of Surgery.

> In addition, Dr. Loyal's love of challenge also drove him to undertake the project. He viewed the task of revision as a test of his organizational abilities, his energy, and his writing talent, the latter of which had been encouraged and refined by his mentor, Harvey Cushing. In short, the Christopher-Davis textbook represented a renewal of his commitment to excellence.

It might also be surmised that Loyal Davis at sixty had spent a great part of his life in the practice of neurosurgery and in the administration of power. His slowly progressive arthritis was beginning to make surgery impossible, and he had become weary of the manipulations of power. He was ready for an intellectual task and challenge. Still, he would later richly enjoy being father-in-law to and having the attentive ear of President Reagan.

By the time Davis was ready to resign from the book, the choice of a new editor was again clear. It had to be David C. Sabiston, Jr., Chairman of the Department of Surgery at Duke University. But this time there were no apprehensions, for Bob Rowan had taken on the responsibilities of medical editorship and was already on friendly terms with the target. Here is part of Sabiston's account of that experience:

In April 1969 when I was first approached about becoming Editor of this classic text, I was enthusiastic about the opportunity and accepted immediately. There were three primary reasons why agreement was reached so rapidly. First, the Saunders Company had a long record of excellence in medical publication, with a reputation for attention to detail and for having a highly responsible group with whom to work. Second, Bob Rowan was well known throughout the entire medical community, and among the surgical group in particular. His depth of knowledge, personal friendships with all segments of the medical profession, and his committed interest in achieving the best were all characteristics for which he was widely known. Bob possessed an enormous wealth of information in multiple fields and was free in responding to one's questions with objectivity and precision. Moreover, his hunches were always on target, and he seldom if ever provided any erroneous advice. Despite this superb record, Bob always allowed his professional colleagues to make the final decisions and he supported them in every detail. Certainly he is due great credit for much of the success of the publisher during his era. All who knew him regarded Bob with great fondness, and he was a loyal and ever-present friend to those of us who had the privilege of knowing him in that capacity. It is very fortunate that even in retirement he continues to have an active influential role in medical publishing. Finally, I had used the text as a medical student, as a resident, and as a faculty member and found it to be a masterful work.

A highlight of being associated with Saunders was the privilege of working closely with Carroll Cann, who had earlier worked with Bob Rowan and who assumed his position at the time of his retirement. He learned much from Bob, a fact which he warmly acknowledged, and has grown in that position during the past several years to an unprecedented height. Thoughtful, exceedingly knowledgeable and possessed of distinct ability to get things done and in the proper way, Carroll has a quiet persuasiveness which is unique. It was his influence which led me to our newest undertaking, *Essentials of Surgery*. He quite systematically accumulated objective evidence from this country and abroad of the need for such a text to be prepared in a format not currently available in other such texts. Although originally I was little stimulated by this challenge, over a period of several years he has brought me to a point of marked enthusiasm for the opportunities associated with his new approach. One recognizes the pleasures of working with an individual whose standards are consistently of the highest level and who has the ability to translate idealism into accomplishment.

As you can perceive, my association with the Saunders Company has been superb, across the board, and I am grateful for the opportunities made available to me as a part of the team. They have been in great measure responsible for the steady improvement in the image and impact of the *Textbook of Surgery*, now printed in seven languages (Spanish, Japanese, Chinese, Portuguese, Italian, and Turkish as well as English). Similarly, *Surgery of the Chest* has had a parallel course with marked expansion of the size and scope of the work in the last edition with Frank Spencer as Co-Editor.

As is obviously clear, the total experience with Saunders has been a highly positive one for which I am most grateful.

As may be imagined from this, the *Textbook of Surgery* has grown not only in influence but also in size, for such a work poses the never satisfactorily answered question of precisely how special surgery is to be handled in it, the contributing authors believing to a man that only extensive treatment can be justified, this necessity arising from the circumstance that in all essentially biologically sciences principles are notoriously reluctant to emerge. Truth is in the details.

However, the Christopher *Textbook of Surgery* and the Maximow and Bloom *Textbook of Histology* were not the only important Saunders books that had their origin in Chicago. It is possible to conjecture that in the early years of this century established Eastern publishers may have imagined that the intellectual world ended at the Appalachians, just as Europeans at one time thought the world ended with an abyss over which spilled the mighty waters of the Atlantic into the ice and fire of damnation. In any event Chicago's ice was no deterrent to Ryland Greene, who assiduously cultivated its schools and people. Here are a few significant books originating from the windy city.

Abt's *Pediatrics* (1923): The definitive reference work in its field whose eight volumes represented a plateau in the progress of pediatrics before which it was no longer necessary for scholars to delve into past literature. Many of its contributor chapters were extensively documented monographic treatises, occasionally the source of other books by other authors. Especially its chapters on genetics and metabolism were hallmarks in the development of these basic disciplines in relationship to pediatrics.

Ranson's *Anatomy of the Nervous System* (1920): The standard reference text in neuroanatomy for half a century. It was fresh in its approach, presenting anatomy not from the static point of view of morphology but from the dynamic perspective of developmental and functional significance of structure. Its later editions were ably revised by Sam L. Clark of Vanderbilt University.

DeLee's *Obstetrics* (1913): The most enduring of all specialty textbooks, superbly illustrated and nicely documented, it was carried on for many editions by Jack Greenhill, of the Michael Reese Hospital, and more recently by Emanuel A. Friedman of Harvard Medical School.

Prentiss's *Textbook of Embryology* (1915): A dynamic far-seeing text carried on for many editions past its first by Leslie B. Arey, it would become the standard text in developmental anatomy and afford for many thousands of students a vivid first picture of the miracles of reproduction, fetal change and birth and their biologic implications.

Jordan's *Bacteriology* (1908): Another reference text that has endured for eighty years in splendid health. Although bacteriology is a subject of primary importance to medical students and physicians, Jordan was one of the first teachers to recognize its immense importance to public health and to preventive medicine; and this character of his book continued in its many revisions, under the later title of *Microbiology*, first by William Burrows of the University of Chicago and later in its twenty-first and twenty-second editions by Bob A. Freeman of the University of Tennessee.

Two unrelated books but alike in their trailblazing influence were Herrick's *Neurology* (1918) and Wells *Chemical Pathology* (1907). The former, although a brief text, placed emphasis not so much on regional localization of nerve cells and fibers as on exposition of the metabolism of the nervous tissues. The latter sought to synthesize the findings of what had previously been but fragmentary studies of the chemical changes that occur in pathologic phenomena. A sense of philosophic skepticism animated both books. Both books too were of such profound personal insight that neither has been carried on by succeeding authors. Giant shoes are not readily filled.

Many years later Jules Masserman would also publish with Saunders a trailblazing text of skeptical turn of mind. The author of hundreds of papers and scores of books, he put his most penetrating insights into his first book, *Principles of Dynamic Psychiatry*. It sets forth the foundations of post-Freudian psychiatry as it has been modified by the later findings of neurophysiology and neuropathology and by the continuing experience of psychoanalysis. Its wide influence was evident in its translation into a dozen languages; but perhaps its erudite polysyllabism impeded its widest domestic use. A reviewer commenting on its many translations wryly asked, "And when will it be translated into English?"

At the opening ceremonies for the Rockefeller Institute for Medical Research in 1906, informed talks described the future work of its laboratories; but not a single reference was made to either the nervous system or mental disease, even though more hospital beds were then maintained at public cost for mentally sick persons than for all other patients combined. Jules Masserman had witnessed the later explosive interest in neurology and psychiatry and their findings; but there is in his *Principles* an implication that psychiatry had failed to keep pace with this interest through neglect of basic research into the origins of personality disorders and the nature and variations of normal development. It was this point of view—so different from that of mere recounting of bizarre case histories—that gave his book a lasting influence on progress in solid psychiatric research.

And from the American College of Surgeons would later come, if not textbooks, surgical guides of splendid teaching usefulness, especially its *Manual of Preoperative and Postoperative Care*, whose editorial committee and board of contributors are a roster of America's most distinguished surgeons. Its directive from the College to provide ready access to recent information in surgical metabolism, nutrition and fluid and electrolyte balance; clotting disorders, infection and shock; and pathophysiology of the cardiovascular, ventilatory and renal systems has been brilliantly fulfilled. "The most important step in any surgical procedure is thinking about it the night before."

11

Rochester, Minneapolis and Boston: Serendipity

Walter Burns Saunders, Ryland Greene and, later, Lawrence Saunders believed in cultivating friendly relationships with the powerful institutions of medicine, among them the American Medical Association, the American College of Physicians, the National Academy of Sciences, the National Research Council, the Rockefeller Institute and the American College of Surgeons, for all of which Saunders published books, sometimes as official publisher. But these were not merely opportunistic acquaintanceships; particularly Lawrence Saunders' friendships with Alan Gregg, Robert Morison, Cushman Haagensen, John Fulton, Robert Loeb, Alfred Kinsey, Max Broedel, Detlev Bronk and others sprang from shared concerns and ideals and not from the purpose of advantage.

Of these many friendships, two of long standing and high mutual respect were those of Ryland Greene with Will Mayo and Frank Lahey, for the three men had much in common. They admired hard work, they relished excellence and esteem and they knew how to seize opportunities; and all three were men around whom legends grow. But the stories of their convivial adventures are probably pure apocrypha, for Greene was a man of somewhat chilling formality who disliked ebullience and impropriety.

At the Clinic it was said that the Saunders Company early in its history fell upon hard times and was unable to raise cash for immediate needs. Will Mayo is supposed to have personally provided money to stave off the crisis with the provision that its repayment be put in a fund to pay for production costs of Mayo Clinic monographs not likely to attract numerous buyers. This too seems apocryphal, for no record supports the idea of such a loan or the disposition of its payment.

However, Saunders did indeed become official publisher to the Clinic with the understanding that Clinic people would do an annual volume of the *Surgical Clinics of North America* and of the *Medical Clinics of North America* and that Saunders would publish yearly the fat *Collected Papers of the Mayo*

Clinic. These understandings endured for more than half a century. It was also anticipated that Clinic authors would want to publish highly special monographs of limited readership such as the later Ogle *Binocular Vision* and Jesse Edwards' extensive atlases of the pathology of *Congenital Heart Disease* and *Acquired Heart Disease;* and a complicated scheme was worked out to cover their probable losses and Mayo Clinic costs of preparation. This arrangement was the cause of some vexation among Mayo authors because their Clinic-generated costs for redaction, artwork and photography not only were high but seemed to rise each year in geometric progression. Skyrocketing editorial costs were due largely to the policies of Dick Hewitt, Chief of the Section of Publications, who insisted that all bibliographic citations in a Mayo book (and sometimes there were thousands) be checked not against reference lists such as the *Index Medicus* but against original publications. He also believed that even the most trivial changes in manuscript required the retyping of each such offending page of typescript. His standards are set forth in his *Physician-Writer's Book,* which offers many useful but sometimes authoritarian advices that contrast with the gentler admonitions of E. B. White's revision of Strunk's *Elements of Style*.

This scheme worked out satisfactorily enough for books that could not possibly be expected to pay their own way; but the authors of more popular books such as Lundy's *Anesthesia,* Krusen's *Physical Medicine,* Braasch's *Urography* (later brilliantly revised and expanded by John Emmett) and the Allen-Barker-Hines *Peripheral Vascular Disease* suffered from it because even best-selling Mayo titles seemed rarely to recover Saunders production and Mayo preparation costs, the point at which the author began to receive royalty. Eventually the arrangement was greatly modified through the intelligent advices of the Clinic counsel, Harry Blackmun, before he became a justice of the Supreme Court.

One Mayo Clinic author who complained mightily about the old scheme was Walter Alvarez, who, like John B. Murphy, stoutly maintained that his style needed no improvement, his books no illustration and his references no checking. After he left Rochester and returned to Chicago, he always employed an editorial aide; but each was more ornamental than functional and had the wisdom not to tamper unduly. In fact, though, one can imagine Dick Hewitt having some qualms about the Alvarez style, which tended to be diffuse, didactic and discursive. When, well on in his remarkably long and vigorous life, Alvarez published his *Neuroses* with Saunders, the Saunders editor was startled to find in its manuscript long passages of advice to the young physician, particularly one that recommended the beginning doctor see to it that the patients in his waiting room were well gotten up. "Walter," said the editor, "this is a nice enough idea about the patients being well dressed; but I think you ought to omit it. In the first place your book is about the neuroses, and, in the second place, how in the world can the doctor be sure his patients are presentable?" "No," said Alvarez, skipping the matter of the book's ostensible subject, "I won't take it out. The point I am trying to make is that the patient should be well dressed. I am not telling the doctor how to do it, only what to do." It stayed in and, if it were to be literally followed, many a novice practitioner should make available in his waiting room two or three spare wardrobes.

In 1876 in his Hopkins address Thomas Huxley had warned that "there is no position so ignoble as that of the so-called 'liberally educated practitioner,' who may be able to read Galen in the original; who knows all the plants from the cedars of Lebanon to the hyssop upon the wall; but who finds himself with the issues of life and death in his hands, ignorant, blundering, and bewildered, because of his ignorance of the essential and fundamental truths upon which practice must be based." In all his books Alvarez occasionally strays into mild eccentricity; but in all he is devoted with percipient understanding to those fundamental truths upon which the wise practice of medicine rests.

During World War II a tall young editor from the Mayo Clinic—a bespectacled, roguish-looking Greek scholar, America's leading authority on early streetcar systems and an avid theater buff—was commandeered by the Army to bring order out of the chaos of a ponderous government-sponsored three-volume work on *Global Epidemiology* that the J. B. Lippincott Company had obligingly whisked away from Saunders, the usual publisher of NAS-NRC monographs. A true Minnesotan, he loved open spaces and found the Lippincott cubbyholes claustrophobic. From the Saunders windows he could often be seen on a park bench in Washington Square poring myopically over distressed orthography, puzzling typescript, impenetrable charts, graphs and maps, frustrating nomograms and obscure symbols. What if he did occasionally nod—so had Homer before him. He was Captain James Eckman, the man who would succeed Hewitt as Chief of the Section of Publications of the Mayo Clinic. A wonderful teller of tall tales and a more flexible sort than his predecessor, he acted as kindly Virgil to Saunders editors on their annual hegira to the Clinic.

Custom is a hard dictator, and custom decreed that the Saunders visit to the Mayo Clinic be made in February, because, it was said, the Clinic was less busy then than usual. If this was so, there was reason for it. In the days before air travel became a necessity in order to preserve the illusion of swiftly moving decision and action, the rail trip from Chicago to Rochester was in February a perilous adventure. Often snow drifts blocked and occasionally derailed the Cannonball Express and, during the night, its toilets would freeze solid when the train's heating system had one of its customary fainting spells. And yet it was a pleasant trip through the lovely snow-blanketed countryside that, on occasion, could be viewed in minute detail while the train stood stock still for hours. It ended with a heart-warming welcome from Jim Eckman, who always managed to act as if he had nothing more pressing on his time or mind than greeting and guiding the Saunders editor, once in a while accompanied by the Saunders president, Harry Most.

It was also a refreshing visit, for many of the Mayo Clinic physicians are cast from a different mold. Scholarly in inclination and astute in diagnosis, they are often physicians of great ability. They work in a framework of order that leaves their minds unencumbered by the extraneous. The Clinic itself, with its marble office tower soaring high above the surrounding plain, has the character of a dream realized. It brings to mind Disney World, for it is the fulfillment in detail of one man's vision and self-belief. In it cleanliness, precision, neatness and a kind of curious formalism are carried to impressive lengths.

It was customary for the Saunders editor on his annual Mayo Clinic visits to take the cramped bus (like so many others, called a limousine) to Minneapolis and the University of Minnesota School of Medicine. There he almost always called on Owen Wangensteen, for each enjoyed the other's company, although on one unpleasant occasion Wangensteen, Loyal Davis, Warren Cole, Evarts Graham and I. S. Ravdin had spent about four hours raking the editor and Vice President Paul Burton over the coals (and they knew how to heat coals) for their lack of zealous interest in the *Surgical Forum*—a volume from the American College of Surgeons that Saunders published annually with considerable loss and some lack of enthusiasm. At one point during their meeting the editor thought of hurling himself from the hotel window but was restrained by the comforting thought that even powerful surgeons may be wrong. He recalled that John Kennedy once asked Cardinal Spellman how he should reply to questions about papal infallibility. "Well," said the Cardinal, "the subject of the pope's infallibility is a complex and difficult one. All I can say is that His Holiness always calls me Spillman."

During one rather rambling visit with Wangensteen in Minnesota, the surgeon produced from his desk drawer and handed to the editor a check. It was three years old and from Saunders in payment for a contribution to the Davis-Christopher *Textbook of Surgery*. It was for thirty-seven dollars. How Saunders' books had balanced three years before is not clear; but "miscellaneous" covers a multitude of oversights. Wangensteen said, "Take this back to Saunders. By any estimate my time is worth more than twenty cents an hour." The editor allowed that this was probably so and asked if a hundred dollars would do. Much to his surprise the peppery surgeon said yes but slyly added, "I suppose that Loyal makes something more than this out of the book." He obviously enjoyed the episode and its discomfiture but all the same instantly cashed the revised check, the editor not suggesting that it be made payable to his department of surgery. Wangensteen later would have neurologic problems that he bore bravely, insisting only that no surgeon be called upon to consider their alleviation.

The editor would also likely call on Sheldon Reed, one of the true pioneers in the study of genetics in medicine whose early researches were supported by the Dight Institute, endowed by bequest from an eccentric who lived on charity in a tree, never paid a dime of income taxes and left an estate of close to a million dollars. In this instance one cannot begrudge the IRS's loss, for it was medicine's gain. Reed also received small dollops of research aid from a lineal descendant of Johann Wolfgang von Goethe who parceled out funds in a fashion he thought would have been agreeable to his great forbear. Later the Rockefeller Foundation generously supported the whole genetics progam of the Dight Institute. Reed's little book *Counseling in Medical Genetics* was wise and elegantly written. It is still an admired and valuable guide.

Boston is far removed spiritually as well as geographically from Rochester, for Bostonians like to imagine that they live at the intellectual hub of the universe. Boston, with its fine medical schools and superb hospitals, is also the only large American city in which medicine is a major industry; and Bostonians are proud of this but sometimes sigh over the uncomfortable fact that medicine is scarcely a paying enterprise. The Lahey Clinic, like its Rochester counterpart, is an exception to the rule of red ink, its profitability arising from highly efficient use of staff and facilities and from the shrewd philosophy that clinics should not run expensive boardinghouses for the ill.

Lahey too published its *Surgical Practice of the Lahey Clinic* with Saunders and also did an annual number in the *Surgical Clinics of North America*. It too had its staff of editors and artists, but its publishing arrangement with Saunders was essentially a standard one and less awkward than that with the Mayo Clinic.

Lahey Clinic books with Saunders have been of a generally marked clinical character, none more so or more skilled than Poppen's *Atlas of Neurosurgical Techniques*. A reticent man, Poppen was intensely devoted to expert surgery of nerve tissue and expert golf, both of which he practiced in concentrated silence. He broke his rule of silence on only one subject—the obdurate dilatoriness and inflated expensiveness of medical artists. During the seven-year-long preparation of his atlas, the Saunders editor listened to a steady stream of excoriations and denunciations of artists and their ways. Finally a call came from Boston. "The artwork," said Poppen, "is finished. Come up and we'll celebrate." The editor heeded this cordial summons, driving to Boston in order to bring back with him the massive drawings. Many of them were displayed effectively around Poppen's office and were genuinely admired by the editor-messenger. "We'll pack them up and I'll take them back this afternoon," he said. "You can't do that," said Poppen. "Why not?" seemed a natural question. "Because," said the author somewhat ruefully, "I haven't written the text yet."

A recent Lahey publication is the Moschella-Hurley revision of the classic Pillsbury-Shelley-Kligman *Dermatology*, itself a kind of extension of the great Stokes *Syphilology*. The revision is typical of the Clinic in its sharp clinical wisdom arising from the wide observation of experience grounded in comprehension of fundamental science. But the *Surgical Practice of the Lahey Clinic*, like the *Collected Papers of the Mayo Clinic*, has faded from use, perhaps because institutionary ways change slowly. The two Clinics are now brought into adventitious relationship by a curious circumstance. John Braasch, son of the Mayo Clinic urologist, is now Chairman of the Department of Surgery of the Lahey Clinic and like his father, the author, with Bentley Colcock, of a fine Saunders monograph—*Surgery of the Small Intestine*.

Just as the University of Minnesota beckons from the Mayo Clinic, so does Harvard University fom the narrower confines of the Lahey Clinic, and no medical editor of any wit would come to Boston without calling on Harvard's Medical School and its associated hospitals. Saunders editorial calls at Harvard have been frequent and remarkably serendipitous.

When the American Surgical Association in 1973 presented its Distinguished Service Medal to Robert E. Gross, he was justly described as "the greatest living surgeon in the United States." During a career of more than forty years the William E. Ladd Professor of Child Surgery at Harvard developed major procedures for correction of congenital anomalies of the heart and great vessels. His most remarkable advance was made in 1930 when, at the Children's Hospital Medical Center, he performed the first successful operation to seal off the patent ductus arteriosus, the duct connecting the fetal lung and aorta whose failure to close is the cause of life-threatening circulatory disability. He went on to develop techniques for correcting constriction of the aorta, openings in the internal walls of the heart, and abnormalities of the esophagus. Through his more than 250 publications he shared his ideas and techniques with surgeons and physicians everywhere, contributions resulting in his twice receiving the Albert Lasker Award. It is interesting that his letterhead has always read "Practice of General Surgery."

Gross is not only a rarely endowed surgeon but also one whose presence is commanding and felt at once upon encounter. In the 1940s it was known that he was at work on the book that would become a world-acclaimed pediatric surgery; but it was also known that he had paused in work on it and had no interest in its discussion with a publisher until it was completed. A Saunders editor decided to call upon him and had the good fortune to become over many years his friend. But the immediate problem was that Gross had become overly concerned that this entirely new book might be considered a revision of the earlier *Abdominal Surgery of Childhood* that Ladd and he had written when he was still a resident at the Children's Hospital. The editor suggested that a rider to an agreement of publication could place all responsibility, legal and other, upon the Saunders Company for the designation of his book as a first edition. The editor had no clear idea what either the meaning or consequence of such a clause might be, but it put Gross's mind at ease. He was also dismayed that another writer had used the title *Pediatric Surgery,* and the editor was quick to suggest the more descriptive and euphonious "The Surgery of Infancy and Childhood." It seemed unlikely that a mind so rich in invention and imagination could be troubled by these trivial concerns; but it was so and their hasty resolution removed a block.

The book was published not long thereafter and made its first appearance at a regional meeting of the American College of Surgeons in Boston. The Saunders Company had the good fortune at this meeting to present brand-new from Boston authors four books: The Gross, Cattell and Warren's *Surgery of the Pancreas,* the Parsons and Ulfelder *Atlas of Pelvic Operations* and Dunphy and Botsford *Physical Examination of the Surgical Patient.* Never have four books been so extensively examined and even read in big chunks at a surgical meeting. Even sales manager Burton, inclined to attribute success to sales skill, acknowledged that the titles themselves probably accounted for setting a meeting sales record that was not to be equaled for many years even at national conventions, although a later assembly of urologists in Chicago would come close when Saunders first presented the three-volume Campbell *Urology* and the two-volume Braasch and Emmett *Urography.*

These books have a characteristic in common that is distinctive of useful observation. Their acute notice of differences and of singularity sheds light on clinical problems. "May I call your attention to the singular incident of the dog in the night time," said Sherlock Holmes. "But the dog in the night time did nothing," said Dr. Watson. "That," said Holmes, "is the singular incident." Conan Doyle (who wrote his first Sherlock Holmes story in April, 1891, while waiting in vain for patients to arrive at his brand-new consulting rooms in Devonshire Place) is said to have modeled his detective's methods on the techniques of diagnosis practiced by Dr. Joseph Bell of the Edinburgh Infirmary.

At about this time too John Behnke became the aggressive editor of the Saunders College Division, an almost inevitable outgrowth from its existing titles in embryology, histology, microbiology and physiology. He developed important reference texts such as the Allee *Animal Ecology*, the Willier-Weiss-Hamburger *Analysis of Development* and the Prosser *Comparative Animal Physiology*; but he never lost sight of the necessary foundation of college publishing in textbooks. He was fortunate in the *Biology: A Human Approach* by Claude Villee, who would later, at the Boston Lying-In Hospital, do work of utmost importance to reproductive biology that would also furnish the philosophic and scientific background for Duncan Reid's *Obstetrics*, the first text integrating the science and practice of its discipline. Under the gentle guidance of Tyler Buchenau, Behnke's successor, Villee's own book would become for many years the leading American text in biology.

Behnke was most fortunate of all in a call made on Alfred Sherwood Romer, Agassiz Professor of Zoology at Harvard and international dean of vertebrate anatomy. Behnke wanted a teaching text in this field and decided to ask Romer's advice about six or so candidates he was thinking of approaching. In a long visit Romer carefully evaluated all the prospects, each an outstanding young figure. The editor thanked him profusely for his advices and, as he was about to leave, Romer said, "Mr. Behnke, it happens that I have here in my desk the almost complete manuscript for a textbook in vertebrate anatomy. I have been working on it for some years. Perhaps you would care to take it along and consider its publication."

Thus Saunders came to publish *The Vertebrate Body* by Alfred Sherwood Romer. The advertisement for it from *Science* shown here was written by Bob Rowan, then advertising director and later medical editor and still later executive vice president at Saunders. Perhaps the fish does not hold up all that well; but the ad is noteworthy for several reasons. It lacks that stereotyped heavy-handed accolade so prevalent in book advertising; it does not even mention the book's color plates; and in small type it reveals that a book of 650 pages exquisitely illustrated with fresh line drawings is $6.00. Could that have been only thirty-five years ago?

Eventually Romer also did a pared-down version of his text, and the two coexisted happily side by side for many years. Although tempted, Saunders wisely refrained from calling his brief book *The Shorter Vertebrate Body*.

The medical editor too was fortunate in a call upon Francis D. Moore, Moseley Professor of Surgery at Harvard Medical School. In the first place, Moore was not an easy man to get to see. Entrance was barred by a very

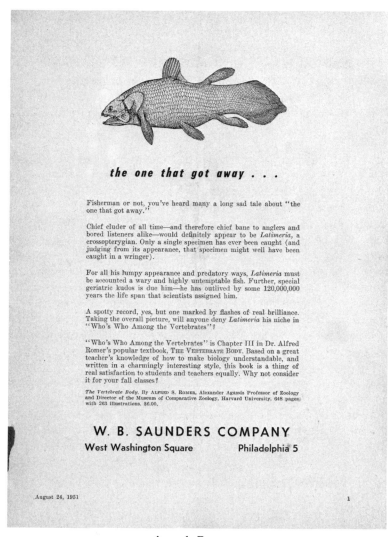

An early Rowan.

pleasant Chief Secretary who regarded it as her primary duty to ward off intrusion. In the second place, the editor, overly impressed by Moore's having available Mildred Codding as an in-house artist, came to suggest that Moore undertake a new depiction of surgical techniques to displace the fabulously popular Cutler-Zollinger atlas. The surgeon listened to this essentially implausible notion with surprising patience and at the conclusion of the visit said in terms almost identical with those of Romer: "But I do have here an almost complete manuscript on metabolism in surgery. Perhaps you would care to consider it." And thus came about *Metabolic Care of the Surgical Patient*—the most influential book ever published on the scientific and theoretical foundations of surgery. But somewhat in the manner of *Global Epidemiology* it abounded in medical shorthand, especially the abbreviations in its charts of water and electrolyte balance. As he looked through its manuscript the editor vainly wondered what sort of potassium balance might

96

be meant by PBBH. It was only after the book was published that he realized it meant Peter Bent Brigham Hospital.

Also, *Controversy in Internal Medicine* came about through hearing Franz Ingelfinger debate with three surgeons the question of the existence of an anatomic gastroesophageal sphincter. Ingelfinger then was a charismatic, scholarly physician and Boston's leading gastroenterologist. That he almost constantly chewed Tums may or may not say something about gastroenterology. He shortly thereafter became Editor of the *New England Journal of Medicine,* in which his engagingly written and witty editorials were a constant pleasure and in which too he exercised a subtle pressure toward publication of papers related to socioeconomic issues of medicine. When asked where the idea for *Controversy* originated, he usually replied, "It just came to me." Actually it came to him in the rotund form of Bob Rowan—metamorphosed from advertising director to managing editor. Ingelfinger and he became fast friends; and on the occasion of Bob's twenty-fifth anniversary with Saunders, the journal editor wrote the book editor a typically Franzian note of felicitation:

The New England Journal of Medicine

10 SHATTUCK STREET, BOSTON, MASSACHUSETTS 02115—TELEPHONE 617/734-9800

OFFICIAL PUBLICATION OF THE MASSACHUSETTS MEDICAL SOCIETY

OFFICE OF THE EDITOR   June 1, 1971

Mr. Robert Rowan
W.B. Saunders Company
West Washington Square
Philadelphia, Pennsylvania   19105

Dear Bob:

     The Saunders enterprise, as I imagine it, resembles a
totem pole, with an aquiline spirit perched on top, and with
a beetle-browed, bespectacled chest-- if such a chimera is
possible. Lower down is a substantial section-- it might be
called Rowanesque. Its solid and respectable dimensions
(see Figure 1) bespeak its 25 years of canny and fruitful
labor. This grand superstructure unfortunately rests on
underpinning of uncertain strength: an amorphous mass of
authors' bodies tangled and intertwined like the statuary of
a well-known Norwegian sculptor (whose name I can't remember.)
From somewhere within this mass, this bit of undifferentiated
tissue salutes you.

                              Sincerely yours,

                              Franz J. Ingelfinger, M.D.

FJI:kk

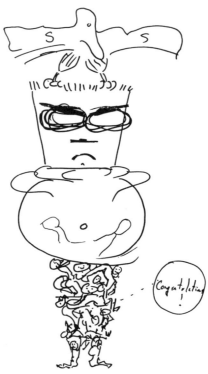

An original drawing by Franz J. Ingelfinger depicting a primitive scheme of the structure of the Saunders Company. Note the prominent gastroesophageal sphincter.

Ingelfinger was joined in the book by Maxwell Finland and Arnold Relman, the latter becoming soon thereafter editor of the *Journal of Clinical Investigation* and then Chairman of Medicine at the University of Pennsylvania. Eventually he would return to Boston to succeed Ingelfinger as Editor of the *New England Journal*.

Serendipity also touched Saunders in the person of Robert H. Williams, of Harvard Medical School, who decided to edit a *Textbook of Endocrinology* at a time when only a handful of American physicians could be identified as endocrinologists. On this account the Saunders sales principals frowned on the idea of the book; but Williams was such a powerful persuader that he prevailed upon Saunders to take his book whether there was any visible audience for it or not. There turned out to be a large and constantly growing readership for it—something Williams had believed in from the outset. After publication of the First Edition, Williams left Harvard for the University of Washington, where as Head of Medicine, he used his persuasive capacities to bring bright and able investigators to distant Seattle, where, according to Williams, the sun always shone (it doesn't) and glorious snow-capped mountain peaks are to be seen from all points of the landscape and all offices of the medical school (they aren't). But he was right in describing the attractions of the school itself—a center for teaching and investigation that, like his book, has always integrated strong fundamental science with skillful clinical perception. Perhaps its great strength in basic science may be ascribed to the circumstance that in its early days there was no University Hospital attached to the school and, when it was finally built, it began as a modestly small structure. But even without his glorious color pictures of the mountains he used to entice the undecided, Williams would have likely had his way anyhow. Granting agencies, colleagues, recruits, publishers, contributing writers, even state legislatures always found it almost impossible to say nay to his stammering enthusiasm. In fact, he could not say no to himself, for after his severe heart attack he scarcely paused in a round of work, commitments and responsibilities that would have taxed the strength of any three men.

One of the notions that a publisher must learn to live with is that the reading public knows what it wants; that there is, in short, little point in publishing books unsuited to the perceived needs of their intended audiences. Yet there is every once in a while a book, brilliant in promise and execution but disappointing in sale, of which the publisher is tempted to believe that its public did not really know what it wanted and that its neglect arose not from a fault in the book but from a mote in the eye of the beholder.

Such a book was the Warren *Surgery*. Edited by Richard Warren, of the celebrated Warren family and himself a meticulous and expert vascular surgeon, it set out to be a new version of the famous Homans *Surgery*, newly illustrated by one artist as was the Homans, and written entirely by members of the Department of Surgery of Harvard Medical School. That it turned out to be nothing at all like Homans was not a failure of plan but a change in execution of a plan—change that seemed, as often is the case, to have improved upon the original idea by deviation from it. The book actually proved to be a fine and careful exposition of the physiologic principles of surgery, seemingly ideally suited to the needs of students and conforming to the new-found belief that surgery does not rest simply on skillful carpentry but on dynamic understanding of the mechanisms, pathologic, physiologic and chemical, of the human body and the process of repair. A century ago William James had said, "Chemical action must of course accompany mental and physical activity, but little is known of its exact nature." Now much is known, and this was to be the foundation stone of Warren's *Surgery*.

And yet the book was a sales failure, although, curiously, its Italian translation was a success. One unduly harsh critic said of it that it was like a B-girl in a bar—much more beautiful at a distance than close up. He may have meant by this that the book had a strangely nonclinical flavor—a character opposite to that of the Homans—none of its illustrations, for example, depicting operating-room situations. The heart and hand of surgery are in the operating room, so that a heavy emphasis on biologic principles may seem approach from an ivory tower.

There was one exception to this character of the book—the chapter on Pediatric Orthopedics. Warren had naturally gone for its doing to William Green, Orthopedic Surgeon-in-Chief of the Boston Childrens' Hospital Medical Center and doyen of his specialty. But Green did not actually write the chapter; it was the work of his young associate, Mihran Tachdjian, later Chief of Orthopedic Surgery at the Childrens' Memorial Hospital of Chicago. Like everything Myke Tachdjian ever did, the chapter was overdue, over-long, over-referenced and perfectly splendid—a fine amalgam of acutely observed experience and far-ranging scholarship. It induced the Saunders editor to ask him to do a *Pediatric Orthopedics*. It appeared in two volumes in 1972 to high praise and extraordinary success. So sure was the editor of its value that he set a sales estimate, for a six-year life, of optimistic dimension, mildly scoffed at by sales manager Perkins. The six-year goal was met in the first six months of sale. *Pediatric Orthopedics* was followed in 1984 by *The Child's Foot*, it too exhibiting that fine quality of rich experience, sagacious reflection and genuine scholarship that make books true representations of the creative mind. Perhaps a small personal note will be allowed: To work with Myke Tachdjian is to experience at once stimulation, exasperation and loads of fun.

But all was not good fortune. Neither Gross nor Moore ever did revisions of their books, again perhaps because the creative mind relishes initiation of ideas, not their rethinking. Chester Keefer never completed his monumental *Medical Diagnosis*, although two-thirds of it was seen by the editor in bulky manuscript; nor did Dameshek ever finish his half-begun *Textbook of Hematology*; and the manuscript of Jean Holzworth's superb work on *Diseases of the Cat* for many years went through the never-ending process of elective change; but by some miracle of feline good fortune its beautiful first volume has now been published. All may have suffered from the vain search for that elusive grail, absolute perfection—"just one case (or one reference) better than the one I have." It may bear noting that by any account one of the most exquisitely imaginative works ever penned by the hand of man is Dante's heretical *Divine Comedy*, in which he says, "I have used up the paper set aside for this canto, and so shall go on to the next." Perhaps containment within the framework of an objective is not quite the suffocating burden it has generally been supposed to be.

12

Hopkins and Saunders:
A School and an Artist

The School of Medicine of Johns Hopkins University and the Saunders Company for many years enjoyed a close and warm relationship centered on the writing and publication of books. The names of Kelly, Cullen, Cushing, Long, Howell, MacCallum, Shackelford, Harvey and Zuidema are all associated with writing and illustration of the highest excellence and with the house of Saunders.

For this reason the Saunders Company decided in 1938 to celebrate its fiftieth anniversary by honoring Max Broedel, America's foremost medical artist and Associate Professor of Art as Applied to Medicine—a chair at Hopkins established primarily through the generosity of Mr. Henry Walters assisted by grants from a few business institutions, including the Saunders Company. At a lavish dinner in Philadelphia a portrait of Broedel, painted by Thomas Corner, was presented to the University. The two hundred guests honoring Max included many of the most influential of American physicians; and the roster of speakers included Ryland W. Greene, Dr. Thomas C. Cullen, Dr. Howard A. Kelly, Dr. Morris Fishbein, Henry L. Mencken and Dean Edward W. Berry. Lawrence Saunders presented the portrait to the University with nice brevity and genuine feeling: "My duty is a very simple, but a very pleasant one. This is a very happy occasion for us. Dean Berry, you have heard tonight from Max Broedel's friends of his varied accomplishments; you have seen the portrait of him painted by Mr. Thomas Corner. Please take back with you another important fact—we have an affection for this man; truthfully it can be said, we love Max Broedel. "Will you, on behalf of the Johns Hopkins University, accept this portrait with the very best wishes of W. B. Saunders Company and the many friends of Max Broedel."

After Dean Berry's acceptance of the portrait, Broedel too responded simply and quietly, concluding with a wish: "I hope the University will find a little corner in the Medical School or somewhere in East Baltimore and hang the picture there, so that I may sneak up to it in my old age, when I am minus teeth and hair and full of wrinkles. Then I shall point to it with pride and say: That's the way I looked when I was only 67 years old and still going strong."

Of the preceding talks some had been long, some short, some formal, some informal; and all paid tribute to the honoree, the Hopkins Medical School, Mr. Walters and the Saunders Company. But in a curious way the passage of fifty years has somehow dimmed their old-fashioned eloquence. Only one of the talks still has real life—that by H. L. Mencken—because it paints in words a picture of a man with the same sure touches Broedel used in giving graphic life to medical ideas, anatomical structures and surgical maneuvers. The talk, otherwise unpublished, is reprinted here in part; it describes Max Broedel as member of what was more or less accurately called a musical club:

> I could give you a list of the compositions we have played since 1910, but it would only alarm you. The club's high point was reached in 1925 or thereabout, when we set out to play the first eight Beethoven symphonies seriatim. We began at 4 P.M., and got through the first two in record time—58 minutes and 12⅕ seconds. But by that time we were growing hungry, so we laid off for dinner.
>
> With dinner we drank a few glasses of beer, and after dinner one or two more. It was very hot weather, and the fiddles shed a great deal of rosin dust. Then we played No. 3—the Eroica. Then we had a few glasses of beer. Then we played No. 4. Then we had a cup of coffee. Then we tackled No. 5—a tough one. But by that time we were hungry again, so after the first movement we stopped for supper.
>
> When supper was over everybody was beginning to be tired, and the cops had the house roped off to keep away the dogs and lawyers of the neighbors. Even so, all sorts of writs were nailed to the door, and a couple of Philistines half a mile away began bombarding us with a one-pounder. So we decided to get the thing over with by playing the Sixth, Seventh and Eighth all together. Max and I took the Sixth, the fiddles and spit blowers ganged up on the Seventh and Raymond Pearl tackled the Eighth as a solo for the *Waldhorn*, with bull-fiddle accompaniment.
>
> I learn for the first time tonight, after thinking of him as a musician all that time, that Max is actually a highly respectable man. It is something to think of. The club will be astonished. But whether it is a fact or not, I am here to say that every member rejoices in the honor you are paying him.
>
> The club is the center of our forlorn and useless lives, and Max is the center of the club. When his epizootic floors him, as it did last Saturday night, we are lost and full of woe. It is like shutting off an airplane motor. We hope to go on playing with him for a century or two to come, and we certainly hope it is true, as you say, that he knows something about anatomy, and can draw a larynx so accurately that it can talk, and even answer questions.

Harvey Cushing, by then at Yale, was one of the guests present at the banquet and wrote a letter about it, that, like Mencken's word picture, confers the gift of vital presence on an occasion that may conceivably have had its dull moments, for Tom Cullen did indeed go on lengthily about the meritorious Henry Walters; but Cushing's account does seem tinged with something more than nostalgia for his days at Hopkins. The letter is addressed to a long-time friend, Arnold C. Klebs, a Swiss physician and medical bibliographer, who was one of the cofounders of the Historical Library of the Yale University School of Medicine.

Dear Arnold:

I went down a week ago on a jaunt to Philadelphia to attend a dinner being given for Max Brödel by the present head of the W. B. Saunders Company, young Lawrence Saunders. It was a delightful affair with a great turn-out of some two hundred people to pay a tribute to the man whose name, I suppose, will outlive most of his Hopkins contemporaries owing to the uniqueness of his contribution to medicine. This is of course debatable and something which time alone will determine; but it was unquestionably a tribute well deserved. Lawrence Saunders, I may add, is a delightful and public-spirited young fellow. He was the person who unwittingly purchased Erik Waller's stolen copy of Harvey's 1628 *ed. princeps*, a book which he without questioning returned to its proper owner.

Tom Cullen presided and told the whole story of his securing from Henry Walters the fund to ensure Brödel's continuance at the Hopkins when the Mayos were making advances to him to go to Rochester at his own price, suggesting $25,000, I believe, as a bid. Max decided to stay at Baltimore for a more or less uncertain $5,000, and he has been very happy there and from his appearance will go on turning out pupils for a decade or two to come. Lawrence Saunders had had a portrait made by Corner, the best in my opinion of the many he has made of Hopkins worthies in years gone by. Howard Kelly, showing his years for the first time, was one of the speakers; also Morris Fishbein, and H. L. Mencken on Brödel as a pianist, very amusing. And then the portrait was presented and Max very modestly and somewhat humorously replied in his own behalf. It was the first time I have seen so many Hopkins people together in many years. I happened to sit by John Finney who must be going on 75 and is still actively engaged in surgery, helped out by two sons, and possibly for all I know as many more grandsons. He ate an enormous dinner while I pecked at my somewhat dubious food, including scrapple, if I am not mistaken, though some of it I did not recognize. John Finney also did well by the champagne, much to my surprise, which made me cast a suspicious eye in the direction of Howard Kelly, but he sat where I could not easily spy upon him.

(From John Fulton's fine biography, *Harvey Cushing.*)

Cushing was no stranger to either exotic foods or institutionary dinners; but scrapple! Certainly not on the menu. Perhaps he, like John Finney, may have fully enjoyed the Mumm's Extra Dry, 1928.

In more recent years Saunders has published other influential Hopkins books. Two of the most important among these were the Shackelford *Surgery of the Alimentary Tract* and the Harvey and Bordley *Differential Diagnosis: The Interpretation of Clinical Evidence.*

Warren Stone Bickham of New York completed in 1924 his monumental six-volume *Operative Surgery;* but the work had exhausted both his physical and financial resources (see also Chapter 6) and he died not long after its publication. In this comprehensive treatise he described and illustrated in detail practically every operative procedure then being performed in the surgical world; but Bickham concerned himself little with evaluation, his emphasis being given solely to description. In this character the work was a remarkable success and to this day is still consulted as an encyclopedic compendium of technical procedure. After Bickham's death Ryland Greene enlisted C. Latimer Callander (author of the successful and similarly exhaustive *Surgical Anatomy*) to undertake revision of the *Operative Surgery*. Callander worked with sustained concentration on the book, providing thousands of new illustrations and mountains of revision notes and first-draft manuscript; but, as is typical of many surgeons, his labors were not systematically organized—he worked on all the volumes at once. Upon his death in 1947, it became apparent that no single volume was complete and the whole far from ready for publication. Several prominent surgeons reviewed the unfinished manuscript; and, although all alleged great admiration for it, none evinced great interest in its completion. For a while the idea was entertained of authorship by a team of specialist surgeons; and names like Blalock and Graham and Ravitch and Gross were, perhaps wishfully, considered. This plan too came to nothing; and the great pile of drawings and manuscript remained unused.

But eventually Lloyd Potter interested Richard T. Shackelford in revising at least the material on the digestive system in a proposed two-volume work to be called the *Bickham-Callander Surgery of the Alimentary Tract*. It was assumed that the task would consist of revision and modest change and that it could be completed within a year.

Dick Shackelford, after serving a Hopkins surgical residency, enlisted in the Army Medical Corps, served with great distinction throughout the war, and in its aftermath was known in Central Europe as "The Angel of Hungary." No more concerned and conscientious surgeon ever took up stylus or scalpel. But, upon his return to civilian life, he found, despite a Hopkins appointment, that it was not easy to find his precisely right niche in the world of surgery. He was an accomplished surgeon and had already made contributions to the practice of vascular and esophageal surgery. Still, time hung heavy on his hands—hence the one-year schedule for revision of part of the original Bickham-Callander. The work would also be a true labor of love, for major royalty shares were to go to the Bickham and Callander estates.

Shackelford soon discovered what Eugene Braunwald intuitively knew from the outset (see Chapter 16): that a thoughtful man may not readily sign his name to the work of another. In the end all of the original text and even hundreds of its illustrations were discarded. After six years of intense labor *Surgery of the Alimentary Tract* was published in three volumes and met with instant success, due in part to the circumstance that in the new work perceptive evaluation was added to description. Technique had become informed technique. Preoperative and postoperative care had been added to operating-room procedure; and indications and contraindications to surgical intervention had been elucidated. A work of very great value undertaken and completed with little prospect of gain but every prospect of worth.

Surgery of the Alimentary Tract has now appeared in its Second Edition in five volumes and has become, in part, a collaborative work under the editorship of Shackelford and George Zuidema, formerly Walter M. Firor Professor of Surgery, the Johns Hopkins University School of Medicine, and currently Vice Provost for Medical Affairs at The University of Michigan. It has again met with great success and, in a curious way, represents the grand scheme of the original—the creation of two fine surgeons working within the framework of the long-ago abandoned plan for the enlistment of specialist writers to bring special expertise to a work of general surgery.

Just as Shackelford and Zuidema complemented each other so well in doing a surgical work of vast scope, so it is unlikely that any two American physicians were better equipped to produce a work on diagnostic decision making based on the clinical-pathologic conference than A. McGehee Harvey and his close friend and associate, Jim Bordley, Director of the Mary Imogene Bassett Hospital and Clinical Professor of Medicine at Albany Medical College.

From boyhood Mac Harvey wanted, above all things else, to become a physician, and he entered the Hopkins Medical School after graduation from Washington and Lee University with the firm intention of returning to his home in Little Rock as a general practitioner. But in medical school he came under the influence of the physiologist E. K. Marshall, Jr., and this kindled in him an absorbed interest in the scientific base of medicine that would lead him into sophisticated laboratory investigation, making him not only a concerned and caring doctor but an academic physician and teacher as well who would hold steadfastly to the conviction that only good science makes good medicine. His early studies with Marshall showed that the loop of Henle was necessary to the action of antidiuretic hormone. This work was done with alligators; and, as Richard Johns suggested in awarding the Kober Medal to Mac, the experience of swimming with sharks would splendidly equip the young investigator to become the youngest Chairman of Medicine in America.

During his Hopkins residency Harvey decided that the study of basic neuromuscular physiology was being overlooked in its relevance to human disease, especially myasthenia gravis, and he delightedly accepted an invitation to work for two years in the laboratories of Sir Henry Dale at the National Institute of Medical Research in London. There he and his colleagues performed experiments that defined the action of curare, quinine, procaine, calcium and tetanus toxin on neuromuscular transmission. Their findings were published in a series of thirteen outstanding papers that appeared mainly in the *Journal of Physiology*. While still a postdoctoral fellow, at the age of 28, Mac Harvey became one of the first foreigners to be elected to membership in the Physiological Society of Great Britain. He still recalls vividly the challenge and excitement of the preliminary presentation of these papers:

> I shall always remember the several occasions on which I presented a paper before the Physiological Society of Great Britain. The presentation was limited to five minutes; breaching that time was not permitted and notes could not be used. The great heroes of British physiology and biochemistry—Dale, Adrian, Barcroft, A. V. Hill, and others—sat in the front row. When the discussion of the paper was completed, the tension of the presenter reached its peak while he waited for a member to propose acceptance or rejection of the paper. A vote was taken, and if favorable, the abstract was published in the official organ of the Society—the *Journal of Physiology*.

The Saunders editor will also always remember the excitement of reading on the then slowpoke train from Baltimore to Philadelphia the preliminary chapters of the Harvey and Bordley *Differential Diagnosis*. He sensed at once that he had before him the beginning of an important book—one that explained the process of differential diagnosis as analytic selection, from a number of possibilities, of the disease or diseases responsible for the patient's presenting syndrome and elucidated the relevant clinical and laboratory findings. Cabot's famous *Differential Diagnosis* had been reborn within the framework of biosience. A letter of reminiscence from Mac recalls the basis of that editorial thrill of recognition:

> I will try to provide as much background as I can about the way in which I got started writing aout clinical decision making. Although this has become the popular term for what I did back in the 50's, the principles that we put on paper at that time are essentially the same as those that are being bandied about now minus modern verbiage and lots of talk about decision theory, decision trees and so forth.

> I served my residency years when the great Hopkins physicians of the second generation were in their prime; namely, Louis Hamman, Charles Austrian and Warfield T. Longcope. They had a systematic approach to differential diagnosis that was the same in principle as the deductive reasoning utilized in the study of a research problem in the laboratory. This was particularly well articulated by Hamman.

> When as a young man of 34 I took on the job as departmental chairman, I had an image problem as most of the leading lights in the department were older and more nationally known than their alleged leader. Dr. Hamman died in 1946 and his clinical-pathological conferences with Arnold Rich had been a center of attraction for students and staff alike. They had a worldwide reputation. I decided to accept the challenge of making or breaking my image with faculty and students by assuming the clinical responsibility for these exercises. It was a severe test and I was at least reasonably successful. As I got more into the intricacies of making the diagnosis in a clinical-pathological conference case, I saw that the principles were really parallel to those involved in clinical decision making, so I decided to do the most difficult of all tasks, trying to explain it on paper instead of merely illustrating it by example at these conferences and in my rounds with students at the bedside. The first book to come out of this was, as you well know, *Differential Diagnosis* with Jim Bordley and then the resurrection of Osler's *Principles and Practice of Medicine*.

In 1973 Mac Harvey retired from his post as chairman of medicine and physician-in-chief to the Johns Hopkins Hospital to become Hopkins' first Distinguished Service Professor of Medicine. Since his retirement he has written forty-five articles and five books conveying the substance and excitement of scientific discovery. Among the books is the Third Edition of *Differential Diagnosis*, in which he was joined in authorship by a long-time friend, associate and astute diagnostician, Jeremiah Barondess.

Mac's has been an extraordinary life; but even in the fullness of its activity he has never forgotten the advice of Daniel Gilman, wise first president of Johns Hopkins, who warned universities against the "danger of losing the elements of repose, the quiet pursuit of knowledge, the friendship of books, the pleasures of conversation, and the advantages of solitude." These he has used to cultivate friendship and learning and to serve the journal *Medicine* as its editor-in-chief and the *Johns Hopkins Medical Journal* as chairman of its editorial board. He has also, under the much earlier electrifying influence of William Henry Welch, embarked on a new research career—that of medical history, the art of putting the past in truthful proper perspective. In this art Jim Bordley and he succeeded brilliantly in their *Two Centuries of American Medicine*, published by Saunders under a tight schedule within the nation's bicentennial year. It is a book of profound significance to the understanding of American medicine, though, like the Garrison *History of Medicine*, it has not in its initial reception been overwhelmingly popular. But perhaps it too, like the Garrison, will enjoy a rebirth in later reprinting and take its rightful place among those few books that penetrate to the innermost meaning of events.

Nelson's Textbook of Pediatrics: The Green Bible

13

In 1896 Appleton-Century published Holt's *Pediatrics,* destined to become for almost fifty years the leading textbook of pediatrics in the world. At that time L. Emmett Holt was Professor of Pediatrics at Columbia University College of Physicians and Surgeons and a commanding figure in the emerging specialty devoted to care of children's diseases. In subsequent editions he was joined in authorship by John Holland, Professor of Pediatrics at Hopkins; and, still later, authorship was assumed by Holt's son and Rustin McIntosh, Chairmen of Pediatrics, respectively, at New York University and Columbia University. Holt and McIntosh was another of those texts, towering above others, that every publisher thought he should somehow be able to displace.

In the early years of this century Saunders also published a respected single-authored *Pediatrics* by J. P. Crozer Griffith, Professor of Pediatrics at the University of Pennsylvania. It was a large two-volume work of personal experience and evaluation of current literature. Perhaps because of its size it was never widely used as a teaching text. In its Second Edition Griffith was joined in authorship by A. Graeme Mitchell, Chairman of the Department of Pediatrics at the University of Cincinnati—the most heavily endowed department in the country with a large full-time staff working harmoniously and productively within the Children's Hospital Pediatric Research Foundation, the gift of William Cooper Procter, the soap baron. At that time too Waldo E. Nelson was a medical student at the University of Cincinnati.

In 1930 Saunders proposed that the Griffith-Mitchell be greatly reduced in size and published as a single volume. The idea was also suggested, arising no doubt from experience with the Cecil *Textbook of Medicine,* that it become a collaborative work. The latter suggestion was never fully realized because of Griffith's objection to it; but single-volume editions, increasingly the work of Mitchell, were successfully published in 1933, 1937 and 1941, none attaining anything like the use of Holt and McIntosh. In the spring of 1941, just when the Third Edition of their book was coming off press, both Mitchell and Griffith died.

Shortly before Mitchell's death, his student and presumed successor, Waldo (Bill) Nelson, had accepted the Chairmanship of Pediatrics at Temple University School of Medicine; and Mac Greene (Ryland Greene's son and a vice president of Saunders) proposed to him authorship of a textbook of pediatrics. Nelson turned down this offer because he was far too busy reorganizing and strengthening the department at Temple and because he felt he owed his career to the helpfulness of Mitchell. But Mitchell's death changed this situation, and Greene now suggested to Nelson his editing a collaborative fourth edition of the Griffith-Mitchell text. Nelson accepted this invitation, and thus was born a new textbook of pediatrics, not displacing but far outselling the Holt-McIntosh.

The Mitchell-Nelson *Textbook of Pediatrics* appeared in November, 1945, as a collaborative thirteen-hundred-page book that was instantly greeted with admiration and affection. Nelson played a significant role in editions four through eleven; but in the 1950s his time available for the book was compromised by the affiliation of St. Christopher's Hospital with Temple University and enlargement of his responsibilities as Medical Director of the hospital. Still, he found time for what had become an important part of his life. Those who knew of his absolute dedication to the strength of St. Christopher's, of his attraction to it of a wonderfully skilled, woefully underpaid staff and of his intense great-hearted concern with the children under treatment at St. Christopher's marveled at his ability to carry out brilliantly both his professional and editorial responsibilities. He even found time to play a fairly good, stubborn game of golf. Only the very busy have time for added duties and pleasures. He would later squeeze into this schedule editorship, reinvigoration and rescue of a badly faltering journal in pediatrics.

But he had help with the book—help of a unique nature. Its doing was from the beginning a family affair. His daughters Jane and Ann assisted in a hundred useful ways, especially in correlation of corrections and cross-references and in preparation of the detailed index ("Birds, for the, pp. 1–1413" was their work). But it was his wife Marge who gave the book her remarkably sagacious attention. After Bill had done whatever compression or rewriting was required, she scanned the manuscript to determine if his editing had altered the author's intent and she imposed upon the whole a style that gave the book an integrity and consistency of expression rare among multi-authored volumes. She also read all galley and page proof with scrupulous care. That she could edit for consistency of style without wounding the delicate sensibilities of contributors complacently satisfied with their own ways of expression can be attributed only to an editorial touch at once firm and light. Especially for the Sixth Edition, which was reduced in manuscript by three hundred printed pages, she undertook the long and tedious task of deleting thousands of unnecessary words without altering meaning. A final paragraph in the Preface to the first edition of the textbook for which Nelson was solely responsible makes her role clear: "Finally, the editorial 'we' must be explained. The task of editing has been shared by my wife. No one has made a comparable contribution. She has read and reread every word in this entire book, save the ones in this paragraph. If there is any evenness and smoothness of construction, much of the credit is hers."

In later editions of the text Nelson would have the help of coeditors: Victor Vaughan, Professor at Temple; James McKay, Professor and Chairman at Vermont; and Richard Behrman, Professor and Chairman at Case Western Reserve and, appropriately, his son-in-law. But for eight editions Bill Nelson played a major role in choice and harassment of contributing writers and in formulating the guiding principles of the work. In early editions, for example, it was only at his insistence that continuing health of the well child was given significant attention in the book.

He endured in his task despite growing academic commitments and single-handedly created and never ceased to cherish the book that became under his deft guidance "the green bible of pediatrics."

14

Conn Current Therapy: Saunders at Work

The natural history of *Current Therapy* is an interesting one, for it demonstrates not only harmony between marketing and editorial ideas but also, on the part of the publisher, far-sightedness and flexibility, the book in creation taking on an architecture and dimension not anticipated in its original planning. Its timing, too, was fortuitous, because by the late 1940s Harry Beckman had grown weary of one of the most successful practical guides to informed medicine ever published—his *Treatment in General Practice*—and *Current Therapy* was destined to fill that gap.

In January of 1947 a young unknown physician visited Lloyd Potter at the Saunders offices. Howard Conn was a likable, attractive person with a rather naive diffident manner but with fairly definite ideas about a book he proposed to put together. The young physician made no secret of the fact that he had been hawking around his idea for a book on treatment for quite a spell and with a good many publishers (Prior, Williams and Wilkins, Lippincott and others). Up to this point, he had had no success although everyone seemed to acknowledge that his ideas were sound.

It may be suspected that his difficulties were in large measure due to his limited qualifications to undertake editorship of so important a project. In the main, his qualifications consisted solely of the fact that he practiced medicine and had visualized a book on therapy quite different from any then being published.

It was his experience that upon release from Army duty his greatest difficulty as a physician was the simple business of trying to keep up with changes in therapy that had been tried and found effective by investigators and clinicians of standing. Not only were changes in therapy too swift for ready assimilation, the dimension of the problem was increased by floods of rumors, newspaper stories, advertisements and fables about new miracle drugs for almost every conceivable disease. Lack of good information was often putting the physician in the unsound and ridiculous position of learning about new chemotherapeutic agents from detail men, *Time* magazine, the Sunday newspaper supplements and even his patients. This was before congressional amendments strengthened effectiveness of the Food and Drug Administration; and untried, sometimes hazardous, new drugs and combinations of existing drugs appeared on the market in flood proportions accompanied by extravagant claims.

The answer? An annual volume in which the current ideas of therapy for each disease would be set forth in detailed but outline form by authorities who were actually working with new methods of therapy and could speak with authority and experience of their results. It is noteworthy that even at this very early date Conn spoke feelingly of the necessity for written statement not only of new treatments but of the validity for existing treatments. He felt that it is just as important for the physician to know what is old and reliable as what is new and good.

Lloyd Potter applauded these ideas and believed that the untried physician could accomplish such a book. It was his faith in Conn's ability that is one of the most striking features of the story of the book viewed in retrospect. Here was a young man with no funds, precious little practice and not even the services of a secretary, situated in a remote town, completely unknown and unassociated with any great medical teaching center, who was preparing to enlist the help of two hundred or so distinguished clinicians who under his editorial secretaryless guidance would actually prepare *brief* statements of therapy in remarkably *little time* for inclusion in a book that was to be published annually and whose content was to be *rewritten by Conn* on the basis of his judgment alone. So formidable were these obstacles that the small fact that the Contributors were to contribute without payment went unnoticed as a trivial detail.

With the central fact of the editor's belief not only in the book but also in its author, the stage was set for acceptance of the basic idea and also for a whole series of evolutionary changes in its development. Among these was a plan to assist getting the work done and to bolster up its authority by inviting a Board of Consultants to help choose suitable authors and to review submitted material. This was Lloyd Potter's idea and can be reckoned a major contribution to the book's value and acceptance. It does the idea no injustice to suspect that its basic purpose was to give the work an air of academic respectability that Conn's name alone could not manage. Potter also undertook to enlist the participation of the Consultants. With only two exceptions (Dr. George Thorn and Dr. Harold Stewart), all the original invitees accepted.

The initial plan for *Current Therapy* was the result of careful thought, hard work, deliberation upon experience in publishing and astute knowledge of the physician's needs. It represented the best of which author and publisher were capable. Someday there may even be a book done like *Current Therapy* as it was originally conceived. However, *Current Therapy* 1949 to 1988 does not in any way resemble that plan. In each particular the plan miscarried.

Phase I (Plan): Each Consultant was to be sent a list of all the "diseases of his specialty, each disease listed separately with spaces for the names and addresses of the investigator or clinician to be contacted for his method of treating the disease," i.e.,

Pneumococcal pneumonia (name)	1. _____ address _____	
	2. _____	_____
	3. _____	_____
Streptococcal pneumonia	1. _____	_____
	2. _____	_____
	3. _____	_____

Phase I (Actuality): The plan was never carried out. The final list of Contributors came rather haphazardly from a few of the Consultants, from Lloyd Potter, Helen Dietz (office editor of the book) and Conn's scrutiny of the *Cecil Textbook of Medicine* and contemporary issues of the *Medical Clinics of North America.*

Phase II (Plan): Upon receiving these names Conn was to send *"detailed questionnaires to each worker mentioned"* and these filled-in questionnaires were "then to be sent to the Consultants for approval and comment."

Phase II (Actuality): The selected contributors were not sent questionnaires—but invitations to write brief statements of therapeutic procedures in specific diseases. These statements were received but never submitted to the Consultants.

Phase III (Plan): Conn was to use the completed approved questionnaires for the purpose of preparing tables of therapeutic procedure. Each table was to be prepared by Conn, including documentation and representing the opinions of several different authorities. Each disease was to take exactly one page (a few very important diseases were allotted two facing pages), and the whole book was not to exceed 350 printed pages of tabular summary of recommended therapy and was supposed to be priced at four dollars.

Phase III (Actuality): Conn simply took the written statements from his Contributors and submitted them to Saunders as final copy. They were often in outline form—never in the tabular form suggested. The book made 704 pages and was priced at ten dollars. The shortest write-up of a disease took 22 lines of type, the longest 24 full pages in a large format.

As the manuscript for *Current Therapy 1949* gradually accumulated at the Saunders offices it was given to Helen Dietz for editing; and the burden of seeing that the book was somehow finished now fell on her. The schedule was, of course, a tight one and reviews were later to comment on the extraordinary up-to-dateness of the therapies described. Nevertheless, tempers remained reasonably calm; the author, office editor and production people kept chipping away at a mountain of obstacles.

Meantime, however, still another major change somehow got itself incorporated into the constantly altering scheme of the book. The original plan had been to present all diseases alphabetically through the book; but suddenly the idea of division into fourteen basic sections (the familiar pegs of knowledge) gained ground mostly through the suggestion of Helen Dietz. The section half titles and their outlines were an afterthought that somehow had to be jammed into the book at the last minute.

Progress was slow and halting. All expedients were being tried as July and August went by and the book still seemed a jumble of disconnected articles. Conn was himself pressed into deeper and deeper service as a Contributor. The Index of Authors discloses him to be an authority on forty-four diseases ranging from Acute Poisoning to Yellow Fever. His most interesting pieces are on Snake Bite and Spider Bite ("The black widow spider—*Latrodectus mactans*—is probably responsible for all cases of spider bite requiring immediate treatment.")

Necessary articles were condensed and rewritten from the *Clinics* and the *Cecil Textbook* and hurried off to their authors for their somewhat astonished approval. One involuntary Contributor said: "All originality and no plagiarism would make Conn a dull book." And things still were a long way from finished. On September 3rd a note of pleading enters the letter of that date, part of which follows. In the second paragraph of Point 2 it will be noted that Dietz is willing to throw standard nomenclature and even the alphabet to the dogs so long as a major section of the book can begin with a real authority:

First some general questions:

1. We have been wondering whether it would not be better to use your name on the articles you have prepared, rather than leaving them unsigned which might be confusing to the reader. Would you want to do this, and if so, how would you prefer to have it worded?

2. Mr. Potter and I both felt that it might be worth while to try to obtain original material from those men whose articles in the Clinics or in Cecil were quoted at some length. He therefore composed a letter which has been sent, with appropriate modifications, to the authors of the Psychoses material and to some of those in the Infectious Disease section, asking them to send in something original. So far we have had two very satisfactory replies and we hope to receive a few more when the vacation period is over. We hope this will meet with your approval.

Re The Infectious Diseases:

3. Since this is the first section of the book, it seems unfortunate that it starts off with two sections that are atypical, that is, they are not written by authorities in the field. This could be avoided by calling Brucellosis Undulant Fever and moving it back to the U's, while Chickenpox could of course be called Varicella and moved accordingly. Then the first article would be the Common Cold, which would be a good one to begin with. If you have no objections, we shall plan to do this.

4. Under Rubella, in the last paragraph, do you think that a more definite statement should be made? As it stands, it leaves the reader quite up in the air and perhaps might better be omitted than left as it is at present.

5. With regard to the synopsis of immunization schedules under Whooping Cough, should reference be made to this under the other diseases mentioned, namely Diphtheria, Tetanus and Smallpox?

Re Diseases of Allergy:

6. After discussion with Mr. Potter, I feel that this is one section in which we might dispense with the alphabetical arrangement of articles. As it now stands, articles based on body systems are mixed in with articles based on the causative allergens, leading to much confusion and duplication. I realize that this presents a very difficult problem in view of the numerous authors involved, but it seems that it might be better to rearrange this section with all the articles based on systems together, followed by the special etiologic agents. I think also that it might be well to combine anaphylactic shock and serum allergy. I should also like to try combining the articles on allergic dermatitis and contact allergy, since as they now stand they are practically duplications. However, I may find that it is not possible to do this.

7. Under Ocular Allergy, the method of Dr. Woods seems unnecessarily detailed and includes material which is really in the province of the ophthalmologist. Could this be modified, or if not, should a warning be included as to consultation with an ophthalmologist?

Re Diseases of the Skin:

8. I notice several omissions from this section as compared with your original list. Most of these do not seem important, but I am wondering if the following should be included: Scabies, Verruca, Tuberculosis cutis.

9. The biggest problem in this section is the inclusion of Dermatitis here, as well as under Allergy. There is some justification for this, of course, but unfortunately the actual articles here deal with allergic dermatitis, as you know, with the sole exception of the article on neurodermatitis. I would suggest moving all of this to the Allergy section, with a cross reference under the Skin section. However, this will of course make the Allergic Dermatitis section quite bulky. What is your feeling on this matter?

10. Folliculitis decalvans seems to be generally classified as a form of Alopecia. Should it be included under this head rather than separately?

11. Under Malignant Growths of the Skin, in the Precancerous section there is considerable mention of diseases which are also treated separately, such as lupus erythematosus. Should cross references be used here, or how would you suggest handling this?

12. Why not omit Pruritus Ani from the article on Pruritus, leaving only the cross reference, since this is covered under the digestive diseases.

I hope you will forgive all these questions. We shall hope to send you some proof very shortly.

Conn remained reasonably unruffled through most of this. He replied urbanely. "I am inclined to agree in general with your comments. They have been very helpful and were much appreciated. Standardization of the material has been difficult because of the great variety of form in the manuscripts submitted."

In the midst of darkening clouds and gathering problems, a flash of lightning streaked across the sky. It was Donald Munro in Boston who had just received his Conn-Dietz–edited and condensed contribution to *Current Therapy*. Conn remained imperturbable:

Dr. Munro, in the enclosed letter, is referring to the long article I had with me when we discussed these matters last week. I believe I mentioned at the time that he would probably be resistant to any change and his letters have indicated that either he does not quite approve of the method or that he has not understood what I have written (giving him the benefit of the doubt). I think he prefers the usual textbook presentation. It is probable that when we tell him there is no financial reward he may lose interest.

In fact, Munro had gone off like an outraged skyrocket; but somehow H. Houston Merritt calmed him down, got him out of *Current Therapy* and pursuaded other people to do his contributions.

As has by now become clear, *Current Therapy* shattered precedents and overthrew established convictions as it went along. Lawrence Saunders took great interest in the cover for the book. He felt that an elaborate eye-catching cover was important but that it should at the same time somehow suggest a feeling of impermanence. The cover should attract and appeal, but at the end of a year it should suggest renewal. Through W. C. Shepard a special artist (Alan Schmidt) was engaged to design the cover. It finally emerged as a background of clouds on which were imposed the world and a gold shield bearing the motto "SAUNDERS." Conn's name was discreetly small and the whole thing somehow did suggest daring innovation.

Thus was planned the first medical book ever published with an offset printed cover. It was in actuality a pretty gaudy affair, but it was eye-catching. Since then the covers have grown more subdued, Conn's name has appeared larger, sales have gone up and the book continues to reflect Conn's astute perception of what physicians really need and his perseverance in achieving it.

In February of 1949 the book appeared. It was an immediate success; reviews were uncommonly favorable, and buyers seemed unusually pleased.

An examination of the records discloses that memory is not always reliable. In thinking back one is liable to suppose the Saunders Company ventured rather timidly into actual publication. There was all the business about whether it was or was not to be announced as an annual volume; and the question of whether Conn's name was to be submerged altogether in promotion of the book stirred up a certain amount of needless anxiety. Anyway, the record clearly reveals that the book was exploded into publication. Certain editorial reservations had apparently not much influenced marketing enthusiasm. A memoir of those early days from Advertising Director Bob Rowan may be of interest.

There was a considerable amount of advance discussion and planning in the Advertising Department for the promotion of *Current Therapy* during the latter few months of 1948. The amount of this activity was considerably greater than attended publication of a "regular" book, and it was obvious to us that this was something important. The line which we ultimately developed to summarize the book's attributes was "the best treatment known to medical science today for every disease you are likely to encounter."

It was made clear to me that the first announcement in the AMA Journal would be subjected to special scrutiny before it was O.K'd. This was rather impressive, because in those days all AMA ads were being subjected to scrutiny by Jack Lutz, W. D. Watson and sometimes Lloyd Potter. The ad was prepared in rather elaborate fashion. The layout was pasted up in an actual copy of the

118

JAMA and done in two colors on the front cover so that everybody could get a good idea of exactly how it would look. When the day of scrutiny dawned, the scrutinizers assembled in the office of L. G. Potter and counted among their number Mr. Potter himself, Howard Conn, Jack Lutz, W. D. Watson, Harry Most, Paul Burton, Mr. Saunders, and myself. I do not recall that there was ever another assemblage of such high-powered scrutinizers for any other piece of advertising. As it turned out, the ad was approved just about as it stood, with the exception that Mr. Watson insisted that the headline on the front cover should read "NEVER BEFORE A BOOK LIKE 1949 CURRENT THERAPY" instead of just plain "1949 CURRENT THERAPY."

After Dr. Conn had left, Mr. Potter stated that in all the advertising we should tread very easily about the phrase "annual volume." He said that we were not certain at all that the book would be published in successive years. After Mr. Potter had gone, Mr. Lutz said that it appeared to him that this was an editorial problem with which we need have no truck and that omission of the annual volume idea would ruin our whole sales story. I set great store by what Mr. Lutz said, because at that time and up until May of 1949 I was on probation in Jack Lutz' care, so far as the job of Advertising Manager was concerned.

The ad eventually pulled about 700 coupons, which is more than we have ever gotten on any other AMA ad excepting Kinsey.

We got our first mailing on the book out on April 8. It was very unusual, as a matter of fact, almost unheard of, to mail a new subscription book so soon after its publication; and it is my recollection that Jack Lutz was rather reluctant to cut into the salesmen's prerogatives in this way, but that the management and particularly Paul Burton felt rather strongly about getting some mail out. It is also interesting to note that in those days very little attention was paid to direct mail—an instrument now as much overused as then underused.

By April it was quite clear that the book had tremendous attraction for the profession, and I was sure that the mailing would do very well. I mentioned my belief to Mr. Lutz, and he said that he thought we might sell a thousand copies through the mail. I bet him a dollar that we would sell 1,500 copies on our first mailing with ease. He took this, and then I bet him another dollar that we would sell 2,000 copies with ease. He took this bet also, and paid both bets on the very first morning that cards started to come back, when we got 700 orders. Altogether we got almost 3,200 orders from the one mailing.

Jack Lutz, pince-nezed loser of the bet, was the former Saunders Advertising Director and the then Subscription Sales Manager. He was a bright, lively pepperpot who was so anxious to maintain his reputation as curmudgeon that he often actually was one; but he was always the champion of fine books and fine people.

Through the following years *Current Therapy* continued as the most successful medical-book project developed in the last forty years of American scientific publishing. More and more, Howard Conn took over completely the planning of each year's volume and securing new Contributors for each issue. Emphasis in office editing was directed toward deletion of unnecessary material, suggestion for minor additions, refinement in the use of headings and insistence on scrupulous accuracy. In 1951 Dwight Hotchkiss (Editor of the *Medical* and *Surgical Clinics*) suggested addition of the Roster of Drugs—the only completely new feature of the book since its first issue.

Schedule and production problems continued to be difficult, but under Eugene Hoguet's production direction the book was kept to a fairly rigid schedule of appearance despite occasional manuscript difficulties and occasional total increases in length. Mostly because of the latter, new typography was introduced but a high degree of legibility maintained. The 1955 issue saw the first serious attempt to persuade Conn to reduce the mere bulk of the book. It fell in 1955 from a 1954 total of 930 pages to 722.

Indeed things went as smoothly as they ever do with big books on a tight schedule, except that in 1951 a new IBM record-keeping apparatus managed to lose the record of all previous Conn purchasers. A fresh subscription start had to be made, but it was a successful one, aided by Bob Rowan's nice phrase "today's best treatment at your fingertips," which has been used more or less regularly ever since.

Current Therapy came along when young doctors returning from service were desperately eager for information. The advent of the antibiotics made need for such information all the more pressing. Howard Conn saw this need and saw how to meet it. From the point of view of its publisher, the book appeared just as the famous *Beckman Treatment* was fading and as the usefulness of the *Yearbook of Medicine* as a specific guide to treatment had begun to decline. Many efforts were made to take away this new healthy business by other publishers. The first and last of these efforts (*Medicine of the Year*, Lippincott, and the Smith-Wermer *Modern Treatment*, Hoeber) have both fallen by the wayside.

In this story the publisher stands out sharply as courageous and astute. In particular Lloyd Potter played a role whose significance can scarcely be exaggerated of planning, encouragement and faith. Helen Dietz did an enormous job of specific helpfulness. The book never would have been finished without the kind of assistance she offered. Robert Rowan wrote brilliantly effective copy for the new work and planned a mail-order campaign of startlng results. In the many spur-of-the-moment decisions that broke sharply with previous policy and notion, the whole management of the Saunders Company displayed flexibility and daring. Mistakes were made, but correction followed hard upon error. There never was any letup on the fronts of editorial action, selling program and production priority.

An early decision suggested by Lloyd Potter was that the Saunders Company advance funds to Conn for his purchase of an airplane. The plane has long since been sold; but it is allowable to conjecture that it once had genuine significance to the book. Back in the early '50s not too many physicians piloted their own planes. The spectacle of young Dr. Conn dropping down from the sky to solicit contributors to his book from landlocked Mayo Clinic people somehow reinforced the concepts of urgency, brevity, up-to-dateness and streamlined presentation.

Through this all, one thing emerged very clearly. It was not simply the ability and attractiveness of Howard Conn—it was his whole character that played the decisive role in creating this fabulous book. He was knowledge-able, stubborn and likeable; but much more important than these character-istics was his astute perception of reality. His almost unconscious recognition of when to accept, when to act, when to bend and when to stand firm underlay the impact of *Current Therapy*. It was *his* book in every sense of the word—planned by him, created by him and maintained by him with some help from his publisher. It is a great book in the sense that it is a starkly useful book. It is an original book in the sense that it is created anew each year. It is a lasting book in the sense that it concerns itself with the essential and never-to-be-solved problems of medicine.

Perhaps it may be said of *Current Therapy* what Thomas Huxley described as the purpose of medical education in his American Address at the dedication ceremonies for the Johns Hopkins University in 1877: "What is the object of medical education? It is to enable the practitioner, on the one hand, to prevent disease by his knowledge of hygiene; on the other hand, to divine its nature, and to alleviate or cure it, by his knowledge of pathology, therapeutics, and practical medicine. That is his business in life, and if he has not a thorough and practical knowledge of the conditions of health, of the causes which tend to the establishment of disease, of the meaning of symptoms, and of the uses of medicines and operative appliances, he is incompetent, even if he were the best anatomist, or physiologist, or chemist, that ever took a gold medal or won a prize certificate." *Current Therapy* is a book of which its publisher may be justly proud, for it assists the object of medical education.

15

The Kinsey Report: A House Divided

There is nothing more annoying than to be hanged obscurely—
or obscurely published.

Voltaire

Alfred C. Kinsey was educated at Bowdoin College and took his doctorate at Harvard University in systematic biology and entomology. In September, 1920, he accepted a post as assistant professor of zoology at Indiana University, becoming full professor in 1929. Shortly after his move to Bloomington he met Clara McMillen, who was doing graduate work in chemistry at Indiana. Their marriage was one of lifelong love and of shared interests and shared work. Together they studied the life cycle, evolution, geographic distribution and speciation of the gall wasp, publishing important papers on what might seem to some an esoteric subject but is, in fact, one of great biologic and economic significance. To collect his 150,000 wasp samples, Kinsey covered vast areas of the United States, Mexico and Guatemala. During summer vacations the whole family would hunt for the scrub oaks in which the gall wasp lay its eggs. In general, wasps are less well adjusted than bees and hence more like humans, being also carnivorous and fierce. Some travel in social communities, others are loners; and their mating habits are various. The success of a Kinsey vacation was measured by the number of gall-wasp specimens collected in bags of unbleached muslin. After nineteen years Professor Kinsey was the world's authority on the gall wasp.

The foregoing suggests that when Kinsey spoke as a scientist he did so on the basis of carefully collected and painstakingly analyzed data. Indeed, he might never have abandoned the insect world if during the course of his biology lectures students hadn't asked rather candid questions about human sexual adjustment and behavior. "I'll look into it," he told them.

He did and found that the most complex, compelling and difficult field of human behavior had never been studied from the perspective not of what

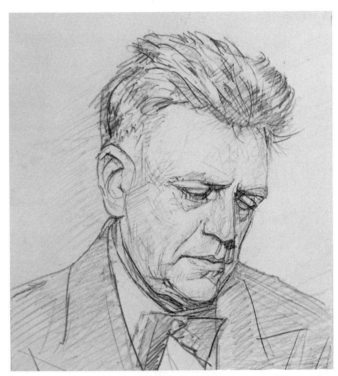

ALFRED C. KINSEY

A charcoal sketch from an unknown artist, made shortly after publication of the second *Kinsey Report*.

people think but of what they practice. It might be said of him as Francis Bacon said of Machiavelli: "We are much beholden to Machiavel and others, that write what men do and not what they ought to do." Like the Renaissance political scientist, Kinsey would begin a construct of human behavior not on the basis of accepted dogma and wishful thinking but on the basis of fact.

From this impulse to look into things before speaking of them evolved the Institute for Sex Research with Kinsey as its Director and with full encouragement from Indiana University and financial support from the Rockefeller Foundation administered by the National Research Council's Committee for Research on Problems of Sex.

Meantime in Philadelphia Lawrence Saunders continued his quiet, enduring friendships with Alan Gregg and Robert Morison of the Rockefeller Foundation and with Dr. Stuart Mudd and Dr. Emily Mudd of the University of Pennsylvania, the latter a marriage counsellor and author of several books on marital relations. Through her Lawrence and Dorothy Saunders met Kinsey and were interviewed by him; and another of the Saunders enduring friendships was formed.

But it was more than friendship that led Saunders to suggest publication of Kinsey's proposed series of books on sexual behavior—it was conviction that this was a study of utmost human importance. His covering memorandum makes this clear:

> These books will probably attract more general notice and attention than almost anything we have formerly published and are likely to be sold through more varied channels of distribution than any of our books. Advertising will differ considerably from that of a college, nursing or medical text, and our efforts should be coordinated and reviewed by a small committee.
>
> I might easily be misunderstood if I did not make clear that Dr. Kinsey's research, which made possible the preparation of these books, is of a fundamental nature and has been carried out objectively and by truly scientific methods. We recognize that the sponsorship under which the research has been done and under which the books will be published could hardly be better.
>
> In spite of this and the potential significance of the volumes, I am mindful of the fact that we are primarily publishers for the medical, nursing, dental and allied professions and that we have 225 books in the current issue of our catalog. I hope what I have said reflects an interest in which you will all join me, in something quite new and very significant. I feel that we have a well-trained organization of sufficient size to handle this without having it interfere with our regular business or the interests of the authors of any of our books.

Well said—and carried. But carried in part, perhaps, because it was what Lawrence Saunders wanted. In any event there was always in the house a certain ambivalence about the Kinsey books, particularly in relation to how vigorously and explicitly they should be promoted. One might expect this division to occur along the classic lines of age, fundamental religious belief and conservatism versus youth, moderate religious commitment and liberalism. But this turned out not to be precisely so. One or two devout Catholics did ask their parish priests about the moral rightness of participation in the Kinsey venture, and the response may be surmised that no blame can be attached to anyone who fills his working responsibilities but had no voice in the decision to publish. Certainly Jack Lutz, far from young, a deeply religious Catholic and a staunch Republican, went right ahead with a vigorous plan of promotion for *Sexual Behavior in the Human Male* with discreetly worded but prominent advertisement in *The Atlantic Monthly, Publisher's Weekly, The New York Times, Saturday Review of Literature, American Bar Association Journal* and many other publications previously unfamiliar to Saunders as media for announcement of its wares. The approved preliminary advertising schedule called also for widespread notice of the book in professional journals, including front cover and three full pages in the *Journal of the American Medical Association*, three full pages in *Science*, front cover and full pages in the *New England Journal of Medicine* and three half pages in *Scientific American*. The total circulation in a heavy early schedule of advertising broke down thus: Professional journals 775,000; newspapers 3,500,000; general magazines 530,000. This could scarcely be called a modest beginning, and in retrospect it appears that Jack Lutz must have pretty much disregarded the sometimes cautionary voices of the coordinating committee or interpreted its timid admonitions loosely, for he also instituted a large mail-order campaign about which not a single word appears in the minutes of the committee.

Nevertheless, the edge of opposition was there, although in part blunted by a genuine feeling among many of the Saunders principals that the book would interest a relatively small number of physicians, psychiatrists, psychologists and sociologists and that the general public would pay it scant heed. Little more than a month before the book went to press, its authorized first print was for 5,000 copies.

As in any opposition, there were different springboards for objection. Lloyd Potter (Editor-in-Chief) seemed to feel that there should be some mechanism for verifying the Kinsey statistics; but how this could be done he never made apparent. W. D. Watson (Executive Vice President) may at heart have been part of the opposition; but always one to accept the inevitable in politic silence he also had a sharp nose for the scent of money and he did not for an instant believe that the book would appeal only to a handful of social-science scholars. A. M. Greene (Vice President in charge of trade sales) felt that the Kinsey books would damage the Saunders name among physicians and he kept constantly distant from it. Jean Hassall (Manager of the International Department) believed that the Kinsey study might adversely affect the high reputation of Saunders among foreign book dealers. Clarence Wheeler (Nursing Editor) was convinced that the Kinsey books would offend and antagonize nurses; and he may have had some reason for his alarm, for the Catholic Hospital Association would indeed ban Saunders representatives from attending their meetings—a prohibition that lasted for many years.

At the same time there was a manifest enthusiasm for the planned publication among most Saunders people—an enthusiasm arising partly from visits by Kinsey. A husky boyish figure in his mid-fifties, with electric blue eyes, a square-cut jaw and an unruly shock of sandy hair, there was something about him exuberant and compelling. There was also in his enthusiasm a strong messianic component. He may not have believed that the truth would set men free; but he did believe with genuine conviction that the great contrast between widely held notions of what sexual behavior should properly be and what his extensive interviews had shown sexual behavior actually to be was a cause of self-destructive guilt, hypocrisy and deceit and that these characteristics were nowhere more evident and vicious than in innumerable state laws whose negligent enforcement was a mask of their acknowledged foolishness and their occasional enforcement a course of willful injustice. Public myth was to be exposed by a sharp look at private reality.

These qualities were also to stand him in good stead with the many reporters and journalists who descended on Bloomington with pleas for exclusive interviews, stories, digests of his findings, excerpts from his book and anecdotes from his surveys. He felt strongly that release of the essential findings of *Sexual Behavior in the Human Male* would prejudice both its acceptance and sale and he handled importunate requests with masterful tact and calm. Many prepublication accounts of the book appeared in newspapers and in magazines such as *Life, Redbook, Reader's Digest, Coronet, Esquire* and innumerable others: but the actual details and conclusions of his study were not fully revealed therein. Nor was it noted that there was already under way in America a revolt against ferocious respectability that Kinsey did not foment but simply discovered.

Meanwhile his publisher struggled with a hundred problems of the book itself. Although Wardell Pomeroy and Clyde Martin were formal coauthors of the work, it was Kinsey who handled its every detail, for the very good reason that the book was his. No more infallible than any other author, he constantly underestimated the time he needed for writing, although one of the many points he insisted upon was advance announcement of a firm publication date and fixed price for the book.

As publication date neared, the storm of publicity became intense; and even the people at Saunders who talked of a 5,000-copy sale began to wonder. For the first time in its history the house employed a marketing-survey organization to discover how many copies of the first volume of the Kinsey Report might be sold. After four weeks of an intensive survey of bookstores and wide public-opinion sampling, the conclusions were forthcoming and are here summarized:

1. If there is one thing the American public does not want and the retail bookstore does not need, it is another book on sex to be sold surreptitiously by the bookseller.

2. Of all the books on sex ever published, the Kinsey Report is by all odds the most cumbersome, dullest and least provocative. Who will have the patience to wade through its hundreds of pages of tables and graphs and understand its inscrutable technical jargon, symbols and abbreviations?

3. However, it is possible the book may appeal to scholarly social-minded physicians, psychologists and psychiatrists and to some sociologists, social workers, anthropologists and biologists. The estimated total sale over five years is no more than 20,000 copies and possibly much less.

Still, the nation's newspapers and journals kept right on giving lavish attention to the forthcoming volume; and the smiling face of Alfred Kinsey became a front-cover familiar. An adventitious lesson to be learned from the Kinsey experience is the desperate daily need of the American press for something new, different, out-of-the-way, daring, and, if possible, titillating. It is a voracious hunger that stimulates its own appetite. Curiously, though, the television networks paid little attention to Kinsey. This may be because there is a profoundly intellectual feel about his writing and because television is largely the chewing gum of the eyes. But more likely telecast disinterest arose from the perception that the Kinsey reports belonged properly to the printed word and not to the visual image.

Kinsey warned his publisher that the idea of a small first print was folly and would be regretted in lost sales. An emergency meeting of the coordinating committee was called. Throwing all caution to the winds, its usually prudent members daringly decided to make a 25,000 first print at Kingsport Press and an immediate backup print at the Saunders plant of an additional 25,000 copies. Miraculously, schedule was kept and publication was achieved on January 10th, 1948.

Within two days the 25,000 copies at Kingsport Press were gone and it seemed likely that the 25,000 at the Saunders plant would disappear in another eight or nine days. There was no emergency meeting this time. On January 14th Lawrence Saunders summoned to his office the Managing

Editor and Production Manager Gene Hoguet. He spoke to them calmly but with a certain chilling finality. "I know," he said, "that there is a severe paper shortage and that we have no Kinsey reprint paper; but I also feel strongly that it would be unwise and a keen disappointment to Professor Kinsey if his book were to be out of print for more than a week, and our present stock seems likely to be soon exhausted. It is therefore necessary to get the book back in print by no later than January 24th. Committees cannot handle problems of this kind; but I am sure you can. Thank you for your efforts on behalf of our company and our author. But let me assure you I am talking about getting this done—not about how much it will cost."

Gene Hoguet was a man who gave every problem his earnest attention. In his long progress from office boy to his later post as Vice President in charge of production he never failed to give every request careful attention and prompt handling—but here was a stunner. Fortunately, he knew of a printing plant in Norwood, Massachusetts, whose dozens of perfecting presses were mostly idle and which also happened to have an enormous reserve of paper being held for distant use by a customer. Within fifteen minutes he had called his friend Walt Alan at Norwood, who agreed to put the book on seven presses and to borrow the needed paper from his obliging customer. It was necessary only to get a first set of plates and part of the binding cloth to Norwood at once. The whole East Coast was at this time paralyzed by a total truckers' strike in which union members took a jaundiced, even malicious, view of anything moving on the roads and carrying what appeared to be commercial freight. Nevertheless, Gene volunteered to bring next day plates and cloth to Norwood in Lawrence Saunders' station wagon.

In the afternoon and night preceding his early Sunday departure the most severe snow and ice storm ever to hit the East Coast struck with violent force. Mountains of snow and sleeting ice covered even the principal highways. It was indeed tough going. Only the weight of the plates kept Gene and the station wagon moving. The latter was a moderately aged rattletrap affair lacking a heater and defroster. Its driver peered through a glass darkly—the ice-encrusted windshield—and shuddered with the cold as he slowly followed snowplows northward. Fortunately, the striking truckers assumed that only a madman would be out on such roads; and madmen traditionally are exempt from usual restraints. At five o'clock on Monday morning Gene, station wagon, plates and cloth arrived at Norwood, where Walt Alan was waiting to get the plates on press. On January 24th the printed copies began to appear at the rate of 5,000 a day, and the 50,000 newly printed copies were soon enough gobbled up—a circumstance of which *Time* magazine took notice in its then breezy and mildly inaccurate way. Here is part of its account.

Manners & Morals

It weighed nearly three pounds, its 804 pages were a dreary morass of technical jargon and statistical charts, it cost $6.50. But last week the U.S. was taking to *Sexual Behavior in the Human Male*, commonly known as "the Kinsey report" (Time, Jan. 5), the way it had once taken to the Charleston, the yo-yo and the forcing two-bid.

Not since *Gone With the Wind* had booksellers seen anything like it. Out less than two months, it had already sold 200,000 copies. Its publisher, Philadelphia's W. B. Saunders Co., a staid old medical-and-textbook house, kept two presses running steadily to stay abreast of the demand.

The itch for the book was most notable among urban intellectuals and college students. But there were plenty of other customers. In Kansas City, a grain merchant bought a copy for his mistress, wistfully wrote on the flyleaf: 'I hope this will help you to understand me better.' In Miami Beach, where no cabana was considered properly furnished without the report, one playboy bought 50 copies and sent them to all the women he knew.

After the Bobbsey Twins. In Hollywood, mentioning Kinsey was one of the few ways to break up a gin rummy game. Radio comedians, ever on the alert against censorship, tested the water with such gags as: He's at the awkward age—you know, too old for the Bobbsey Twins and too young for the Kinsey report.

Hoosiers began to call Kinsey's base of operations at Indiana University The Sex Center. Hotter than the Kinsey report became a common figure of speech. At Harvard, the chorus of a student song featured the lines:

> I've looked you up in the Kinsey report
> And you're just the man for me.

Successor to Darwin? Sexologist Alfred C. Kinsey was not taken aback by the uproar. He had predicted three years ago that his book might sell a million copies (all royalties would go back into the project). Journeymen book reviewers took a quick look and promptly hailed Kinsey as one of the greatest scientists since Darwin. He appeared to have found that some 85% of U.S. men had premarital intercourse, nearly 70% have intercourse with prostitutes, between 30% and 45% have extra-marital intercourse and 37% have some kind of homosexual experience.

Last week the Gallup poll reported that the U.S. people were agreed (by a 5-to-1 majority) that it was a good thing rather than a bad thing to have this information available. But how good was the information? And was its popular acclaim a healthy sign? Almost unheard amid the general hubbub, a few expert faultfinders began to ask questions.

How did Kinsey, in his interviews, make allowances for boasting, covering up and lapses of memory? With adults, he depended largely on looking an individual squarely in the eye, and firing questions at him with maximum speed. To many psychiatrists and pollsters, this seemed amazingly naive.

The storm of protest some expected upon publication of Kinsey Volume I did not materialize. Instead, Kinsey and the Institute for Sex Research received hundreds of letters of approbation and gratitude, many of them touching in their pictures of a needless guilt and of suffocating deceit. But there were, of course, letters of objection and criticism. These were answered—never by a form letter—and here is an odd sample and the rejoinder to it from Jack Lutz:

Dear Sirs:

My sister thought the Kinsey book might be a good one, so I bought it. I never felt so "cheated" all my life and am spreading my understanding of this stupid book which gives no definite information and tries to prove all of God's laws are wrong.

Last month's Reader's Digest included many prominent persons' views on the subject of this book. It's a shame some money was spent but thank goodness not very much will in the future. Because peace is the aim and end of every individual. The thing which *all* in this world are seeking. Only one emotion brings this wonderful state, the Riddle of the Sphinx; this emotion is called "love."

Since love brings peace—send Kinsey and his book where he belongs and read a book called "The Married Woman: A Practical Guide to Happy Marriage" published by The World Publishing Company. Only after you have read this book and put it in practice would I care to hear from you.

Thank you.

Mrs. E_____ F_____

Dear Mrs. F_____

I have just read your letter of June 28 regarding the Kinsey volume and your purchase of it.

I am afraid, Mrs. F_____, that you bought this book under a misapprehension. The book is strictly a scientific report, a collection of data with no clinical application whatsoever. None was intended. It is simply a factual book published primarily for professional people who could and are making application of the data thus recorded.

Now I do not want you or anyone to keep any Saunders book with which she or he is not completely satisfied in every way. Therefore, you would do me a favor if you would return the book to this office and upon its receipt here I will immediately mail you our check for $6.50, the price which you paid for the book. I am enclosing a gummed stamped label for that purpose.

Insofar as I am not married I cannot very well advantageously read "The Married Woman: A Practical Guide to Happy Marriage" and put it into practice, so despite your request that I not write you until I have, I am doing so anyway because I do not want you unhappy because you have bought a Saunders book and have been disappointed in it.

Sincerely yours,

W. B. SAUNDERS COMPANY

J. A. Lutz

To a few irrational letters no meaningful reply was possible. Several of these not only expressed violent aversion to the book but also were overlaid with a fanatical anti-Semitism that could only be construed as a lunatic reaction.

If it is possible to speak of a conservative faction at Saunders disinclined to either publish or promote the Kinsey books, it had its way in one particular—the matter of bookstore discount. This too was a source of endless discussion; and the final decision was to stick to the 20 percent discount commonly offered bookstores on technical books and not to offer the 40 percent traditional in trade publishing. Certainly book retailers resented and fought this decision; and perhaps it was hoped by some at Saunders that in this way the book would never reach the general public. Nevertheless, *Sexual Behavior in the Human Male* was indeed available almost everywhere—and the low discount probably had no important effect, except in respect to appearance of the book on best-seller lists. It was felt at Saunders that somehow the book was not appearing on such lists although its sale was much in excess of that of many "best sellers." Therefore a letter was addressed to all book wholesalers asking them to request their retail clients to submit sales figures to appropriate best-seller lists. This reply from a Chicago bookstore clearly expresses the attitude that kept the Kinsey volume off the magical lists:

```
January 22, 1948


Mr. J. A. Lutz
W. B. Saunders Company
West Washington Square
Philadelphia 5, Penna.

Dear Mr. Lutz:

We have just received a letter asking us to include
SEX BEHAVIOR IN THE HUMAN MALE on our best seller
list.

This certainly is a ridiculous request as you have
done everything possible to make it unprofitable
for us to sell this book.  Our cost of doing busi-
ness is over 30% and we, therefore, lose 10% on
each copy of this book we sell.  We certainly would
be stupid to do anything to promote its sale.

This is a trade book and you are advertising and
handling it as such and we certainly are entitled
to the regular trade discount.

Very truly yours,
```

The hubbub of frantic production, diverse attitudes, difficult translations, serializations, condensations, paperback versions, publicity, international distribution, book awards, pirated editions, unlawful borrowings and irate booksellers and occasional irate buyers finally settled down and *Sexual Behavior in the Human Male* assumed its place as an important and wise social document. Whether all who bought it read it and whether all who read it understood it must be unanswered questions. The Saunders Company profited from and was not harmed by its publication. Its royalties supported the work of the Institute for Sex Research, and a substantial part of its publishing profit was given at Lawrence Saunders' suggestion to the Fund for Medical Education. A rich and exciting publishing venture built around a book whose meaning to its author and to its perceptive reader is summed up by Alfred Kinsey in the last two paragraphs of its text:

> Viewed objectively, human sexual behavior, in spite of its diversity, is more easily comprehended than most people, even scientists, have previously realized. To each individual, the significance of any particular type of sexual activity depends very largely upon his previous experience. Ultimately, certain activities may seem to him to be the only things that have value, that are right, that are socially acceptable; and all departures from his own particular pattern may seem to him to be enormous abnormalities. But the scientific data which are accumulating make it appear that, if circumstances had been propitious, most individuals might have become conditioned in any direction, even into activities which they now consider quite unacceptable. There is little evidence of the existence of such a thing as innate perversity, even among those individuals whose sexual activities society has been least inclined to accept. There is an abundance of evidence that most human sexual activities would become comprehensible to most individuals, if they could know the background of each other individual's behavior.

> The social values of human activities must be measured by many scales other than those which are available to the scientist. Individual responsibilities toward others in the social organization, and the long-range outcome of behavior which represents the individuals' response to the stimuli of the immediate moment, are things that persons other than scientists must evaluate. As scientists, we have explored, and we have performed our function when we have published the record of what we have found the human male doing sexually, as far as we have been able to ascertain that fact.

As publication time for Kinsey-Pomeroy-Martin-Gebhard on *Sexual Behavior in the Human Female* neared, a change in the atmosphere surrounding the book was readily apparent. Volume I had established the work of Kinsey and his associates as that of scientists, not fanatics; and at Saunders there was less uneasiness about the book. Prepublication publicity in the press, all approved by and emanating from Kinsey's office, was even more intense but more specifically informative; and there was a feeling that Volume II would far outsell its predecessor and that Saunders had not only a right but a responsibility to promote its sale vigorously. A change observed but not much commented on at the time was that Kinsey's robust health had begun to fail. His work on the manuscript for the forthcoming study had been unremitting and was constantly beset by the usual inroads of reporters and journalists. His death three years later may well have been hastened by overwork.

Also there were many more satellite projects of one kind or another to consider. The bandwagon of opportunity attracts hangers-on; and many who had once come to scoff remained to prey. These, too, kept the authors and their publisher constantly engaged in negotiations, many of which in the end came to little.

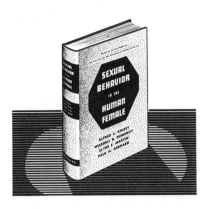

SEXUAL BEHAVIOR IN

THE HUMAN FEMALE

By *Alfred C. Kinsey, Wardell B. Pomeroy, Clyde E. Martin, Paul H. Gebhard, Research Associates;* and others on the Staff of the Institute for Sex Research at Indiana University.

W. B. Saunders Company

West Washington Square   Philadelphia 5

Nevertheless, things were calm, and there were genuine changes both of attitude and action. Principal among these was a revised discount schedule applicable to orders from all bookstores:

Number of copies	Discount
1–4	25%
5–49	30%
50–99	31%
100–249	32%
250–499	33%
500–999	34%
1000 or more	35%

In addition, the publisher allowed a privilege unprecedented in its history—the unrestricted right of bookstores to return unsold copies. Small wonder that there was eventually an oversupply of books.

Book wholesalers were to have a uniform discount of 40 percent regardless of quantity; and there was a euphoric belief that these measures would greatly assist visibility and availability of the book.

Perhaps even more important was a change in the book itself. It was less rigidly statistical, more freely expressed, and more humanly interesting than its predecessor. The simple circumstance that in the new volume tables were grouped at the end of each chapter made it possible to read the findings themselves without interruption; and these findings included analysis of the social and biological factors that influence sexual behavior and of the factors that account for the similarities and differences between female and male patterns of behavior. It was a more readable, interesting and socially significant book.

This was to be told in an early intensive campaign of professional advertising as well as unprecedented later promotion in general publications. The plan for the principal nonprofessional media follows:

The New York Times: every Sunday, beginning October 4th, until book is on their best-seller list, then every week for a month at least while it is on top, then every other week

New York Herald Tribune: every Sunday, beginning October 4th, until book is on best-seller list, then every other week for probably a month, then every three weeks

Saturday Review of Literature: every week until book is on best-seller list, then every week for probably a month, then every three weeks

San Francisco Chronicle: every Sunday, beginning October 18th

Chicago Tribune: every Sunday, beginning October 18th

Atlantic: one ad per monthly issue

Harper's: one ad per monthly issue

New Yorker: ads in November and January

Time: one ad in November

Newsweek: one ad in November

Publisher's Weekly: one ad per month

The Reporter: every issue, beginning October 27th

Nevertheless, all was not going forward expeditiously, for preparation of manuscript dragged on far beyond Kinsey's projected completion date. Finally, Helen Dietz, who had been the office editor for Volume I and whose abilities Kinsey respected, was sent to Bloomington to help correlate last-minute changes and put the manuscript in finished form. Her recollections of work on both the Kinsey volumes recall sharply the careful consideration Kinsey gave to his writing.

> I remember sitting with Dr. Kinsey in the old library of the Seventh Street building and going over the manuscript for Volume One. I informed him that we indicated portions to be set in small type by drawing a vertical line down the left-hand margin. He wanted us to do this immediately on the whole manuscript, so we sat there into the evening drawing lines. What impressed me most was that, whereas I drew the lines freehand in my usual sloppy manner, he insisted on using a ruler to make sure each line was absolutely flawless. Thus I saw for the first time his attention to detail. Nothing was too small to require his attention, from the schedule of the little airline between Indianapolis and Bloomington to the quality of the soup at meals at the Indiana University Union. I believe he suffered greatly at seeing the inevitable markings

I made on the manuscript, but the typescript was in such good shape that it required little change on my part.

Although I had contributed little to the first volume, I was in the unique position of being probably the only person at Saunders who had read every word of it. I therefore became something of a house authority on the subject, and was called in for consultation on various occasions. I remember being sent to attend a symposium in New York City at which various authorities were on the platform. It was my first and only sight and hearing of Margaret Mead, who was "for." I also saw and heard for the first time Frank Beach, the authority on animal behavior and strong ally of Kinsey. I also was called upon by Mr. Saunders and others to advise about questions that arose as part of the general furor caused by the volume.

As I look back on this, I see the total absurdity of my position in this matter, and the incongruity of the Saunders Company in general being faced with this challenge. On the whole, we probably did as well as could possibly have been expected.

As any publisher would have anticipated, the female volume took longer to prepare than had been planned. Publicity began to mount in advance, and the pressure was great on the people at Bloomington. I suppose it was in response to this that I was sent to work with the group, in the hope probably of saving editorial time.

I spent about three months living on the Indiana campus and working every day in a small cell-like room in the crowded basement quarters of the Kinsey staff. The details of just how we went about the editorial and publication process escape me now, but I recall lots of telephone calls back and forth to Philadelphia, and I made a few trips back during this time.

My stay in Bloomington was not all work. I shared in the famous Sunday night record-playing sessions and had many pleasant lunches and dinners with Kinsey and his staff. A staff picnic, toward the end of my stay, was a very happy occasion. I continually was impressed by the warmth of feeling among the staff and by their devotion to ACK, in spite of some inevitable minor bickering.

ACK's attention to detail was always in evidence, and I remember entering his office several times to find him reading the manuscript aloud to himself. It was his belief that the sentences must have rhythm and cadence, and he insisted that the entire manuscript be read aloud before final copy was made.

The clamor for publication increased, and in May of 1953 a few days were set aside for representatives of the press to come to Bloomington and have an opportunity to examine proof of the book. People from *Time*, *The New York Times*, and numerous other prominent publications were on hand. A reception was given, and hospitality was laid on fairly lavishly. Bob Rowan, the Advertising Manager, came out for the occasion.

Preparing the index was in my hands. I went over the matter with ACK and his helpers, of course, but did the final work after I came back to Philadelphia. Unfortunately Kinsey was not satisfied and raised quite a fuss.

Kinsey's final decision to remake the already-set-in-type index seemed at the time catastrophic in its effect; but somehow it was managed. The printing and binding schedule entrusted to Kingsport Press seemed sensible and well within expected needs. Kingsport completed printing of 175,000 copies on September 16th and first bound books were available on September 22nd—a date that had been hoped for but that no one had expected to meet.

Initial demand was tremendous and reception of the book enthusiastic. But something happened—abruptly sales fell off sharply. Exactly what happened is difficult to say; but it is possible that the hundreds of articles and new accounts about the second Kinsey volume at once satisfied curiosity and deadened interest. A letter of October 27, 1953, from Alan Hood of the Baker & Taylor Company is typical of many: "On October 22nd we have 9596 copies of *Sexual Behavior in the Human Female* on hand. Since our stock room gets pretty congested at this time of year we would like to return 7500 copies now. I am sorry to report that we are selling only about one hundred a week, which disappoints us almost as much as it must you." In the reply from E. E. Craig, Manager of Saunders Trade Department, a note of despair creeps in: "We will be perfectly happy to have you return the books to us; but I'd appreciate it if you would hold them for another week or so until I let you know where they are to be returned. We are rather pressed for space in the building at this moment and wouldn't be able to handle them here." Neither a liberal discount policy nor Art Buchwald's imaginary interview with Gina Lollabrigida about Kinsey in Europe seemed to help. Buchwald: "But statistics are important." Gina: "I object to people taking the beautiful idea of life and saying 50% do this and 45% do that. Love should be left alone without percentages in the way."

In any event, 45 percent of expected buyers of Kinsey Volume II seemed to have gone away. Here is President Most's memorandum of September 27, 1954, on the matter:

> At the end of 1953 we charged off 50,000 copies of Kinsey II. As of today, we have destroyed 33,600 and we have, therefore, decided that we can go ahead now and destroy the remaining 16,400 of the 50,000 already charged-off.
>
> I should imagine that you will want to do this from the quantity now stored at Kingsport, Tennessee.
>
> We hope that at the end of the year we can authorize the destruction of additional copies and so substantially reduce the remaining balance at Kingsport.

In the end 140,000 copies were destroyed; but this, like many another publishing decision, may have been hasty, for eventually Volume II settled down to a remarkably steady, if unspectacular, sale, and before long it would have to be reprinted again. The later Pocket Book Edition of the book had a similar initial sales pattern—taking off like a sizzling rocket but soon fizzling.

In the end the Saunders hardbound editions of the two Kinsey volumes had close to equal sales, with a total of more than three-quarters of a million copies. Their steady sale may well be the fulfillment of the Saunders early view that these were books for scholarly social scientists and physicians. Their sale in translation seems to bear out this character, for of the translations listed below only one sold more than ten thousand copies.

Kinsey Translations

Volume I

French	Editions du Pavois
Spanish	Editorial Interamericana
Swedish	Ljus Company

Volume I—continued

Italian	Casa Ed. Valentino Bompiani
Dutch	Bigot and Van Rossum
Japanese	Cosmopolitan Sha
German	S. Fischer Verlag

Volume II

French	Amiot Dumont
Hebrew	Achiassaff
Portuguese	Livraria Athenau
German	S. Fischer Verlag
Spanish	Ed. Medico Quirurgica
Norwegian	J. W. Cappelen
Finnish	Valokirjat Publ. Company
Dutch	Bigot and Van Rossum
Japanese	Cosmopolitan Sha
Italian	Casa Ed. Valentino Bompiani

Objection to Volume II was far less than to Volume I but more organized and vociferous, as suited the changed times. Representative Louis B. Heller, Democrat of Brooklyn, tried to introduce a congressional resolution barring shipment by mail of the new Kinsey volume. *The New York Times* thus summed up its interview with Heller:

> Mr. Heller said he had not read the book, but in a letter to Arthur E. Summerfield, Postmaster General, he declared that advance information released to the press and other news media had resulted in extensive reports that had led him to suspicions such as follow:
>
> That Dr. Kinsey had drawn conclusions that were highly questionable, if not downright ridiculous, on the basis of interviews with fewer than 6,000 women, many of them frustrated, neurotic outcasts of society.
>
> That through these fewer than 6,000 interviews Dr. Kinsey was accusing the bulk of American womanhood of having sinned before or after marriage.
>
> That under the pretext of making a great contribution to scientific research the doctor-author is hurling the insult of the century against our mothers, wives, daughters and sisters.
>
> That Dr. Kinsey's report was contributing to the depravity of a whole generation, to the loss of faith in human dignity and human decency, to the spread of juvenile delinquency, and to the misunderstanding and the confusion about sex.

Even in England, where the first volume had been published independently by Saunders' London company without any adverse public opinion, there was the possibility that the Director of Public Prosecutions might ban the sale of Volume II. This seemed to subside upon written opinion from Sir Frank Soskice (formerly Director of Prosecutions) upon the issue. His memorandum follows:

> In my opinion, the book Sex Behaviour in the Human Female is not obscene.
>
> It must, of course, be borne in mind that there is nothing to stop proceedings being taken before Magistrates in any part of the country in which the book

may be on sale under section 1 of the Obscene Publications Act 1857, and it may always be the case that individual Benches of Magistrates may conclude that the book is obscene. If this should occur I think it would be right to appeal. When the book is published, and on sale, questions may be put to the Attorney General in the House of Commons urging him to give instructions to the Director of Public Prosecutions to institute a prosecution. In the event of proceedings being launched, in my opinion they would fail; but in any case, I should doubt very much whether in the case of a book of this character there is any real risk of proceedings being launched.

In the nature of things, there is no certain test by which the question whether a book is or is not obscene can be answered; but in view of its general make-up, purpose, and the readers for which it is intended, I think the risk of it being held obscene is small.

Publication of *Sexual Behavior in the Human Female* did not end a cordial continuing relationship between Alfred Kinsey and his associates with Saunders; but it did mark the end of further publishing agreements between the Institute for Sex Research and the Saunders Company. Kinsey had projected a series of perhaps twenty volumes in which topics such as *Sexual Behavior of Confined Criminals, Sex Offenses,* and *Sexual Behavior of Captive Primates* would appear. It was the view of many Saunders principals that these books would be beyond the interests of the professional groups Saunders best served—those actively concerned in the social, mental and physical well-being of people.

This opinion was given to Kinsey by Lawrence Saunders on September 28, 1955, in a letter typical of him in its friendly dignity and forthright honesty:

> I have been waiting to reply to your last letter until you were back from your field trip to California.
>
> Just as you appreciate the help, and realize the importance of having had Saunders publish Volumes I and II, so also we here at Saunders have always taken a pardonable pride in having been your publishers and in having participated, in our way, in your great scientific adventure. For these reasons, as well as for the many and pleasurable contacts we have had with you and your associates over the years, we regret that your forthcoming books will go to another publisher. At the same time, it is apparent to us that considering the subject of some of these forthcoming titles, you will be happier to see them in the hands of a general publisher.
>
> I understand Harry Most told you in July that it seemed unlikely to him that we would want to participate in any sort of joint imprint venture. All of us here agree with Harry in that statement—and in so saying we do not mean in any way to be critical of McGraw-Hill Company, which in every sense is an excellent publishing firm. We have such a proprietary interest and pride in the two volumes which we have published that we prefer to continue to sell them as our own titles and under our own imprint as heretofore. This, of course, does not mean that McGraw-Hill should not bring out the remaining books in similar format to Volumes I and II. In other words, what we visualize from here on, is the continued sale and distribution of Volumes I and II by us, and the publication and distribution by McGraw-Hill of your succeeding titles.
>
> I feel sure that there will be opportunities to talk this over at greater length before your next Volume is ready for the publisher.
>
> With kindest personal regards and best wishes for the continued success of your important research, believe me
>
> Sincerely yours

In the actual event, future volumes did not go to McGraw-Hill but to Harper's. The reasons for this change are obscure. They may have been connected with the circumstance that Kinsey and his coauthors felt at home in the Hoeber Medical Division of Harper's or with the unexpected separation from McGraw-Hill of Edward Aswell, the man who had been conducting its discussions of future Kinsey volumes. In any event, the long list of books was not completed, owing in part to the death of Kinsey, and those published seemed to attract little notice and relatively small sale.

The great adventure was at an end—an adventure in which Saunders made its way in unaccustomed waters and in which effective publication was achieved of books that by any standard of measurement are among the most influential works of our times. Opinions as to their merits and effects vary; but those whose concern is with health would almost unanimously agree that the Kinsey volumes served good purpose. They released men from mindless guilt, morbid anxiety and hypocritical deceit. Their character was eloquently evoked in Alan Gregg's Preface to *Sexual Behavior in the Human Male*.

> Seen from the four points of the compass a great mountain may present aspects that are very different one from the other—so different that bitter disagreements can arise between those who have watched the mountain, truly and well, through all the seasons, but each from a different quarter. Reality, too, has many facets—some too readily disputed or denied by those who rely only on their own experience. Nor can science itself rightly lay claim to finality or the complete comprehension of reality, but only to honesty and accuracy of the additional facets it may be permitted to discover and report. I say may be permitted since the human race is familiar with the suppression of truth in both small matters and great. The history of science is part of the history of the freedom to observe, to reflect, to experiment, to record, and to bear witness. It has been a perilous and a passionate history indeed, and not yet ended.

> Living creatures possess three basic characteristics or capacities—growth, adaptation, and reproduction. In human biology, the reproductive function has been the least and the last studied, scientifically. To the National Research Council's Committee for Research on Problems of Sex belongs the credit for sponsoring a more significant series of research studies on sex than has been accomplished perhaps by any other agency. Among these studies the findings of Dr. Alfred C. Kinsey and his associates at Indiana University deserve attention for their extent, their thoroughness, and their dispassionate objectivity. Dr. Kinsey has studied sex phenomena of human beings as a biologist would examine biological phenomena, and the evidence he has secured is presented from the scientist's viewpoint, without moral bias or prejudice derived from current taboos.

> Certainly no aspect of human biology in our current civilization stands in more need of scientific knowledge and courageous humility than that of sex. The history of medicine proves that in so far as man seeks to know himself and face his whole nature, he has become free from bewildered fear, despondent shame, or arrant hypocrisy. As long as sex is dealt with in the current confusion of ignorance and sophistication, denial and indulgence, suppression and stimulation, punishment and exploitation, secrecy and display, it will be associated with a duplicity and indecency that lead neither to intellectual honesty nor human dignity.

> These studies are sincere, objective, and determined explorations of a field manifestly important to education, medicine, government, and the integrity of human conduct generally. They have demanded from Dr. Kinsey and his

colleagues very unusual tenacity of purpose, tolerance, analytical competence, social skills, and real courage. I hope that the reader will match the authors with an equal and appropriate measure of cool attention, courageous judgment, and scientific equanimity.

16

Friedberg and Braunwald: The Heart of the Matter

In 1948 on a chilly autumn day of torrential rain, Charles K. Friedberg arrived at the offices of the Saunders Company. Perhaps he had been unable to get a cab at Thirtieth Street Station; but for whatever reason he had taken a bus instead and had had to walk three or so blocks in the downpour. He wore a drab dark raincoat of the kind all Russian men then wore as a uniform of the Soviet Union; his hat, soggy with rain, had already been misshapen for years; he carried two water-logged cardboard suitcases heavy with typescript and wetness; and he had a look about him of a man who expects a record-breaking deluge when he is carrying a weighty manuscript.

He came to Saunders at the suggestion of Harold Hyman, with whose manuscript for the monumental *Integrated Practice of Medicine* Lloyd Potter was struggling daily—and nightly too for that matter. Perhaps this experience had soured his normally sanguine temperament, for he seemed unduly wary about what threatened to be a book of considerable dimension by an author distinguished but not well known—a book in direct competition with Paul Dudley White's classic text that had dominated the study of cardiology for years. He had asked his managing editor to attend the session with Friedberg; and the manager, ignorant enough of cardiology, nevertheless perceived that this was a different kind of book, one in which the manifestations and therapies of cardiac disease were seen in relationship to physiologic mal-function or structural disturbance. Potter somewhat reluctantly agreed that this seemed to be so and that Saunders should offer to publish Friedberg's *Diseases of the Heart*—a single-handed work of absolute brilliance and forward-thinking concept.

Friedberg was one of those rarely endowed people to whom the word genius may be aptly applied. He had a marvellous capacity for the synthesis of data and for the lucid formulation of ideas. He also had an incredibly capacious memory. In his spacious apartment he worked on the book in a tiny office cluttered with thousands of pieces of paper. These were his notes on the current literature of cardiology; but merely writing them had impressed their words—even their specific citations—indelibly on his mind; and in fact he

141

seemed rarely to consult the slips, once they had been written. Perhaps the little pieces of paper carelessly strewn here and there were his defense against intrusion, like Proust's cork-lined bedroom. Friedberg was also a physician of ultimate skill and uncanny diagnostic acumen. Anyone with him late at night who witnessed his caring concern with calls from anxious patients knew that he understood too the physician's cardinal role—to comfort and reassure.

He was born into a poor immigrant background, and even his birth date was not certain, for he was delivered by an unlicensed doctor. At the age of fifteen he matriculated at Columbia University, and it may be imagined that being an impoverished young prodigy is itself not an easy experience. Perhaps because of his background he was at once suspicious and envious of power and affluence. One of his associates once said, "Charles will never be truly satisfied until a universal plebiscite unanimously names him the greatest man who ever lived." He was, in short, a sometimes difficult person; and he found, as other original thinkers have, that the process of revision is not nearly so exciting or stimulating as the process of first exposition. But his book was never far from his thoughts, and his sometimes acerbic commentary to his Saunders editor was generally in jest. Once he wrote him: "What a powerfully persuasive and beautifully expressed letter you have written. A joy to read. Too bad it is wrong-headed in every particular."

While he was at work on a new edition of his by then world-acclaimed book, Friedberg was tragically killed in a cab accident. His death left a gap not only in the field of cardiology but in the hearts of his patients and in the hearts of those at Saunders who had come to know the real man behind the saturnine mask.

As is so often the case, there was only one man to turn to—Eugene Braunwald, then Hersey Professor of the Theory and Practice of Medicine at Harvard. But this was another invitation the editor was apprehensive about, for the life of the mind is lonely and demanding, and Braunwald neither cared for fruitless discussion nor bothered to put on the face of politic agreeableness. But many creative people wear a mask of aloofness lest their energies be frittered away in the demands of trivial affairs. He listened to the proposal to revise Friedberg and said, "I am honored to have this invitation, for I deeply admire Friedberg's book. But I cannot revise it, for I am not Charles Friedberg—I am Eugene Braunwald. If you were to ask me to do a book of my own, which I shall not even be able to begin for another three years, I should be glad to listen to such a proposal." The editor made this proposal and Braunwald accepted it, eventually creating an altogether new *Heart Disease: A Textbook of Cardiovascular Medicine*, like Friedberg in the esteem it at once won, different from it in its foundations in basic science and fundamental research. Here is Braunwald's own account of his book and its character:

> I wanted to write the book and was delighted to receive the invitation from Saunders because it had been a secret ambition of mine to prepare a comprehensive cardiology text since 1951 when as a medical student I became interested in cardiology. It took 29 years to realize this dream.

Whenever the book is compared to Friedberg in a not unfavorable manner, and is considered as a successor to Friedberg, I am thrilled because, as I wrote in the Preface, the Friedberg was my bible and was the book on which all cardiologists of my vintage—and older ones—cut our teeth. My own personal contacts with Charlie and my enormous admiration for this extraordinary man all served to enhance this feeling.

My book differs from Friedberg in many ways. Leaving aside the fact that he was a far better writer than I, that his book was "better" and a one man job, there are some obvious differences which reflect the changes in cardiology that are also reflected in differences between Friedberg's professional background and mine. Friedberg was a master clinician who spent most of his time in the practice of internal medicine; actually, when I was at Mt. Sinai he did not even have an appointment in the Cardiology Division. Obviously, upon publication of his book, he saw many cardiac patients in consultation but never lost his roots in internal medicine. He was basically a clinician, a keen observer of patients, and somewhat of a skeptic about "new-fangled technology." His book, which I still consult frequently, is always "patient-oriented" and the improvement of patient care is the bottom line. Friedberg's training other than his straight clinical training involved two years of *pathology*—not physiology or biochemistry. Thus, when he thought of a cardiovascular disorder, he must have visualized the abnormalities in the structure of the valve or the coronary vessel, etc.

My background and training were entirely different. After my clinical training—which included some contact with Friedberg—I spent 12 years in the Intramural Program at the National Heart Institute. Although I saw many patients with heart disease there, perhaps 75% of my time was spent in bench research. Thus, the frontiers in cardiology between the 1930's, when Friedberg trained, and the 1950's, when I did, moved from straightforward descriptions of disease to an appreciation and emphasis on the pathophysiology and the mechanism of disease. I would have to regard the work which I carried out at the NIH and subsequently as being on the physiology, pathophysiology, applied biochemistry, and pharmacology of the heart and circulation. My training and early work were directed toward gaining an understanding of the mechanism of disease and exploiting the new technology for the cardiac patient which became available during the postwar period. Obviously, a comprehensive book reflects the state of the field and both Friedberg and Paul Dudley White's texts reflected the state of cardiology at the time they were published and I hope that *Heart Disease* does the same thing for the current era.

My relations with W. B. Saunders have been extremely positive. As you know, I have been (or am) involved with three other publishers and I can say with all sincerity that the support, understanding, professionalism, courtesy and colleagueship which I have received from W. B. Saunders is in a class by itself.

Those who might wish to pursue the subtleties of this difference further will find them precisely set out in Braunwald's *Thirty-Five Years of Progress in Cardiovascular Research* published as a Supplement to *Circulation* in October, 1984. They will also find there that lucidity of thought that has made his book a new classic. In a thoughtful and laudatory review of the first edition, the *British Medical Journal* mentioned that there had been but four great textbooks of cardiology: Levine, Wood, Friedberg, and Braunwald—all of them in their time expert distillations of current knowledge and individual wisdom and three of them published by the Saunders Company.

17

Robbins and Guyton:
Two Authors and Their Ways

The United States is often said to be a chauvinist country; but in its use of textbooks in the basic medical sciences it has been above all else eclectic. For many years the Grant *Atlas of Anatomy*, the Best and Taylor *Physiology*, and Boyd's *Pathology*, all by Canadian authors, were stalwart giants that every publisher wanted to topple from their lofty place, but none could. There are other Canadian texts too of profound influence on medicine everywhere, and Saunders has had the good fortune to publish more than its fair share of them. They include the Fraser and Paré *Diagnosis of Diseases of the Chest*, the Thompson and Thompson *Medical Genetics*, the Leeson and Leeson *Histology*, Bates, Macklem and Christie on *Respiratory Function in Disease*, the Cherniack and Cherniack *Respiration in Health and Disease* and Moore's *The Developing Human*. Eventually, with even greater good fortune, Saunders would publish texts in pathology and physiology preeminent throughout the English-speaking world. Only Grant would defy its three unsuccessful attacks.

In the mid 1950s Jim Hughes, a textbook representative in Boston, reported that Stanley Robbins was writing a textbook of pathology. How many times editors have heard this or a similar phrase; but the disillusionment of experience never stifles hope in the editorial heart. An editor went to see the author at the Mallory Institute, the site of origin of important work in the morphology of disease from the Mallory brothers but also the city morgue of Boston with that scroungy, woebegone look of all municipal structures whose maintenance is farmed out as part of an entrenched system of patronage. Nonetheless, many a bright young resident has spent time within its unkempt corridors, including that wittiest of all surgeons, J. Englebert Dunphy, who said of the place, more realistically than wittily, "If you haven't learned to spit on the floor at home, you'll learn it here."

There Robbins disclosed that all textbooks of pathology were too large and that he would write a new text of seven hundred pages or less that would be sharply focused on teaching needs and omit extraneous matter. This too the editor had heard often enough; but there was something about the boyish enthusiasm of the author that inspired belief. The great adventure had begun.

After a while the manuscript arrived in Philadelphia looking considerably more bulky than one might anticipate for seven hundred pages. An estimate revealed that, even in a large format, the book would make thirteen hundred pages. "Too big," said Robbins, "I'll come to Philadelphia and cut it." And he did, spending three weeks of constant paring and pruning. The goal was achieved. In reading galley proof in Boston, the master cutter restored all the deletions he had made in Philadelphia, for Boston still lives within a Victorian tradition of hard work and longish books. The pathology was published in 1350 pages; but a brief note from a Temple University medical student restored faith. "I have begun reading," he wrote, "my new Robbins textbook. I know now that Someone up there loves me."

The book would indeed become the best in a hotly disputed field; and its author worked diligently in keeping it so and in writing with Marcia Angell a condensed version coming in roughly at the seven hundred pages originally aimed for. He should have saved the cut-down manuscript from the First Edition. The whole story of that beginning and of what followed is best told by Robbins himself:

> I know I have gotten old when I look back wistfully to the bygone years and I certainly have nostalgia for the WBS I knew 30 years ago. How to capture it?— urbane, relaxed, classy, an aura of quiet efficiency and commitment to excellence, a pervading impression of quality individuals committed to excellence and, above all, a gentility that reached out to this young author and embraced him with warmth, respect, and in fact made him feel good about himself and his work. The offices gave more of the impression of an elegant club than of a business. As you walked in you had the sense that the receptionist had been notified of your arrival and you were treated with TLC. Yes, you knew that making money was important but it almost seemed like a pleasant by-product of the pursuit of excellence. I was part of that old company and was made to feel an important part. All these reactions began almost from Day One. You recall that jovial, extroverted Jim Hughes said to me one day: "I'm going to tell the home office that you're working on a book. I know they will be interested." I thought to myself, "Good old Jim—nice guy, but they will probably laugh at him in Philadelphia." To my surprise, a young editor called, wanted to see some material, sent out some sample chapters which were damned—no, excoriated—but then had the courage to come to Boston and say "We are going to publish it." I thought to myself, "He's either a renegade like me and can't resist taking on his consultants or he's starving for titles and willing to gamble." And then when the manuscript was completed you came to Boston personally to carry back the couple of hundredweights of paper in a string-wrapped carton box. You told me not to worry because if the plane went down, you'd throw the box out the window and it would not get destroyed in the exploding plane. I will never forget your last words as you walked through the door of my office. Arm around my shoulder, you said, "Stan, I don't know whether this book is going to sell or not, but I promise you that either way, we will go into a second edition."
>
> Well, I have talked enough but let me just say a few words about why I wrote and something about revisions. As you know, I have always been first and foremost a teacher. I have always felt that it is wrong to expect students, when entering a subject, to use the same book that serves as a reference to experts. "All you need to know is 25 percent of what is in there." But which 25 percent? So I decided to take a crack at a nonreference teaching book. Only my youth

146

made that possible because an older Stanley would have known a dozen reasons to hold him back. But I loved the initial writing and fed on the challenge of producing a book that students would enjoy. I find that same challenge in every revision. I have been approached dozens of times by middle-aged clinicians who can't remember a bit about the pathology but they "loved that wisecrack about——." I must also say that revisions come less easy with each passing year—the volume of literature, the volume of garbage, the growing complexity of our knowledge, the need to learn methodologies and science that didn't exist 10 years ago and the challenge of what to include and what to leave out. It would be so much easier to write so much more.

It was an immense labor but one shared in spirit by Stan's wife Elly—a lovely person, gracious hostess, splendid cook and keen appreciator of art—who had the forbearance to let her husband write when he needed to and the insight to know that traveling editors despite their busyness are often lonely and deeply relish dinner in a home whose atmosphere is one of concern for the human spirit and for the creative mind.

Stanley Robbins and Arthur Guyton have certain characteristics in common. They are both masterful teachers who know how to make details meaningful and memorable. Both know how to unfold the complex story of a scientific idea from its beginning elements to its astonishing conclusion. Neither is a reciter of long lists and dull facts. Each is a writer who follows his own impulse.

Saunders editors have not depended much on expert reviews of manuscript, for reviewers, however expert, can be biased and often raise alarums over the excessive use of semicolons or the inability to distinguish between that and which. In the instance of both the Robbins and the Guyton manuscripts reviews were taken. They turned out to be of a severity equal to that of the early review of Gray's *Anatomy* quoted earlier. Sparing them some of the more grisly commentary, the editor gave the substance of the criticisms to both authors, who acknowledged their vigor and helpfulness and went on their separate ways undaunted. The editor, not quite so dauntless, kept his fingers crossed and failed to distribute the reviews to his colleagues in marketing. No sales effort has ever been helped by visible apprehension.

But there are differences. Arthur Guyton is a more reticent person than Robbins, more inner-directed and intense in his goals, a man of firm opinions but never disputatious. In 1946 he was a graduate of Harvard Medical School and a surgical resident at Massachusetts General Hospital who was already doing experimental surgery of the greatest promise. "I had been on duty for 120 hours of the past week," he recalls, "and was running a high fever. I became too weak to work and was placed in isolation. One night I discovered I couldn't move one of my arms, and I knew I had polio." His wife Ruth, no less remarkable in her bravery and determination, remembers it well: "At first I couldn't accept it. My husband was six-foot-two, a powerful man with muscular legs. He ran up stairs two at a time. Now I was told he might never walk again. It took a while to believe that somehow we would pull our lives together and raise a family, as we had planned."

Guyton returned to Mississippi, to his beloved home town of Oxford, with his wife and two children. They lived near his mother and father, the latter an ophthalmologist and dean emeritus of the University of Mississippi School of Medicine. It was clear to Guyton that he could not be a surgeon; but that only meant that he could devote himself to the two lodestars of his life—his family and his research.

He remained partially paralyzed but began to regain strength and to recover his zest for living and his capacity for doing. Always inventive and adept at things mechanical, he designed braces and hoists and built the first motorized wheelchair—inventions for which he received a Presidential citation. And in 1948 he became Chairman of the Department of Physiology and Biophysics of the University of Mississippi School of Medicine, which the Guytons would follow to Jackson. There his emphasis on solid research, especially in his own work on the circulatory system, and his absolute dedication to teaching attracted to the university other bright and able investigators who together gave the school a new strength and character. Research has been the guiding pole of his life and has earned him esteem from the world and honors from the American Association for the Advancement of Science, the American Heart Association, and the Royal College of Physicians.

His family has been the other pole around which his life revolves. The ten Guyton children have learned from the example of their father how to accept and meet challenges. One of his boys says, "I learned most from his disability. He showed me that the intellectual life can be as vigorous as the physical one." They all have pursued the intellectual life vigorously. The first four Guyton sons all graduated from the University of Mississippi and Harvard Medical School and have become distinguished teachers and investigators. The two girls graduated summa cum laude from Radcliffe and have also become physicians. Of the next four boys two followed the family tradition of undergraduate work at Mississippi and medical training at Harvard. The younger two are still undergraduate students who may well follow a course that has been forced on none of the children but in which all excel.

The Guytons live in a sprawling, poured-concrete, twenty-room house that Arthur Guyton designed and built with unskilled labor working under his supervision. It is built upon the shifting subsoil of the Jackson area on which it is impossible to erect a poured-concrete structure, but Arthur Guyton has spent his life doing what everyone else thought was impossible. Its construction was one of many shared projects that helped shape the character of the Guyton children. They installed its heating plant—just one of a hundred enterprises in their busy lives that embraced the delights of building electric motorcars, gasoline go-carts, model airplanes, homemade computers and original laboratory equipment.

Somehow there was also time for writing. The *Textbook of Medical Physiology* began as the voluminous lecture notes Guyton prepared for his students, and they reflect another of his extraordinary gifts—the ability to explain. Arthur Guyton is probably the only person in the world who could explain to the Saunders editor so he really understood it how a computer works. In his textbook he explains how the body works with the same subtle but accurate simplicity around which he built his own life and guided the lives of his children.

Again a Saunders textbook representative, Jim Ross, called attention to the lecture notes, clearly the basis for a textbook, and added the caution that other publishers were looking at them. Author and editor met first in Philadelphia and soon thereafter at a Federation meeting in Atlantic City. In a recent letter Guyton tells why he selected Saunders as his publisher: "I chose Saunders over several other publishers, especially Macmillan and Blakiston, because Saunders seemed really to want the book, while to the others it was simply a business proposition. You perhaps remember taking me through all the processing plant, and this was a major element in the selection process. In essence, therefore, you were the real factor in my decision to go with Saunders." In an earlier delightful visit with Arthur and Ruth in Jackson, the editor heard the author say: "I think once in a while about our conversation in Atlantic City at the meeting where I also talked with other publishers. You talked with me about my book. They talked with me about hunting and fishing and football, and they were not the things I wanted to talk about."

Eventually Guyton would publish with Saunders four research monographs and three separate texts in physiology geared to different purposes and levels of teaching. Each of the latter is the outstanding text in its field and together they have sold more than three times the number of copies of the two Kinsey Reports. This pleasant reward is but a trifling part of the Guyton story, at whose heart is the cry of King Henry: "We are in great danger;/The greater therefore should our courage be."

18

Nursing Education: An Encyclopedia/Dictionary of Nursing and its Genesis

A book is a mirror; if an ass peers into it, you can't expect an apostle to peer out.

Lichtenberg

A significant achievement of ancient Indian medicine was provision of public-health services. Vital statistics were collected; dangerous diseases reported; and, above all, hospitals established. They were the first in world history, nothing like them appearing in Europe until the Middle Ages. Early Indian surgery was skilled and thoughtful, and it was the surgeons who felt the need for institutional facilities—especially in the postoperative care of their patients. Hospitals were constructed by government order, staffed by government-paid physicians and provided by government with necessary supplies, equipment and medicaments. Thus early on the stage of world history state medicine appeared in answer to a perceived need.

Thus also appeared early in history and in answer to need a special group of health-care professionals—nurses—for the existence of hospitals made auxiliary-care personnel necessary. Consideration had to be given to two problems that have ever since been basic to all nursing programs: How to secure devoted service from nurses and how to train them effectively to carry out this service. The first is a matter of moral or spiritual ideals, the second a teaching objective. These goals in turn involved questions concerning the relationship of nurses to patients, to physicians and to basic medical knowledge that persist today, for in modern times it is only within recent years that nursing educators and nursing texts have given emphasis to the scientific underpinning of practice.

It was clear in Indian antiquity that achievement of neither the moral nor the scientific ideal alone would be sufficient to the purposes of intelligent care. Neither devotion without knowledge nor learning without sympathy can constitute effective nursing. Indian medicine approached this problem with matter-of-fact insight, as shown in the *Charaka Samhita:*

> In the first place a mansion must be constructed, spacious and roomy. . . .After this should be secured a body of attendants of good behavior, distinguished by purity and cleanliness of habits, attached to the person for whose service they are engaged, possessed of knowledge and skill, endowed with kindness, adept at every kind of service the patient may require, and accomplished in waiting upon one that is ill.

How different from the picture of the disreputable Sairey Gamp in *Martin Chuzzlewit*—in time but a stone's throw away from the present.

The *Sushruta Samhita* sums up the matter thus: "The physician, the patient, the medicine, and the attendants are the four essential factors in a course of medical treatment," and it adds the advice—so often unheeded—that "drugs should be helpful but at the same time pleasant and harmless even in overdose"; and the physician should be a "benignant friend of all created beings."

Twenty-five hundred years later there appeared the first edition of *The American Pocket Medical Dictionary* (Saunders, 1898), later called *Dorland's Pocket Medical Dictionary*, a book that has almost certainly had a greater influence on the education of nurses and other allied health personnel than that of any other published volume. It was the personal creation of Ryland W. Greene, and in its long life has sold more than two million copies. Hence one may reflect that if sale in tens of thousands is the mark of success of a medical title, nursing success can be reckoned only in hundreds of thousands.

Its influence can be laid to the circumstance that knowledge of the vocabulary of a discipline or science is vital to its understanding and that the Pocket Dorland defines the whole vocabulary of medicine and nursing with extraordinary clarity and concision. Its definitions are always scientifically accurate but never simplistic. Here is a typical example: "**abscess** (ab'ses) a localized collection of pus in a cavity formed by disintegration of tissues." There then follows less than half a column describing briefly twenty abscess subtypes. Although this is in contrast to the usual medical dictionary entry of three to five pages of congested type, it omits no essential information.

It is a curious circumstance of Saunders history that for the first ninety-odd years of the company's life only four persons were charged with the development of nursing books: Ryland Greene as senior editor and Clarence Wheeler, Robert E. Wright, and Helen Dietz as nursing editors. Each was associated with books of great usefulness and appeal, but each also devoted unusual care and thought to a single nursing title of paramount importance: Greene—*Dorland's Pocket Medical Dictionary*; Wheeler—Marlow's *Pediatric Nursing*; Wright—the Miller-Keane *Encyclopedia and Dictionary of Medicine and Nursing*; and Dietz—the Luckmann-Sorensen *Medical-Surgical Nursing: A Psychophysiologic Approach*. It is noteworthy that each of these titles so important to learning and so successful put sharp emphasis on the scientific objective of nursing education; but here our concern will be with the Miller-Keane *Encyclopedia/Dictionary*.

In 1940 the F. A. Davis Company published Taber's *Cyclopedic Medical Dictionary*, a reference source that appealed immediately and specifically to nurses in training and in practice and from the very outset of its life enjoyed a phenomenal sale. It was the creation of Clarence Wilbur Taber, the F. A. Davis senior editor, who for ten editions thereafter gave its revisions shrewd care. Subsequent revisions have been in the capable hands of Clayton L. Thomas of the Harvard School of Public Health. The Taber is distinguished by fine detail; but it also occasionally includes irrelevant terms. However, obsolete or even unnecessary terms in a dictionary are no real disadvantage to its usefulness, for the user seeks only the entry in which he has immediate interest; he does not read surrounding entries. To some extent the Taber succeeds on the realistic principle of dictionary making that more is better, the appendices alone of its current edition running to 225 pages.

Instant success in publishing always attracts envious competition. A nice question might be whether the competitive instinct of publishers is aroused by the impulse to serve better or by the well-known tendency of bank robbers to go where the money is; but in either event books competing against an established title can succeed only by their superiority to or valid difference from their target. The question then posed was why Taber was so successful. Like all one-man creations, it had certain peculiar characteristics, but it also had marked virtues. It excelled in richness of detail, and its most distinguishing feature was elaborate attention to nursing procedures— a feature altogether missing from the *Dorland Pocket Dictionary* and from other abridged medical lexicons. The Taber did many things but it was unique in addressing itself to the techniques and maneuvers of skilled care that the ancient Indian writers found so important an element of nursing.

Saunders eventually made three attempts to publish books that would compete with or even supplant the Taber *Cyclopedic Medical Dictionary*. The first two were solid, reasonably successful books that never attained anything like the sale of Taber; but this failure was in part due to Saunders' own myopia as publisher. The first—Price's *American Nurses Dictionary*—was published in 1949; the second—Petry's *Encyclopedia of Nursing*—was published in 1952. Each was in its individual way a work of real worth; but the Price was handicapped by failure to appreciate the genuine value of the Taber, and the Petry was disadvantaged by a curious lack of enthusiasm at Saunders for an inherently different and useful lexicon whose meager promotion never did reflect the specific merits of the book, especially its nicely done material on historical aspects of nursing and on the rationale of nursing procedures.

In 1964 Bob Wright, then the Saunders Nursing Editor, received from Dr. Benjamin F. Miller a proposal to create a new encyclopedia/dictionary of medicine intended primarily for the nursing market. It presented a new opportunity to compete with the Taber; but experience had already demonstrated that although opportunity may knock, it does not open its own door.

But there were good reasons for heeding this knock. Ben Miller graduated from the Massachusetts Institute of Technology in 1928 with a degree in chemical engineering, followed by a year of study in physical chemistry at

Harvard and three years at Harvard Medical School. His career as a scientist and teacher was interrupted when, at the age of thirty-five, he became seriously ill with sarcoidosis. Long hours spent in hospitals and at home in bed made his previously difficult work impossible. He had to find means less arduous with which to support his family and use his skills. He decided to write in clear and understandable style a medical book for laymen. The result was his *Complete Medical Guide*, which became a Book-of-the Month-Club selection, was translated into a dozen languages and sold in its original edition well over a million copies.

When his sarcoidosis finally burned itself out, Ben returned to full-time medical teaching and research. He became deeply involved in the development of kidney transplantation while he was serving on the staffs of the Massachusetts General Hospital and the Peter Bent Brigham Hospital, and his scorn of accepted but empty dogma was shown by his research in atherosclerosis, which he found to be more likely a disorder of carbohydrate rather than fat metabolism in the artery wall. These investigations led to his appointment as Director of the May Institute, where he dynamically applied research findings to the practice of internal medicine.

But writing had by now become part of Ben Miller's life. He was above all a bookish man, agreeing that "a good book is the best of friends, the same today and forever." When he proposed his dictionary to Bob Wright he had already done for Saunders with his wife Zelma a highly successful hygiene text, *Good Life*, later revised with John Burt; and he had just completed his editorship of the multivolume *Modern Medical Encyclopedia*, whose publisher, the Golden Press, had given him permission to use material from the encyclopedia in the proposed dictionary.

In fine, Ben's offer was simply too promising to suggest rejection; but Bob Wright was informed and cautious enough to know that the real strength of the Taber was in its rich detail and the specificity of its sections on Nursing Procedure (see, for example, its entry "dressing"). He came up with the suggestion that would make the new book not simply a competitor of Taber but a work of unparalleled usefulness in its own right. He suggested that Claire Brackman Keane become its coauthor.

Claire Keane brought to the work long and thoughtful experience in nursing education, nursing service, and textbook authorship. She had long ago resigned herself to the conviction that the only way to overcome the temptation to do books is to write them. Her Saunders texts (*Essentials of Medical Surgical Nursing, Saunders Review for Practical Nurses*, and, with Sybil Fletcher, her programmed text *Drugs and Solutions*) had already demonstrated a forthright and informative style and a sensitivity to the needs of nursing education that would become the qualities of the new Miller-Keane encyclopedia/dictionary. Here is her account of its beginning:

> In 1965, when we were living in St. Louis, I received a phone call from Bob Wright asking if I would be interested in working on a dictionary. It was my task to write all of the encyclopedic entries, especially those under the Nursing Care heading, and to revise and up-grade the material used from the *Modern Medical Encyclopedia* so that it was more appropriate for the professional reader.

Additionally, I reviewed and rewrote as needed the entries from both Dorlands; i.e., the illustrated and the pocket editions. It was my impression that Dr. Miller approached Saunders with the idea for the encyclopedic dictionary, but I do not know how he envisioned it or the market for which he originally intended it.

The selection of items in addition to those in the above mentioned works was, for the most part, done by myself, Helen Dietz, and Bob Wright. John Friel, Kitty McCullough, and others in the Dictionary Department at Saunders also provided lists of items to be included in the first edition. I wrote entries from these lists.

To some extent all lexicons depend upon existing dictionaries, a notable exception being Johnson's famous *Dictionary of the English Language*, 1755, which drew almost entirely upon its author's capacious memory and vast knowledge for its definitions and in whose preface he ruefully reflected that "Language is only the instrument of science, and words are but the signs of ideas: I wish, however, that the instrument might be less apt to decay and that signs might be permanent like the things which they denote." The "signs of ideas" of the Miller-Keane came from many sources; but stitching them together to form a cohesive and consistent whole was no mean task— one in which thoughtful editing of the manuscript was vital. This was entrusted to Betty Taylor, who brought to redaction the same quality of insight that Ben Miller and Claire Keane brought to creation. Here are her recollections of the book and its problems:

The Miller-Keane *Encyclopedia and Dictionary of Medicine and Nursing* was conceived as an attempt to introduce an authoritative, attractive competitor for *Taber's Cyclopedic Medical Dictionary*, a work that had dominated the market for nursing dictionaries for 30 years. The Miller-Keane was not Saunders' first attempt to capture this market, but it has been the most successful. Its basis was three other works. Most of the brief dictionary entries were drawn from *Dorland's Pocket Medical Dictionary* or *Dorland's Illustrated Medical Dictionary*. The encyclopedic entries—comprising an extended discussion of an organ, for example, with its anatomy and physiology as well as disorders and treatment of them—were provided by the *Modern Medical Encyclopedia*. Melding of this melange was done by Claire Keane, who added a nursing focus and supplied sections on patient care to the encyclopedic entries, and by the Saunders editorial staff, who smoothed the seams.

The dictionary was published in March 1972 at the price of $9.95. A well planned marketing effort announced the book. The goal of this effort was to ensure that every nursing instructor and every practicing nurse knew of the book's existence. Several thousand complimentary copies were distributed. Full-page advertisements were placed in all the nursing journals; the one in the *American Journal of Nursing* was accompanied by a tear-out mail-order card. Mail-order circulars were sent to all nurses who could be identified. The theme of the campaign was the suggestion that the reader compare particular definitions with those in the dictionary she already owned.

Sales of the first edition over its six-year life totaled 588,000 copies. A less expensively produced, soft-cover version was made available in 1976 to provide an alternative to the original book, whose price had risen to $14.50. It sold 64,000 copies.

That the Miller-Keane was an instant success is true; but it by no means displaced the sturdy Taber. This is because the Saunders entry in the crowded field of lexicography found a place of its own in the front ranks. This was due to its emphasis on the basis in science of all health professions and to its skillful formulation of sophisticated concepts. Terms in metabolism and immunology, in genetics and neuroscience, are defined with a just attention to their substrates in the biosciences and in their researches based on molecular biology. The healing art may have little enough to do with ability to remember the names of the cranial nerves; but, all the same, care and healing can no longer be understood without intellectual recourse to basic science. The Miller-Keane realizes the ancient Indian ideal of dedicated practice informed by learning and knowledge It instructs its readers but demands careful attention from them.

It is this difference that has made the Miller-Keane not only a successful but a highly influential teaching instrument. This difference has been intensified in the second (1978), third (1983) and fourth (1987) editions. Further, these later issues of the book have given greater attention to the educational needs of non-nursing allied health professionals. This involved securing extensive reviews of the first edition, changing the Nursing Care heading to Patient Care, providing detailed information relevant to the clinical practice of all allied health personnel and even modifying the book's title to *Encyclopedia and Dictionary of Medicine, Nursing, and Allied Health*.

Responsibility for all editions past the first has rested solely on the strong head and shoulders of Claire Keane, for Ben Miller died after he had completed his work on the manuscript of the first edition but before he could see it brought to print. He would have relished seeing the printed book, for it was beautifully designed and produced; and he would have enjoyed reading the hundreds of letters of commentary from its pleased readers, perhaps finding this one of the most pleasant:

W. B. Saunders Company
West Washington Square
Philadelphia, Pennsylvania 19105

Gentlemen:

I am just writing to tell you how much I am enjoying and using the *Encyclopedia and Dictionary of Medicine and Nursing* written by Benjamin F. Miller and Claire Brackman Keane and published by your company. I have been an R.N. nursing student for about three months and this book has been by my side during all of my studies. I have found it invaluable. Everything is written very clearly and concisely and it is very rarely when I cannot find what I am trying to look up. I really wish I had had this book in college when taking Biology and Zoology as it would have made my studies much easier. Many was the time I was totally frustrated because my textbooks had used terms for which I could not find a meaning. I have since found many of those terms in this dictionary and encyclopedia. I do hope you will tell the authors that I appreciate their work.

Not only this but I feel the book is very attractively bound and printed. I have never written a letter like this before but as I enjoy this book every time I pick it up which is often I feel that you should know.

Perhaps, too, he would have agreed with Johnson that "The value of a work must be estimated by its use; it is not enough that a dictionary delights the critic, unless at the same time, it instructs the learner."

19

The Selling of Saunders Books

by Robert B. Rowan

Walter Burns Saunders was, after all, a bookseller before he became a book publisher; and it is therefore not surprising that he carried over into his publishing philosophy a strong sense of the importance of advertising, selling and marketing efforts.

Very early on, when the Company was only about ten years old, he signaled this conviction by two striking actions. First, in 1898, he contracted to take as advertising space one half the front cover of the *Journal of the American Medical Association* on an every-other-week basis. Then, two years later, he opened an office in London to insure good distribution in the United Kingdom and on the Continent, as well as to develop editorial contacts.

The original overall marketing plan embraced five main areas: advertising in journals in the United States and abroad; direct selling to American doctors by commission salesmen; selling to both doctors and individual bookstores, also in the United States, through regional book wholesalers and jobbers; direct sales to bookstores in the United States (mostly in medical schools); and direct sales to bookstores around the world (except for those in the United Kingdom and on the Continent, which were handled through the London office).

Note that direct mail selling was not even considered in the original marketing plan. It was believed by the founder, and by John A. Lutz, who served as Sales Manager of the company for more than half a century, that the primary and most important channels of sales to doctors were first the commission salesmen; then the bookstores; and then journal advertising, which early on began to incorporate direct-return order forms.

The Messrs. Saunders and Lutz considered that direct-mail sales efforts to doctors would vitiate the salesmen's effectiveness and determination; as a matter of fact, this same philosophy prevailed at the company until after World War II.

That was the master plan.

JOURNAL ADVERTISING AND THE FRONT COVER POLICY

Sensing that the great early success of the company was partly due to the *JAMA* front-cover advertising, Lutz embarked on a startling policy. He attempted to get advertising space on the front cover of every leading medical journal in the English-speaking world.

As a matter of fact, he refused to advertise in a journal unless it would agree to rent front-cover space to Saunders. Astonishingly enough, this seemingly too bold and perhaps shortsighted approach succceeded. At one point the Saunders Company advertisement appeared on the front covers of

> *Journal of the American Medical Association*
>
> *New England Journal of Medicine*
>
> *Surgery, Gynecology & Obstetrics*
>
> *British Medical Journal*
>
> *Lancet*
>
> *Science*
>
> *American Journal of Nursing*
>
> *Postgraduate Medicine*
>
> *Indian Medical Journal*
>
> Texas and other state journals
>
> *Journal of Medical Education*

One reason why the front-cover policy was so successful was that Saunders held the distinction of being the heaviest advertiser in medical journals and could command special attention and concessions—especially in the Depression era, when all business, including the journal business, was sluggish. In the *JAMA*, for instance, each week Saunders took half the front cover, the inside front cover and page one. In special issues, like the Education Issue, the Saunders ad ran to four, six, eight or, occasionally, twelve pages.

But the winds of change were blowing.

In the 1930s and 1940s, a number of successful journals closed their covers to advertising—including *Surgery, Gynecology & Obstetrics, Science* and the *Lancet* and the *British Medical Journal*. And in the immediate post-World War II period, the cascade of new pharmaceutical products, led by antibiotics, tranquilizers, and new cardiovascular agents, resulted in equivalent cascades of journal advertising. Saunders was no longer a vital source of advertising income, especially to the *JAMA*, and in 1952 confidential word reached Lawrence Saunders from friends of his among the Trustees of the American Medical Association that the *Journal* planned to close its front cover to advertising. In due course Dr. Austen Smith, Editor of the *JAMA*, requested and was granted an interview in Philadelphia, purpose supposedly unknown. He arrived on a Saturday morning of the early spring and met in

Lawrence Saunders' office with W. D. Watson, Jack Lutz and Bob Rowan, the young Advertising Director. Smith was clearly surprised that the purpose of his visit was already clearly understood by the Saunders people and that defenses and alternative approaches had already been devised.

After a couple of hours Saunders agreed to study a plan according to which its space on the front cover would be reduced by one half but that it would continue to occupy each week the inside front cover and page one. In another year or two, naturally, the front-cover space was again reduced by half and the final step was total elimination of front-cover advertising. *The New England Journal* soon followed suit, and over a period of a few years all major journals closed their covers. Still, in retrospect, it was remarkable that a single publisher could have such a dominant position in the world's journals for more than half a century.

THE COMMISSION SALESMEN

By 1900 the company already had a force of traveling salesmen who called on doctors in their offices and in hospitals and sold Saunders books to them on a straight commission basis: no salary, no expenses, just a percentage of the list price.

One of the early salesmen was Dr. J. A. Majors of Dallas, who had been a great football player at Centre College and picked up a medical degree during his considerable stay there. In 1909 he founded the J. A. Majors Company in Dallas and later opened offices in Houston, New Orleans and Atlanta. The business was capably carried on by his sons John and Bill and, until his untimely death, his son-in-law Jack McClendon. In the early part of this century Northern publishers were still reluctant to extend credit to doctors in the South because of financial problems associated with Reconstruction. Dr. Majors solved the dilemma incisively by guaranteeing all accounts serviced by his organization; he kept funds on deposit in Philadelphia to back up his guarantee. The relationship with Majors flourished for more than 50 years.

The Saunders commission sales force reached a high of 65 representatives, and these agents were largely responsible for the great success of the many *Clinics of North America* and of the larger, expensive and often multivolume sets that marked the Saunders line—like Hyman's *Integrated Practice of Medicine*; the Campbell-Harrison *Urology*; the Emmett-Witten-Myers-Utz *Clinical Urography*; the Bockus *Gastroenterology*; the Braunwald *Heart Disease*; and many others.

These large works were expensive and were difficult to sell in quantity through the mail. By this time, it should be noted, Paul Burton had been named Vice President in charge of sales and he had rescinded the old custom of not allowing promotion of a book through the mail until it had been published for two and a half years. His decision was based on two factors. First, in 1949 Saunders published the first issue of Conn's *Current Therapy*, and while the series was at first not prominently identified as an annual

The Men
Who Sell Saunders' Books

Here are portraits of some of the men who sell Saunders' Books.

They are the men behind the books—not in the bookstores or in the office, but on the road. They are our personal representatives, calling on physicians all over the land.

Moreover, they are experts, with a life-long experience in selling medical books.

These men, and many others like them, are personally carrying Saunders' Books to every part of the English-speaking world.

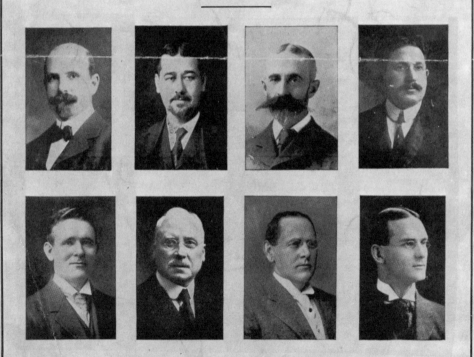

SEE ALSO THE TWO PAGES FOLLOWING

A Saunders advertisement in the JAMA, c. 1902. Dr. J. A. Majors is at lower left.

160

volume, its success was immediate and a new edition has been published every year since. Clearly, one cannot wait two and a half years to do mail promotion on an annual volume. The second mind-changing event was an experiment designed at that time by the mail order department. Careful records were kept of salesmen's sales of Meschan's *Normal Radiographic Anatomy* over a period of three months, and then an aggressive mailing was made to all internists and general practitioners in the United States. Salesmen's sales of the book immediately increased sharply and continued at the higher level for four months. End of no-direct-mail program, and mail order sales increased steadily. Good salesmen soon realized that, far from hurting them, direct-mail activity helped them: for every 100 physicians who received a direct mailing, only one or two returned the order card but perhaps 40 or 50 more looked at the brochure and might be more inclined to order from a salesmen on his next call. Eventually Saunders' retail sales just about evenly divided between salesmen and mail order.

Sales at Medical Meetings. From its earliest days the company made it a policy to have a manned exhibit at just about every medical meeting in the United States, right on down to the level of county medical society meetings and state chapters of national specialty societies.

There was a beneficial side effect from this blanketing of small meetings: the astonished gratitude of authors. A distinguished physician-author would agree to present a paper at a small county medical society meeting in his state, generally out of a feeling of loyalty. As he strolled through the ten or twelve commercial exhibits, inevitably there would be the familiar Saunders booth, with his book prominently displayed. The writer would often know the salesman on hand who would speak glowingly of the reception the book was having. Authors would almost always report these experiences to other would-be authors, and so grew the legend "Saunders really pushes its books."

REGIONAL BOOK WHOLESALERS AND JOBBERS

J. A. Majors distributed Saunders medical books to medical-school bookstores in its territory and, beginning in the 1920s, college textbooks also. But the principal wholesaler of medical, college and nursing textbooks in the United States was the J. W. Stacey Company of San Francisco. Stacey had no commission salesmen calling directly on doctors but it did have its own textbook marketing representatives calling on medical and nursing schools (teachers *and* bookstores). So Saunders had no textbook marketing representation in the thirteen western states. This role was played by Stacey and in return it was given a compensating discount. Other important distributors were T. H. McKenna, which had four commission salesmen in New York City and also exclusive wholesale distribution rights to bookstores in New York—up until the early 1950s; Brown and Connolly in Boston with two New England salesmen and exclusive bookstore rights, until 1965; Chicago Medical Book Company, probably the oldest and certainly one of the largest until the postwar era; Matthews of St. Lewis; and later Login Brothers, starting out in Chicago but branching out to various locations; and Rittenhouse Distributors, an offshoot of the Rittenhouse Bookstore on Rittenhouse Square in Philadelphia.

THE TEXTBOOK MARKETING REPRESENTATIVES

Known in earlier, simpler times as "travelers" these persons called on professors in schools—medical, dental, veterinary, nursing, allied health— and colleges and attempted to convince teachers to adopt, or at least recommend, Saunders texts for their classes. They also kept their eyes open for likely manuscripts (for example, Jim Ross originally discovered Arthur Guyton at Mississippi, and Jim Hughes found Stan Robbins at Harvard). Their role became more important in the mid 1920s when Saunders went into college textbook publishing in earnest, after observing that many of its basic medical school texts were being used in undergraduate courses in better colleges. Some examples were Howell's *Physiology*, Arey's *Embryology* and Maximow and Bloom's *Histology*.

The textbook marketing representative could definitely influence adoptions in nursing schools and colleges. Some marketing managers were skeptical of their selling effectiveness in medical schools, where outright adoptions were less frequent and where students paid more attention to the advice of upperclassmen as to what books they needed "to pass the course" than to the recommendations or commands of professors as to what they *must* read.

Since the 1970s the respective roles of the textbook marketing people and the commission salesmen have become increasingly fuzzy and less well defined. Also, textbook promotion by telephone has become more important, especially in smaller and less accessible schools.

DIRECT SELLING TO DOMESTIC BOOKSTORES

From the time of the founding of the company there were many sales directly to bookstores from Philadelphia. These became somewhat fewer with the founding, growth and greater influence and importance of the major wholesalers. Clearly these were regional distributors that could maintain large inventories and provide prompter service and delivery to local customers than could the Philadelphia office. But as transportation facilities improved and as the Saunders Company grew to the point where it could maintain a West Coast Distribution Center, it was felt that special arrangements with wholesalers were no longer required.

And so, in 1970, arrangements with wholesalers were terminated, except for nursing books. At that time, most nursing schools had a fixed curriculum and a correspondingly fixed list of required textbooks—almost always from a variety of publishers. The jobber would assemble as many of these textbook "packages" as a school required, deliver them in bulk and send the school a single invoice for all textbooks being used—regardless of publisher. This represented a very worthwhile service for the schools and many of them still avail themselves of it today.

SALES TO BOOKSTORES OUTSIDE THE UNITED STATES

As has been mentioned, from the time of opening of the London Company in 1900 sales of Saunders books to bookstores in the United Kingdom and on the Continent were handled through London. (There were no direct sales from publishers to physicians in those areas; by tradition, doctors bought their books from bookstores and the only Saunders effort to breach that tradition, by sending an English-accented Canadian to England to call on doctors in their offices and in hospitals, was unsuccessful and caused considerable resentment.) London also handled sales to India and to some parts of Africa. Actually, the African countries had the option of ordering from either Philadelphia or London. A later, bizarre development was that after the Cuban missile crisis the United States imposed an embargo on trade with Cuba, and this meant that books destined for customers 90 miles away were shipped first to London and then to Cuba.

Canada. Early in the twentieth century the company made an arrangement with McAinsh and Company, Ltd., of Toronto for exclusive distribution rights to Saunders books in all provinces of Canada. McAinsh ultimately hired its own commission salesmen and operated very much as did the wholesalers in the United States, except that McAinsh had also a textbook marketing force calling on schools.

In 1967, in line with the general restructuring of wholesale distribution, Saunders formed its own Canadian company, headed first by James Cornwall and then by Walter Bailey. Saunders Ltd. did some publishing of its own and handled some other publishers' lists (e.g., John Wright of Bristol) before being absorbed into Holt-Saunders, Ltd., a CBS International Publishing division, in 1978. McAinsh continued in business through these periods of change.

The International Department. This was organized just after World War II under the direction of Regina (Jean) Hassall, the first female department head at Saunders. She was responsible for all sales outside the United States and immediately directed the creation of an international catalogue designed with air mail rates in mind: it listed fewer books, with less descriptive copy on each, and was printed on lighter paper than the Saunders domestic catalog. It also bore a patriotic red, white and blue cover. Jack Gramling, who had been a textbook marketing representative in the Southeast, was brought into the office to act as assistant manager and he immediately undertook to carry the Saunders flag to the four corners of the earth. He was the first Saunders employee to visit India on company business.

Growth of the overseas market was rapid as American medicine became recognized as the world leader. Soon there were major distributors like Westdene and P. B. Mayer in South Africa; Ramsay in Australia; Peryer in

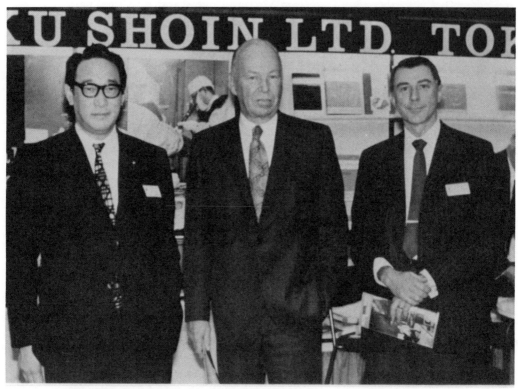

Igaku Shoin and Saunders at the Frankfurt Book Fair in 1971. Standing left to right: Hajime Kanehara, Harry R. Most, and Jack Gramling.

New Zealand; Lawyer's Cooperative in the Philippines; and Domingo Delgado in Puerto Rico.

Igaku Shoin in Tokyo assumed a special role in addition to distributing Saunders publications in Japan—they translated a great many Saunders books into Japanese and also created a new concept in international medical book publishing. The product became known as the Asian Edition and was actually an offset-printed, reduced-size version of the original Saunders book, printed on lightweight paper, priced at about half the cost of the original and available in many countries of the world. Some notable Asian Editions were the *Dorland Dictionary*, the *Cecil Medicine* and the Guyton *Physiology*. Under the leadership of its founder's son, Hajime Kanehara, Igaku Shoin became the most influential medical publisher of Asia, publishing translations and important indigenous titles in both Japanese and English.

PIRACY. In the Far East, especially, piracy, or unauthorized production and sale of important medical books, became a major problem. There was no return to the original publisher or to the author. Some of the pirating was done in countries that did not subscribe to the International Copyright Union. Other pirating was just plain illegal, but in either case it was a very difficult practice to eradicate. In 1968 Bill Feullian was appointed the permanent WBS representative in the Far East and he worked to control piracy.

For many years the state publishing houses of Russia translated and published whatever English language books struck their fancy. Sometimes they notified the original author and told him that royalties were awaiting him in Moscow if he chose to come and pick them up—and, presumably, spend them there. In recent years the Soviet Union has subscribed fully to the Geneva Convention.

SPANISH TRANSLATIONS. Saunders had old, pleasant and productive ties with Salvat of Barcelona (and some other lesser houses) for translation and sale, in Spain and Latin America, of its books. A loose alliance of publishers in South America handled indigenous distribution and translation until Eulogio Ripol and his wife Marjorie founded Editorial Interamericana in 1947, which grew quickly and soon was more important to Saunders than was Salvat. After Ripol's tragic death in a plane crash in 1962 the company was taken over by his nephew Jorge De la Vaga, who ran it very successfully until the company was acquired by CBS Inc.

One may say of Saunders marketing that it has been both shrewd and aggressive and perhaps reflected Johnson's opinion that "promise, large promise, is the the soul of an advertisement." But Saunders sales principals have also always been conscious of the fact that promise, large promise, can be held forth only in the instance of a worthy product. This gave to successful selling an edge of concern and understanding.

20

Beyond Philadelphia

At the very outset of establishing his own publishing house Walter Burns Saunders was intensely interested in marketing his books outside the United States and in the importation of books from abroad, perceiving that German reference monographs based on morphology and elegantly illustrated would be attractive in translation to the American market. This interest was shared by his son Lawrence and by Harry Most, Lawrence's successor in presidency of the company.

In 1900 Walter Saunders went to London and opened an office there, primarily for distribution of books in the United Kingdom and in continental Europe. However, all did not progress as smoothly as had been hoped, and Saunders returned to London to consult with solicitor A. E. Leonard and chartered accountant Herbert J. Page, both of whom remained steadfast friends of and advisers to W. B. Saunders Ltd. for more than half a century. The upshot of these discussions was that Ryland Greene came over from the Philadelphia home office to manage the London Company. In less than two years he made it a thrifty branch of the parent tree. He not only knew the specific function Saunders books were meant to serve but he also instituted large-scale advertising in *Lancet* and the *British Medical Journal;* and this attracted British authorities to become Saunders authors, among them Berkeley Moynihan, whose *Abdominal Operations* found immediate international acclaim. In 1903 Greene returned to his editorial duties in Philadelphia, leaving the London Company in charge of W. A. Pierce.

All proceeded nicely until the outbreak of World War I, when restrictions on imports, lack of shipping, German submarine activities and a dearth of able manpower made management of the business extremely difficult. At one point Pierce, John F. Brown (Pierce's eventual successor) and one packer, William Gorman, were the complete staff of the London house.

In 1932 John Brown succeeded Pierce as Managing Director and made it his aim to expand business in Europe. He was able to report on his first visit to America in the spring of 1939 amazing success in continental distribution of Saunders books. But by September England was at war again, and once more import and export restrictions, fivefold increases in the cost of marine insurance and lack of able help made for tough going. Bombings struck close to home several times, one attack completely destroying Bill Gorman's home and another knocking out all the windows and extensively damaging the storage area of the office at 7 Grape Street. By 1944 things had begun to return to normal, and 1945 saw the end of the war and record sales for the London company. But these years had been hard on Manager Brown, who often had had to stay late at night in the darkened office to pack books that otherwise could not have been shipped. Ill health now forced his retirement.

In 1945 William Carter succeeded Brown as Managing Director, but the coming years were not to be easy ones. Especially the acute shortage of dollars in England cut seriously into existing import quotas. Nevertheless, Carter, who had served as an officer in the British army in the terrible Normandy fighting, was not daunted. He made it his business to capitalize upon the partial exemption from quotas extended to scientific books, and he made it his practice to know well every book dealer of any significance on the continent of Europe. He always attended the Frankfurt Book Fair and there visited cordially with book agents who respected his knowledge, his honesty and his good judgment. They may even have respected his inflexibility in the matter of discounts.

When Lawrence Saunders visited the office in 1949, Carter could report not only thriving business but a renewed interest by British authors in either Saunders publication or distribution of their books; and, through his past connection with H. K. Lewis & Co., he was able to arrange a meeting between S. Cochrane Shanks and the visiting Saunders, who promptly signed an agreement for exclusive distribution in America of the great Shanks and Kerley *X-Ray Diagnosis,* which continues some editions later as a preeminent and successful reference source in radiology.

Of those who played a major role in the influence of Saunders books beyond the boundaries of the United States none played a more vital part than Lawrence Saunders. His interest in the London company was cordial and well-informed; he instituted with Harry Most the separate Saunders distribution agency in Canada; and he maintained the friendliest of relationships with the world's leading medical and scientific publishers, notably the Salvat Company of Barcelona, Interamericana of Mexico City, Igaku Shoin of Tokyo and Masson of Paris. Each of these houses from time to time sent executive trainees to the offices in Philadelphia to learn the Saunders way of doing things. They also experienced the warm hospitality of the Saunders family and its instinctive knack for making the foreigner feel at home abroad.

With the help of his knowledgeable secretary, Kathryn Pfister, Lawrence Saunders alone managed the whole difficult program of translations of Saunders Company books, conducting all negotiations and handling the exacting details of joint production ventures. It is not too much to say that, though a shrewd businessman, he was, like Walsh McDermott, interested primarily in the dissemination of sound and helpful medical information throughout the world and he was interested too in the pleasure Saunders authors took in translations of their books and in finding their original editions in unexpected places. He enjoyed quoting a letter from Bill Boyd, who wrote to him about an extended trip to Europe in 1955 (The Book, of course, is the *Surgical Pathology*):

> I thought you might be interested to know that three weeks ago, my wife and I were walking along a street in Florence—that enchanting city. We passed a bookstore, in the window of which there were lovely copies of books on Michelangelo, Dante and other famous citizens of this incredible place.
>
> My wife, who is more psychic than I am, suggested that they might have a copy of Boyd. I said "Absurd!" However we went in. The book man could not speak a word of English, but my wife produced her driver's license, whereupon the fellow's face lit up and he at once produced a copy of The Book!

At this very time Saunders books were enjoying unprecedented use throughout the world and hundreds of Saunders titles were available in translation, some of them achieving remarkable sales records, notably the Bockus *Gastroenterology* in Italian, Spanish and Portuguese editions and the *Cecil Textbook of Medicine* in many languages. But it was more the idea of translation than return from translation that appealed to the son of the founder of the company, and he not infrequently counseled friendly foreign publishers against overly ambitious or rash translation projects.

Prosperity begets privilege, and a privilege that Saunders Company officers greatly enjoyed was a kind of rotating visit to the London office and the Frankfurt Book Fair. Frankfurt itself is neither a festive nor a beautiful city, having a certain stolid German air combined with a typical capacity to enjoy excessively crowds, beer and noisy singing. Nevertheless, the Fair itself has a companionable and mildly extravagant flavor of its own. Here Russians speak with Chinese and Cubans with Americans—all in the interest of books and of course in the interest of turning a shrewd penny. Perhaps both interests tend to dispel cultivated animosities.

The annual visit to the London office was a thoroughly enjoyable, somewhat formal affair. Things were humming along so nicely that at the meeting of the Board of Directors the home-office editor could never think of anything to say except "Well done, chaps." By this time complacency permitted annual visits by the editor to Europe and alternate visits by the president or executive vice president. On one such visit the editor and Harry Most met with an old friend of Harry's, the cheerful Willie Macmillan, then of the Longman Group Ltd. Out of this meeting came an agreement for Saunders distribution of the thirty-fifth Edition of *Gray's Anatomy*, edited by Roger Warwick, Ph.D., M.D., and Peter L. Williams, D.Sc., B.Chir., both Professors of Anatomy at Guy's Hospital Medical School, University of London. Its 1,500 large pages of densely packed detail and thousands of minutely drawn pictures of human structure scarcely make it a primer of anatomy or a lazy student's delight. But it is by all odds the most highly respected and widely used textbook of medical science ever published. (However, see the review of its First Edition quoted in part earlier.) Even the unauthorized, unprotected-by-copyright American reissue of its Seventh Edition enjoys a huge sale in the discount book houses that stock only best sellers.

How did it come about that this rich plum still hung unplucked on the tree of opportunity? The first Gray was published in 1858 and in 1859 Lea & Febiger acquired its American distribution rights. But Lea & Febiger also gradually developed a distinctive American edition of Gray that, of itself, became a markedly successful textbook. Among its American editors were J. Chalmers DaCosta and Charles Mayo Goss, the latter supervising the Americanization of Henry Gray over many editions. The American parallel version ceased to refer to itself as a reprint as long ago as 1896, though continuing to preserve the name of Gray on its title page. What this in practice meant was that Lea & Febiger (quite properly, too) neglected in its promotional efforts the British forbear and concentrated its attention on the American offspring. For several editions previous to the thirty-fifth it had sold no more than five hundred copies of each issue of the original Gray.

So in 1973, for the first time since its beginning in 1858, a direct descendant of the British Gray was made widely available in the United States side by side with the American scion. The time had come to see whether the Thirty-Fifth Edition of *Gray's Anatomy* could sell more than five hundred copies in America. It did, selling in fact 65,000 copies, along with an added pleasant sale of its separately reprinted Neurology section. For the first time the London office said to the Philadelphians, "Well done, chaps."

A somewhat similar circumstance had attended the editor's first visit to the Frankfurt Book Fair, where his polite, even flattering, conversation with the Russian delegation was taped and appeared in full in *Izvestia*. Fortunately, Senator Joseph McCarthy either did not see it or regarded editors as prey too trifling for pursuit.

At that time Urban & Schwarzenberg published Eduard Pernkopf's *Topographischen und Angewandten Anatomie des Menschen* in seven thick volumes illuminated by full-color figures anatomically precise and pictorially elegant but accompanied by a somewhat discursive text taking off from the Creation and gradually inching forward. This was in the United States a greatly admired but little-used work; and the Saunders editor had the notion that maybe the Creation should be left to King James's bishops and the Pernkopf drawings reproduced without their cumbersome text.

He suggested this to young Michael Urban and found a ready response, with agreement that, if it all came about, it would be published in two volumes to be called an *Atlas of Topographical and Applied Human Anatomy*. Urban said that if Saunders would supply translation of the illustration captions, he would print both German and English editions and would allow worldwide distribution of the latter by Saunders. He also soon came up with a quotation for folded printed sheets in lots of a thousand. The quoted figure seemed to the editor astronomically high; but, carried away by the beauty of the drawings and of the plan itself, he then and there agreed to take four thousand sets of sheets.

On the crowded economy flight back home he began to wonder whether he might have been more foolhardy than sagacious; and thoughts of the Anson *Atlas of Anatomy*, also strong on anatomic variations but weak in sales, added to uncertainty. Nevertheless, he presented the idea to the Tuesday Editorial

170

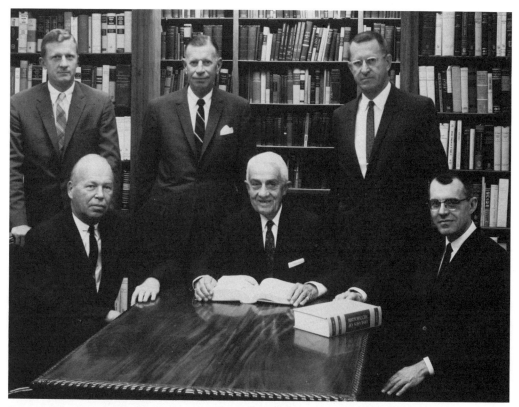

Senior officers of the Saunders Company, 1964: standing, left to right, Sherman Perkins, Paul Burton, Ted vanden Beemt; seated, Harry Most, Lawrence Saunders, John Dusseau. Each looked at publishing and its problems in individual ways, but all shared a common purpose.

Conference with a show of vigor and with a display of some of the exquisite Pernkopf drawings.

Comptroller vanden Beemt led off with the observation that the price seemed almost as exquisite as the drawings. Sales Manager Burton allowed that the *Atlas* seemed to be far too complex and expensive to compete with Grant. Advertising Manager Brauckman mentioned that it was difficult to sell costly books by mail. Vice President Rowan recalled that emphasis on variations was supposed to attract surgical interest but this had not proved to be so with the Anson atlas. Subscription Sales Manager Perkins added that the salesmen loved expensive books—expensive clinical books, not expensive or any other kind of books in the basic sciences. A theme of universal sorrow had been sounded, and a subdued silence fell upon the room. Finally, Lawrence Saunders asked if the editor had actually committed the company to purchase of four thousand sets of sheets. Upon an affirmative response, he cleared his throat apologetically. "Well," he said, "if we only sell two thousand we won't lose much and publication will be recognized as a service to anatomy in its finest exemplification. Let us go uneasily ahead with it."

Harry Monsen, of the University of Illinois College of Medicine, did a careful and prompt translation, but the project somehow dragged on for quite a spell—a spell mostly of trepidation. The volumes were published in 1963 in time for the annual meeting of the American College of Surgeons, where their sale was a pleasant augur. In the end fifty thousand sets of the English edition were sold—a welcome variation on a theme.

Similar ventures arranged with Günther Hauff of Georg Thieme Verlag of Stuttgart, especially the magnificent Frieboes-Schönfeld *Color Atlas of Dermatology*, also worked out very well. They seemed to reinforce Walter Burns Saunders' early belief in translation of superbly illustrated German monogaphs dealing essentially in morphology. This is not to say that every Saunders translation or import succeeded—of course not—but it is to say that the Saunders editor worked in a generally relaxed atmosphere in which recriminations were rare and in which informed hunches were respected without the benefit of elaborate calculations whose impressive computation conceals what is at the heart of publishing—guesswork.

This atmosphere changed with acquisition by the Columbia Broadcasting System. The house of Saunders had been not only an autonomous but a self-contained and self-sufficient unit. It was not to remain so. Its centers of distribution abroad were small, but they were manned by people who had an awareness of their function and of the use and worth of Saunders books. CBS Inc. had at its command an international network of large distribution agencies dealing in the many products of a communications conglomerate that included diverse publishing enterprises. When the Saunders foreign outlets were incorporated within these broader groups, the feeling in Philadelphia was that a certain pride in and knowledge of Saunders books were lost. When one deals in large figures, the sale of a couple hundred medical monographs in English to European specialists or academicians—a thing in which Pierce or Brown or Carter would have taken great pride—no longer seems worth expenditure of time, money or effort.

The program of importing and translating books has undergone its own changes in recent times. Varying in large part with the fluctuating international value of the dollar, the import program still contributes substantially to sales, both in anatomic texts and atlases and in those clinical reference works, magnificently illustrated in color, that originate from the renowned German and Spanish houses.

Also the interest of foreign publishers in translation of Saunders' books has continued to be lively. As manager of the international division, John Scott pursued this interest vigorously. Even today, some years after his retirement, handsome and imposing volumes in a variety of languages are received from abroad. Though their words may not be familiar, the books themselves seem to have a familiar character. They somehow resemble their originals and make the Saunders library a symbol of worldwide interest in American medicine and its books.

PART III

PROGRESS AND PICTURES

Where is the wisdom we have lost in knowledge;
Where is the knowledge we have lost in information?

T. S. Eliot

In the chronology to follow, the descriptions of events and publications important to the Saunders Company are accompanied by brief listings of significant advances in the progress of medicine. In compiling this material emphasis has been placed on the contributions of American medicine, and the Garrison *History of Medicine* (Fourth Edition, Saunders, 1929) and the Bordley and Harvey *Two Centuries of American Medicine, 1776–1976* (Saunders, 1976) have been liberally used. However, the author's knowledge of either the Saunders Company or the great world of medicine after 1976 is not very solid; therefore this chronology will terminate with that year, but its substance is resumed in Al Meier's chapter, A Decade of Change. Unless otherwise specified, the year of publication is that of the first edition of a book or the first issue of a journal. Subsequent editions of books of fundamental importance appear only when there is a change in authorship. Even in this summary, it is intended that emphasis be placed not on what happened but on the people who made things happen.

Walter Burns Saunders founds the publishing company that bears his name and still follows the principles upon which he built a flourishing and respected publishing house. Its first home was modest—scarcely a thousand square feet of floor space at 33 South 10th Street, Philadelphia; but it was soon to outgrow its humble beginnings (see Chapter 4). **1888**

Publication of Hobart Amory Hare's *Quiz Compend in Physiology*, a question-and-answer primer. It was the initial and successful title in a line of similar compends, uniformly priced $1.00, called the "Blue Series"—forerunner to the Haldeman-Julius little blue books. By 1901 Hare's *Compend* had been replaced by Budgett's *Essentials of Physiology*, and the page opposite its title proudly announces success.

SINCE the issue of the first volume of the
Saunders Question=Compends,

OVER **200,000** COPIES

of these unrivalled publications have been sold. This enormous sale is indisputable evidence of the value of these self–helps to students and physicians.

Small triumph.

Roux and Yersin isolate toxin of diphtheria. Chantemesse and Widal introduce vaccines against typhoid fever. Osler describes hereditary form of angioedema. American Association of Anatomists founded. Marine Biological Laboratory at Woods Hole established.

1890   A new, more comprehensive series begun, the "Saunders Manual Series." DaCosta's *Surgery* and Gleason's *Nose, Throat and Ear* were among the early distinguished books of the series.

Behring and Kitasato develop antitoxin treatment of diphtheria. Koch announces discovery of tuberculin and observes that tuberculous animals resist reinoculation. Maffucci isolates avian tubercle bacillus. Schleich introduces infiltration anesthesia. Babcock develops method for estimating fats in milk. Bowditch demonstrates nonfatigability of nerves. State Institute for Experimental Medicine founded in St. Petersburg.

1891   The cramped confines of the Saunders office prove insufficient to accommodate growing pains, and the company moves to larger quarters on Walnut Street, whose garret had housed the famous physician Chevalier Jackson while he was a student of Jefferson Medical College—the source of many fine, early Saunders books.

Waldeyer formulates the neuron theory. Quincke introduces lumbar puncture. Von Bergmann standardizes aseptic procedures in surgery. Welch describes the bacillus of gas gangrene. Hedin invents the hematocrit. Copeman introduces glycerinated lymph for smallpox vaccination. Association of American Medical Colleges founded.

1892

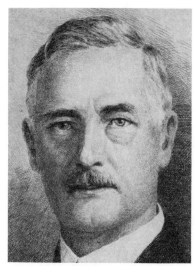

G. E. DeSchweinitz.

An American Textbook of Surgery is published. A collaborative work by W. W. Keen of Jefferson and J. William White of the University of Pennsylvania, it was the first of the influential "American Textbook Series." Its Second Edition (1895) would incorporate detailed description for use of the Murphy button in intestinal anastomosis (see Chapter 5). The year saw too publication of the first definitive American treatise on ophthalmology—the DeSchweinitz *Disease of the Eyes*. This writer's grandmother journeyed every five years to Philadelphia to have her eyes refracted by her distant kinsman, the great DeSchweinitz. The glasses she wore she bought at Woolworth's, picking out from a large pile those comfortable and comforting. So much for the fame of relatives.

Halsted successfully ligates first portion of the subclavian artery. Smith and Kilbourne demonstrate tick transmission of Texas fever. Kossel and Neumann discover pentose in vegetable substances. Sternberg first describes viral neutralizing antibodies. Ivanovski identifies mosaic tobacco virus. Galton introduces identification by fingerprints. Hartley resects gasserian ganglion for relief of trigeminal neuralgia. Buckner demonstrates effect of sunlight on self-purification of streams. Van Jaksch establishes value of leukocytosis in diagnosis. Wistar Institute of Anatomy and Biology incorporated in Philadelphia. American Psychological Association founded in New York.

1893

Publication of the two-volume *An American Textbook of the Theory and Practice of Medicine*, edited by William Pepper of the University of Pennsylvania, an internationally celebrated figure who devoted his great capacities to improving medical education at the medical school he ably served, having become its provost in 1881.

Haldane invents apparatus for estimating respiratory exchange. Gilbert discovers paracolon and parathyroid bacilli. Fowler performs pulmonary decortication. Anderson describes first mechanical water filter. Halsted removes infected kidney. Freud defines anxiety neuroses and develops the concepts of psychoanalysis. Ewing describes what is now known as complement. First Army School of Public Health opened. Society of Anesthetists founded in London.

1894

Publication of DaCosta's collaborative *Modern Surgery*. An immediate success, it would go through many editions and in its Tenth Edition (1931) become essentially a single-authored work, DaCosta writing, "The making of a revision is always an irritating, a difficult, and in a certain sense a hopeless thing. It is particularly hard to get rid of old impressions. In the present edition we have taken the course of revising the difficult sections ourselves instead of having them looked to by friends and associates. The only section that stands untouched is that of Dr. Chevalier Jackson, the eminent bronchoscopist."

Kirstein devises direct laryngoscopy. Kitasato and Yersin discover plague bacillus. Banti describes splenic anemia. The Wellcome Physiologic Research Laboratories are established in London.

A TEXT-BOOK

OF THE

THEORY AND PRACTICE

OF

MEDICINE.

BY

AMERICAN TEACHERS.

EDITED BY

WILLIAM PEPPER, M.D., LL.D.,

Provost and Professor of the Theory and Practice of Medicine and of Clinical Medicine in the University of Pennsylvania.

IN TWO VOLUMES—ILLUSTRATED.

VOL. I.

PHILADELPHIA:

W. B. SAUNDERS,

913 WALNUT STREET.

1893.

The equal of Keen and White *Surgery* in esteem and sale.

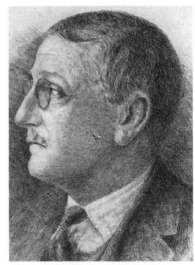

John Chalmers DaCosta.

Publication of the *Year Book of Medicine and Surgery,* an annual digest and appraisal of current literature edited by George M. Gould for ten years and then somewhat abruptly dropped by Saunders; but the idea was to be successfully revived and amplified by Year Book Medical Publishers of Chicago; and Gould crossed the street to Blakiston and compiled a medical dictionary.

1895

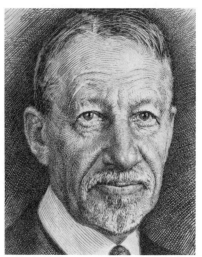

William H. Howell.

1896

Publication of *An American Textbook of Physiology*, edited by William H. Howell, the first of a long line of important texts and monographs to come from the Johns Hopkins University School of Medicine (see Chapter 12). It was also the first collaborative text in physiology—an idea Howell defended in his preface: "Perhaps the most important advantage which may be expected to follow the use of the collaboration method is that the student gains thereby the point of view of a number of teachers. The different standpoints assumed, and the differences in emphasis laid upon the various lines of procedure, chemical, physical and anatomical, should give the student a better insight into the methods of science as it exists today." A plausible notion and the foundation upon which many towering structures have been built—and yet also one Howell would abandon, for in preparation of a planned Second Edition he found it easier to write the book himself than to coordinate the work of writers of differing and sometimes conflicting points of view. He had found a team of a hundred strong-willed, often intransigent horses difficult to manage. He began afresh and admonished himself that "the author must assume the responsibility of sifting evidence and emphasizing those conclusions that seem to be most justified by experiment and observation."

Gruber discovers bacterial agglutination. Casper employs ureteral cystoscopy in diagnosis of renal disease. Welch founds the *Journal of Experimental Medicine*.

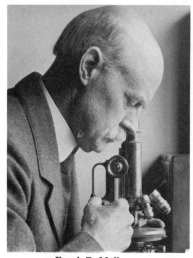

Frank B. Mallory.

1897

Publication of *Pathological Technique* by Frank B. Mallory and James H. Wright, the former Pathologist to Boston City Hospital, the latter Director of Laboratories of the Massachusetts General Hospital, and their book a forward-looking presentation in unusual detail of the bacteriologic, histologic and chemical aspects of the methodology of pathology.

Nuttall demonstrates fly transmission of plague bacilli. Horton Smith shows the health hazard of chronic typhoid carriers. MacCallum demonstrates sexual conjugation of parasites of avian and human malaria. The cancer research facility at Roswell Park is established by the University of Buffalo.

178

Walter Burns Saunders goes to Europe to observe at first hand the exceptional printing results being achieved by color lithography in Germany and returns with an agreement for translation and publication of the eighteen "Lehmann Hand Atlases," beautifully depicting the morphology of disease (see Chapter 4). All of the volumes were published in German and translated and published in English within less than five years, although, as one of the authors said, "imperfections in the skiagraphs presented extremely difficult problems of reproduction." Publication of the *American Pocket Medical Dictionary*—later titled *Dorland's Pocket Medical Dictionary* and, like its subsequent fat scion, credited to W. A. Newman Dorland but actually written by Ryland W. Greene (see Chapter 4).

Ramón y Cajal publishes his treatise on texture of the nervous system, elaborating his histologic discoveries in all nerve tissue and extending knowledge of the terminal arborization of the brain and cord. The Curies discover radium. Fischer isolates the purine nucleus of uric acid transformation. Dreser introduces heroin. Simmonds demonstrates transmission of bubonic plague by fleas.

Extensive advertising had already become a hallmark of the Saunders Company and it now signed the following agreement with the *Journal of the American Medical Association.*

This contract, with some upgrading of its financial considerations, was to continue in effect for sixty years (see year *1960*).

Publication of *Nervous and Mental Diseases* by Archibald Church and Frederick Peterson—an influential but rather curious work consisting of two independent sections—600 pages by Church on nervous diseases and 300 by Peterson on mental diseases. In the words of its preface, "This is not the joint work of two authors, but each author has contributed to the making of a single volume what might have made a separate monograph." The year also saw publication of the first true *International Textbook of Surgery*, in two volumes, edited by John Collins Warren of Harvard, who gave the first public demonstration of ether anesthesia, and by A. Pearce Gould, Surgeon to the Middlesex Hospital and Council Member of the Royal College of Surgeons.

Killian introduces direct bronchoscopy. Porter demonstrates that ventricular fibrillation is not irreversible. Vincent describes spirillobacillary angina. Bordet and Tsistovich demonstrate agglutinins, hemolysis and precipitins in blood serum treated with alien corpuscles. Jacques Loeb produces chemical activation of sea-urchin egg. Nuttall summarizes the role of insects as vectors of communicable diseases. Kossell states theory of protamine nucleus in protein transformations. Abel isolates epinephrine. Society of American Bacteriologists founded. London School of Hygiene and Tropical Medicine founded.

1900   W. B. Saunders, Ltd., organized and opened for business in London, and shortly thereafter, Ryland Greene dispatched to England to straighten out the tangled affairs of the British office (see Chapter 20).

Publication of the *American Illustrated Medical Dictionary*—twenty-seven editions later still the world's leading medical lexicon (see Chapter 4). Publication also of the *Treatment of Fractures* by Charles L. Scudder, Orthopedic Surgeon to the Massachusetts General Hospital, whose work was to endure as a wise and practical guide through eleven editions. He had the notion that an author of any book should set out in detail why he is entitled to write it; so his preface to the First Edition provides a year's calendar of cases with their complications and fees. The latter for routine procedures were slight; but he did manage some extremely difficult and prolonged forty-dollar cases.

Landsteiner sets forth his ABO blood-group system. Theobald Smith describes hypersensitivity reaction to foreign protein. Solis-Cohen introduces epinephrine in the treatment of asthma. American Association of Pathologists and Bacteriologists and the American Roentgen Ray Society founded.

1901   Publication of the first volume of translations of the monumental Nothnagel *Encyclopedia of Practical Medicine*, eventually running to fourteen very thick tomes. General editorship and responsibility for appropriate American additions were entrusted to that otherwise unoccupied physician William Osler, and translations were carried out under the supervision of Alfred Stengel, Professor of Medicine of the University of Pennsylvania and Saunders author. These were completed with remarkable speed and accuracy; but the names of those who performed this herculean task are not given, competency apparently conferring its own recognition. The Nothnagel volumes contained the first writing by Sigmund Freud to appear in English. The year also saw publication of Torald Sollmann's *Textbook of Pharmacology*, the first comprehensive scientific examination of the action of drugs made possible, as the author says, "by recourse to animal experimentation; by methods analogous to those on which the modern science of physiology is built; by replacing accidental observation by well-directed research." Curiously, though, the First Edition lacked that extensive painstaking documentation that was to distinguish and make famous other editions. These later bibliographies were set from cards in the author's crabbed handwriting and were called by one critical reader "the most valuable, most judiciously selected, and most inaccurate list of references ever compiled by one man."

Frazier introduces section of sensory root of trigeminal nerve for neuralgia. Nuttall founds the *Journal of Hygiene*. Rockefeller Institute for Medical Research established.

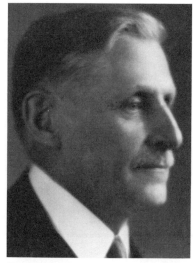

Torald Sollmann—pharmacologists' pharmacologist.

Publication of *Diseases of the Pancreas* by A. W. Mayo Robson and B. G. A. Moynihan, both then surgeons at the Leeds General Hospital. Their book was the first work on pancreatic disease attempting to integrate surgical procedure and prognosis with developing knowledge of function of the pancreas, especially in relation to the significance of the islands of Langerhans.

1902

A young Alabama surgeon, Luther Hill, called upon to operate on a boy who had been stabbed five times in the chest, finds that a stab wound had penetrated one of the heart chambers. Hill successfully sutured the wound and the boy recovered. The procedure was performed by the light from two kerosene lamps on an old kitchen table in a slum shack. Hill had come under the influence of the great English Quaker surgeon, Joseph Lister, and named his first son after him—the future Senator Lister Hill, father of the Hill-Burton Hospital Construction Act.

Hugh Young performs first perineal prostatectomy. (His later *Urology* with Saunders described in detail this and other innovative, then-daring procedures.) Stenbeck treats cancer with roentgen rays. Leishman and Donovan discover the pathogenic protozoon of kala-azar.

Publication of the original one-volume Bickham *Operative Surgery*, the precursor of his later monumental seven-volume work of the same title (see Chapter 6) and of the Peterson and Haines *Legal Medicine and Toxicology*, in two volumes—an important pioneering work not revised until 1923, when Ralph W. Webster joined its authorship, bringing to its inherent value his extensive experience in medical jurisprudence.

1903

Bruce demonstrates transmission of sleeping sickness by the tsetse fly. Von Pirquet outlines the concepts of hypersensitivity. Carrel introduces new methods of vascular anastomosis and organ transplantation. Jensen propagates cancer through several generations of mice. Emil Fischer devises method of synthesizing polypeptides. American Society of Clinical Surgeons organized. Henry Phipps Institute for Study of Tuberculosis opened. American Genetic Association founded.

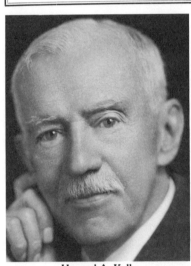

Howard A. Kelly.

A fine book whose authority was made greater in revision.

1904

Publication of the classic *Vermiform Appendix and Its Diseases* by Howard A. Kelly of the Johns Hopkins University—the first of many fine clinical monographs from Hopkins that Saunders would publish (see Chapter 12). Its Preface concludes, "Lastly I would call attention to the index of names. It has been one of the pleasantest features of the work to realize, as I culled these from the text, the truth of that inspired declaration of the great Apostle to the Gentiles: 'Others have labored, ye have entered into their labors.'" The year also saw publication of a fine import: H. D. Rolleston's *Diseases of the Liver, Gallbladder and Bile Ducts*. It culminated Rolleston's twelve-year study, at St. George's Hospital, of liver disease and was the first truly authoritative monograph on a subject of ever-increasing importance and complexity in modern medicine.

Pschorr and Vongerichten demonstrate phenanthrene nucleus of morphine and codeine. Stolz determines composition of adrenalin. Atwater devises a respiration colorimeter. Construction of the Panama Canal begins, with Gorgas heading its disease-control division. National Tuberculosis Association founded.

1905   Upon the death of Walter Burns Saunders, W. D. Watson assumes responsibility for management of the business, although Mrs. W. B. Saunders becomes its nominal President. Ryland Greene is summoned back to Philadelphia to become formally what in fact he had already been—Senior Editor—a role in which he attracted to the Saunders Company the authors of textbooks and monographs that are still, many editions later, the foundation stones of its success and of the respect in which it is held—one of them, published that year, Berkeley Moynihan's *Abdominal Operations* (see Chapter 4).

Schaudinn discovers *Treponema pallidum*, the causative agent of syphilis. Vassale employs parathyroid extract in tetany. König describes osteochondritis. Winter resuscitates the heart by injection of epinephrine. Einhorn discovers Novocaine. Dutton and Koch demonstrate tick transmission of African relapsing fever. Wilson uses first frozen sections in surgical diagnosis. German Röntgen Ray Society founded in Berlin. American Child Health Association organized. American Sociological Society founded in Chicago.

The publisher is formally incorporated as W. B. Saunders Company and begins its entry into the nursing field by the publication of textbooks, typical of them the finely illustrated Millard and King (later King and Showers) *Anatomy and Physiology*. Only much later would it begin publishing clinical books for the practicing nurse.

1906

The year saw publication of the famous *Atlas and Textbook of Human Anatomy*, in two volumes, by Johannes Sobotta of the University of Würzburg. The American translation was considerably modified, especially in respect to terminology, by J. P. McMurrich of the University of Michigan, and the volumes were independently copyrighted by Saunders. The German Sobotta continued for many editions as a classic depiction of human anatomy; but, for obscure reasons, no second American edition was ever published, although the idea was from time to time discussed and explored. In that year too was published a *Textbook of General Bacteriology* by Edwin O. Jordan of the University of Chicago. It became at once a standard reference text and was to remain so through many subsequent editions by William Burrows and later by Bob A. Freeman.

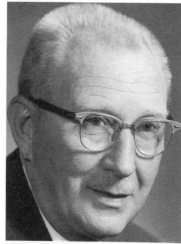
William Burrows. He brought a classic text into the age of electron microscopy.

Wasserman introduces serum diagnosis of syphilis. MacDougal demonstrates heredity of experimentally acquired characteristics in plants. Howell demonstrates presence of amino acids in the blood. Flexner and Joblin transplant a rat epithelioma. Ehrlich develops arsenical therapy for syphilis. American Society of Biological Chemists founded. Federal Food and Drug Act passed.

1907

Publication of the pioneering *Chemical Pathology* by H. Gideon Wells of the University of Chicago (see Chapter 10) and of an enduring

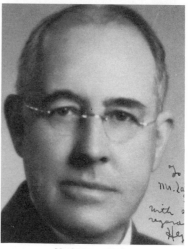
H. Gideon Wells.

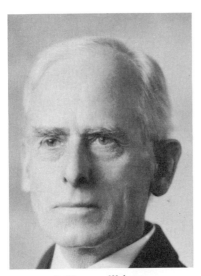

J. Clarence Webster.

standard in gynecology, *Diseases of Women* by J. Clarence Webster, also of the University of Chicago.

Theobald Smith suggests use of toxin-antitoxin in diphtheria. Ricketts demonstrates tick transmission of Rocky Mountain spotted fever. Flexner develops an antiserum for cerebrospinal meningitis. Von Pirquet introduces the tuberculin skin test.

1908

Publication of Thomas Cullen's *Adenomyoma of the Uterus*, another classic monograph from the Hopkins School of Medicine, to be followed in 1909 by the Kelly-Cullen *Myomata of the Uterus*. The year 1908 also saw publication of one of the longest-lasting of all medical texts, the Todd *Clinical Diagnosis* (see Chapter 7).

Finlay produces experimental rickets by deficient diet. Bernstein investigates temperature coefficients of muscular energy. Buerger describes thromboangiitis obliterans. Cushing operates on the pituitary gland. Landsteiner transmits poliomyelitis to monkeys. Garrod interprets pattern of inheritance of alkaptonuria in mendelian terms (see Chapter 9).

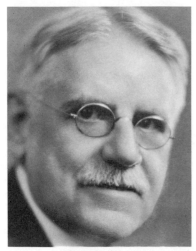

Henry V. Arny.

1909

Publication of the Arny (later Arny and Fischelis) *Principles of Pharmacy*—a text that would act as definitive guide to two generations of pharmacists. It was an altogether original work intended neither to displace nor to compete with the official *Pharmacopeia of the United States*, begun by Lyman Spalding in 1817, or the *National Formulary*, published by the American Pharmaceutical Association.

Russell begins vaccination of U.S. Army personnel against typhoid fever. MacCallum and Voegtlin clarify the relationship of parathyroid-gland activity to calcium metabolism. Marine and Lenhart standardize iodine treatment of endemic goiter. American Society for Clinical Investigation founded.

1910 Publication of *Dislocations and Joint-Fractures* by Frederic J. Cotton—a highly individual but wonderfully graphic account of the intelligent management of dislocations. In a disarming preface the author says, "It has occurred to me in reading the completed text that references to the literature are not very full. This is because my voluminous notes on the 'literature' were used for verification of fact and perspective, not for incorporation in the text. Perhaps this is not the right way to work, but a reaction from the benumbing German scholasticism in which I was trained has led me to adhere to this plan." He later adds, "A review such as this may be modified by the *clinical records* of preceding generations, *but is in no way concerned with their opinions.*" In fact, Cotton had secure opinions of his own, noting elsewhere that in his long medical experience he had observed that his surgical friends had a lot fewer surgical scars than his nonsurgical friends.

Flexner publishes his revolutionary *Medical Education in the United States and Canada*. Vedder shows the amebicidal effects of emetine. Auer and Lewis demonstrate bronchial spasm in acute anaphylaxis. Rowntree and Geraghty introduce the phenolsulfonphthalein test for renal function. The Hospital of the Rockefeller Institute is opened.

1911

Publication of the famous two-volume *Differential Diagnosis* by Richard C. Cabot of Harvard. The plan of the book was to study medicine from the point of view of presenting symptoms analyzed and illustrated by actual cases—the forerunner of many a similar book. Its author says simply that diagnosis is often faulty either because "physical signs are not recognized or because we do not think correctly."

Morgan and Wilson associate the pattern of inheritance of hemophilia and color blindness with the X chromosome. Rous publishes his studies of viral cancer in chickens. Van Slyke develops method for estimating amino nitrogen. McCoy and Chapin isolate bacillus of tularemia. Gullstrand receives the Nobel Prize for his optical studies.

1912

The present main Saunders building on West Washington Square is completed. The architect had previously been employed by the American Telephone and Telegraph Company, and the building has the familiar look of a telephone office. Its site was selected because it was the publishing center of Philadelphia and because the square had been dedicated to the public in perpetuity by William Penn. The two upper floors of the building were for many years occupied by the pressroom, and the whole building swayed gently back and forth in tune to burgeoning demands on overscheduled presses. Occasionally visitors were made motion-sick by the rhythmic rocking; but old Saunders hands would miss it when the pressroom moved to Callowhill Street.

Publication of the first issue of *The Surgical Clinics of John B. Murphy* (see Chapter 5) and of the first volume of the *Collected Papers of the Mayo Clinic* (see Chapter 11). The Murphy Clinics were the forebear of the *Surgical Clinics of North America* and the *Medical Clinics of North America*, and these two bimonthly book-journals were the only periodicals published by Saunders until 1954.

Nicolle, Anderson and Goldberger produce experimental typhus in the monkey. Pavlov investigates conditioned reflexes. Von Behring employs toxin-antitoxin immunization

against diphtheria. Cannon begins work on the effect of adrenal secretions on the emotions. Osborne, Mendel and McCollum discover vitamin A and study the effects of deficient diet. Schloss introduces scratch test for human hypersensitivity. Nobel Prize awarded to Alexis Carrel for his pioneering work on vascular suturing and organ transplantation. Act of 1912 creates the United States Public Health Service. National Organization for Public Health Nursing is founded in the United States.

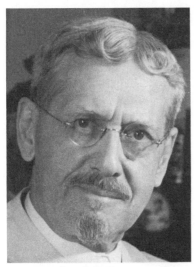

Joseph B. DeLee.

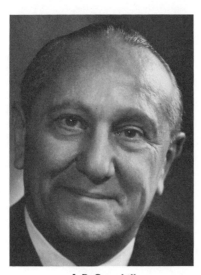

J. P. Greenhill.

1913

Publication of the *Principles and Practice of Obstetrics* by Joseph B. DeLee of Northwestern University Medical School. It became a necessity for medical students, practicing physicians and obstetricians in training or in practice. DeLee, an imposing figure, would conceal his name tag at meetings and ask some novice salesman if Saunders published anything in obstetrics except the book by that scoundrel DeLee. Almost always the salesman would reply that, scoundrel though he might be, Dr. DeLee had written the world's best book on obstetrics. It was to be continued successfully in later editions by DeLee's pupil J. P. Greenhill and by his pupil Emanuel A. Friedman, Professor of Obstetrics at Harvard Medical School. It is now a volume slimmer in size but more heavily weighted toward the biology of reproduction. In its various editions the book has been widely translated, and Jack Greenhill keenly relished seeing his work in Spanish, Portuguese, French, Italian and Serbo-Croatian. The year also saw publication of *An Introduction to the History of Medicine* by Fielding H. Garrison of the Surgeon General's Office. The most scholarly of all medical histories published up to that time, it won immediate recognition and praise; but through its life of four editions its sale was slight. It was not until its reprinting in 1960, after a long out-of-stock period, that it came into its own as an indispensable reference. Continuing reprints have sold substantially more copies than the total sale of the four original editions. "The history of medicine is, in fact, the history of humanity itself, with its ups and downs, its brave aspirations after truth and finality, and its pathetic failures." The book too has had its ups and downs, and its proper revision has been difficult to achieve. More than one (including John Fulton, knowledgeable bibliographer and sage medical biographer) has tried without success; but there is yet hope that someday it will be expertly done. In 1913, too, Salvat Editores of Barcelona published its first translation of a Saunders book, Keen's multi-volume *Surgery: Principles and Practice.*

Schick introduces susceptibility test for diphtheria. Dakin and Dudley investigate intermediary metabolism of carbohydrates and proteins. Holst and Fröhlich postulate vitamin C. Rockefeller Foundation chartered. American College of Surgeons incorporated. Association of Experimental Pathology founded. Institute for Cancer Research established in New York.

Publication of the *Principles of Pathologic Histology* by Frank B. Mallory, Pathologist to the Boston City Hospital—a profusely illustrated and sophisticated study of pathology from the point of view of cellular elements and changes that give rise to pathologic lesions. To many students of medicine the morphology of pathologic states is difficult to understand because they cannot visualize the active process of cell modification. This was the first of technical books in pathology to elaborate cell changes such as the exudative and proliferative elements of inflammation.

1914

Christiansen, Douglas and Haldane investigate carbon-dioxide carriage by the blood. Slye studies hereditary susceptibility to and immunity from cancer. Margaret and Warren Lewis study mitochondria. Dandy and Blackfan demonstrate pathogenesis of hydrocephalus. Association of Immunologists founded.

1915

Publication of the forward-seeing *Introduction to Neurology* by C. Judson Herrick and of the *Textbook of Embryology* by Charles W. Prentiss, both authors representing the dynamic attention to bioscience distinguishing the leading medical schools of Chicago. The *Embryology*, carried on in subsequent editions by Leslie B. Arey, was to become the standard reference text in developmental anatomy and, for many thousands of medical students, a first glimpse into the miraculous field of reproduction, fetal growth and birth. The year also saw publication of the Braasch *Urography* from the Mayo Clinic—a work later amplified and brilliantly revised by Braasch's pupil, John Emmett. In 1915 pyelography had scarcely come into existence, and few could have foreseen that this would become the single most influential book in roentgenology written by a nonradiologist. Braasch, even as a young man, was peppery and opinionated, so that many years later John Emmett must have faced with some trepidation the prospect of his performing surgery on the now indomitable old man. Fortunately, all turned out well, and Braasch could applaud his student not only as writer but as surgeon too.

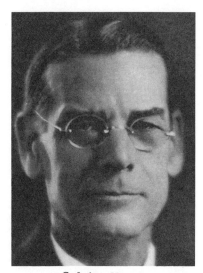

C. Judson Herrick.

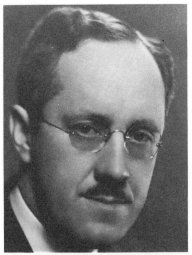

Leslie B. Arey.

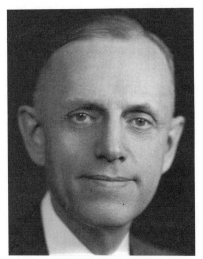

William F. Braasch.

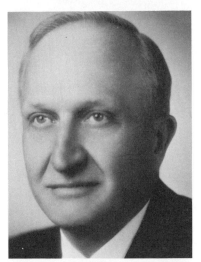

John L. Emmett.

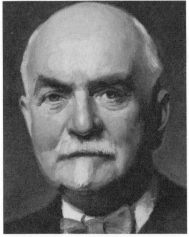

Thomas S. Cullen.

Kendall discovers and investigates thyroxin. Futaki and Ishiwara discover the parasite of rat-bite fever. Simmonds describes pituitary dwarfism. Hunt describes progressive cerebellar dyssynergy. Goldberger demonstrates that pellagra results from nutritional deficiency. Rous develops method for isolation of individual cells from tissue for study. The American College of Physicians is incorporated.

1916

Publication of two important Hopkins books. The first: Cullen's *Embryology, Anatomy and Diseases of the Umbilicus*, illustrated by Max Broedel. (See also Chapters 4 and 12.) The preface to the work—a monolithic monograph still of immense value—begins and ends in typical Cullen style: "During the summer of 1904 I saw a case of cancer of the umbilicus. Up to that time I had thought hernia was practically the only lesion to be found in this locality. No autopsy was obtained; but examination of the umbilical growth showed that it was an adenomatous carcinoma. I could not rid myself of the desire to find out just how an adenocarcinoma could exist in the umbilicus. . . I trust that this work may help the general practitioner, the pediatrician, and the surgeon to treat more satisfactorily lesions of this heretofore relatively unknown region—unknown, although up to the day of birth the main

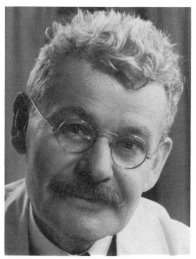

Max Broedel.

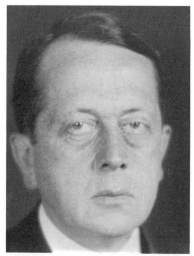

W. G. MacCallum.

highway between the mother and child." The second was MacCallum's *Textbook of Pathology*—an outstanding student and reference text that was to have a curious effect on the later fortunes of both Saunders and Lea & Febiger (see Chapter 4).

Heparin discovered by McLean and Howell. Bull introduces antitoxin for gas-gangrene. Kasmelson treats pupura hemorrhagica by splenectomy. The National Research Council is organized in Washington.

1917

Publication of Cushing's *Tumors of the Nervus Acousticus*—a monograph written while the author was a youthful neurosurgeon at Hopkins—and of the great Norris and Landis *Diseases of the Chest*—a valuable text in internal medicine also written with youthful enthusiasm and a zest for speaking out and containing an extraordinarily prescient chapter on "Electrocardiography in Heart Disease" by Edward Krumbhaar, Professor of Research Medicine of the University of Pennsylvania.

Dandy introduces ventriculography. Avery and Dochez describe specific soluble substance of pneumococcus. Stockard and Papanicolaou demonstrate vaginal epithelial changes during estrous cycle. Gray and LeMaître establish principle of wound excision. Windaus extracts vitamin D from

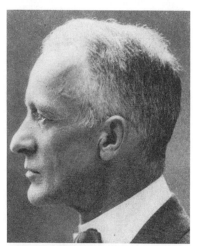

Harvey Cushing.

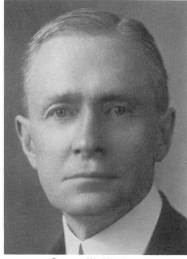

George W. Norris.

189

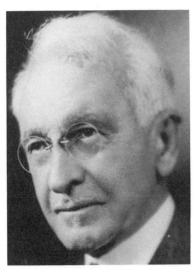

James P. Warbasse.

cod-liver oil and formulates it. *Annals of Medical History* begun in New York.

1918

Publication of *Surgical Treatment*, in three volumes, by James P. Warbasse. Unlike other surgical encyclopedias of the times, its emphasis was not on the techniques of procedure but on complete management of the surgical patient. Some of its brief paragraphs discussing surgical judgment are not unlike modern "decision trees" without the extraneous foliage.

Ellerman establishes transmission of leukemia by virus in chickens. Benedict devises basal metabolism test. Fahraeus introduces erythrocyte sedimentation test. Sachs-Georgi introduces flocculation test in syphilis. Harkness Commonwealth Fund established in New York.

1919   Publication of the great Ewing *Neoplastic Diseases* and of the Griffith *Diseases of Children*, in two volumes—the former a classic in the literature of pathology, the latter to become in later manifestations the world's leading textbook of pediatrics (see Chapter 13).

Krumbhaar describes leukopenia and dissolution of lymphoid tissue by mustard gas. Loeb induces mammary cancer by ovariectomy in mice. Blake and Trask demonstrate viral origin of measles. Huldschinsky demonstrates curative effect of sunlight on rickets. Dale and Laidlaw investigate histamine shock. International Bureau of Labor established at Geneva.

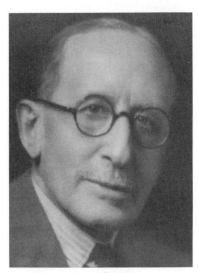

James Ewing.

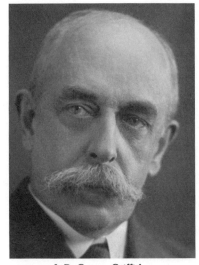

J. P. Crozer Griffith.

1920

Publication of the Ranson *Anatomy of the Nervous System*—to be revised in later editions by Sam L. Clark and to remain for many years the standard teaching reference in neuroanatomy but eventually to succumb to the modern notion that the fine details of anatomy are not necessary to the understanding of medicine. The copyright book also lists for 1920 Einhorn's *Duodenal Tube and Its Possibilities* with the cryptic notation: "Book destroyed, not published." Perhaps this should be the unkind fate of more books; but in 1922, the past apparently forgotten, Max Einhorn did publish with Saunders his *Lectures on Dietetics*.

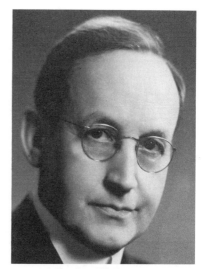

Stephen W. Ranson.

Cutler performs surgery on the mitral valve. Allen rediscovers use of salt-free diet in the treatment of edema. Saxl introduces mercurial diuretics in treatment of cardiac edema. National Child Health Council organized.

Publication of Crile's *The Thyroid Gland*—an important book because it brought together metabolic and chemical considerations that should govern management of thyroid disease. It stated unequivocally, "Endemic goiter is a geologic deficiency disease due to lack of iodin in the organism. By proper administration of iodin to the pregnant mother and to the child through the period of adolescence, endemic goiter may be prevented." The year also saw publication of Gaston Labat's famous *Regional Anesthesia*. At the time of its publication Labat was at the Mayo Clinic; but he was from the Faculty of

1922

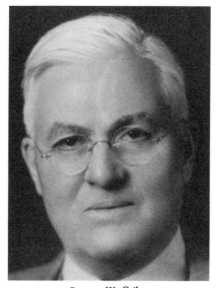

George W. Crile.

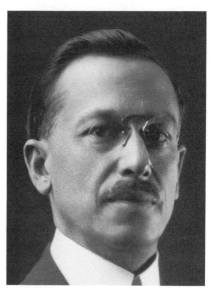

Gaston Labat.

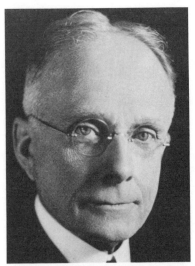

Chevalier Jackson.

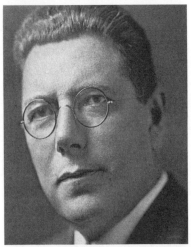

Raymond Pearl.

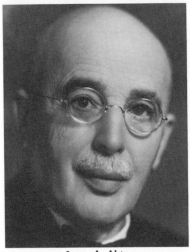

Isaac A. Abt.

Medicine of the University of Paris, and when he died it appeared that he had been living in an "Anesthesiologist's Paradise." The tangled skeins of his estate never did get straightened out, and it was only after the mists of time had shrouded them in obscurity that John Adriani was able to revise the Labat. Crile and Labat were colorful figures; but the great Chevalier Jackson was a peacock to their sparrow. His *Bronchoscopy and Esophagoscopy,* also published in 1922, was one of his many Saunders books setting out the careful techniques and varied uses of what were then new tools of medicine.

McCollum and Steenbock discover vitamin D. Whipple shows regenerative effect of liver on experimental anemia in the dog. Banting and Best report the results of their experiments with insulin in dogs and in diabetic patients. Association of Clinical Pathologists founded.

1923

Publication of Pearl's *Medical Biometry and Statistics.* Although called "An Introduction," the book was the first American text to provide rigorous analytical methods for the compilation of medical statistics. As Pearl said, "Whether the mathematician likes it or not, there are now and there will continue to be many biologists and medical men who are going to use biometric methods in their work whether they have any mathematical training or not." At the time he wrote his book, Pearl was Professor of Biometry and Vital Statistics at Hopkins; and perhaps the experience of playing in a musical club with H. L. Mencken and Max Broedel gave the theoretician pragmatic insight (see Chapter 12). The year also saw publication of the great Abt *Pediatrics* (see Chapter 10).

Dandy evolves a method for localizing brain tumors. George and Gladys Dick discover the hemolytic *Streptococcus* of scarlet fever and devise its susceptibility test. Graham and Cole introduce cholecystography by use of an opaque dye. Avery and Heidelberger show that the specific soluble substance of the pneumococcus is a polysaccharide. Murlin and Kimball discover glucagon. Plummer introduces iodine therapy before surgery for Graves' disease. The Nobel Prize is awarded to

Banting and McLeod for the discovery of insulin. The Society for Advancement of Applied Psychology is founded in Berlin. American Society of Parasitologists founded in Baltimore. History of Science Society founded in Boston. American Society of Plant Physiologists established in Chicago.

1924

College publishing was a natural outgrowth from the influential texts Saunders already published in the biological sciences; but now specific attention was focused on college publishing, and within the next five decades the list would grow to over three hundred titles. Among the early fine texts was the Frobisher *Bacteriology*, author and book to experience a half century more of fruitful life. However, although the Saunders imprint was continued on its college texts, the list and its care were eventually absorbed into the CBS large college publishing program.

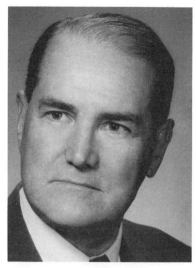

Martin Frobisher.

Publication of the Bickham *Operative Surgery* (see Chapters 6 and 12) and of the Draper *Human Constitution*—a forward-thinking effort to see disease as a derangement of the mechanics of the living organism. Sir Arthur Keith said in his introduction to the book that he shared with Draper a zeal for understanding the human body in its morphologic and functional interrelationships; and, he added, "It will probably fall out that the machinery of the hormones and endocrines will prove to be infinitely more complex than we now think."

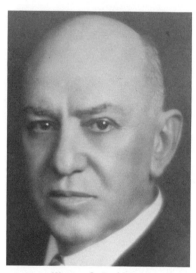

Warren S. Bickham.

Calmette vaccinates children against tuberculosis with B.C.G. (bacille Calmette-Guérin), a nonvirulent bovine culture. Steenbock and Black treat rickets by irradiating food with ultraviolet light. Chen and Schmidt introduce ephedrine. Libman and Sacks describe atypical verrucous endocarditis.

Publication of Boyd's *Surgical Pathology* (see Chapter 4) and of Lilienthal's *Thoracic Surgery*, in two volumes, a work of rich surgical acumen arising from close observation of experience amplified by a keen reading of the literature devoted to diseases of the chest. A single-handed creation, it contained two important contributor chapters—one on respiratory physiology by Evarts Graham and the other on pulmonary tuberculosis by J. Burns Amberson.

1925

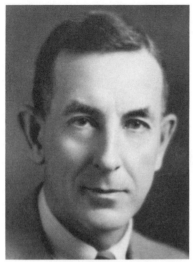

William Boyd.

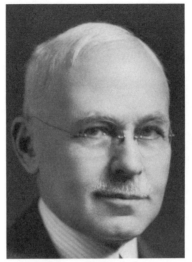

Howard Lilienthal.

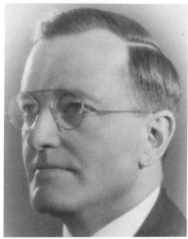

John H. Stokes.

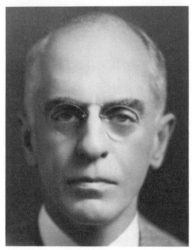

Russell L. Cecil.

Parker and Nye grow vaccinia virus in tissue culture. Rowntree and Adson report first sympathectomy for hypertension. Hess and his associates demonstrate antirachitic properties of cholesterol. Foerster investigates hyperventilation epilepsy.

1926

Publication of *Modern Clinical Syphilology* by John H. Stokes, Professor of Dermatology at the University of Pennsylvania. Its fine drawings and detailed tabular outlines of data were the hallmarks of a universally admired work. Stokes in subsequent editions would be joined in authorship by Herman Beerman and Norman R. Ingraham. The advent of antibiotics made the vast detail of the work no longer necessary; and Stokes would say in his preface to the Third Edition (1944), "We take comfort and courage in the way in which a book like this records the impending extinction of a centuries-old plague in the short space of two decades." But in a curious way the book would have its continuation in the Pillsbury-Shelley-Kligman *Dermatology* and in its successor, the Moschella-Hurley *Dermatology*.

Minot and Murphy report liver treatment for pernicious anemia. Abel isolates insulin in crystalline form. Cushing receives Pulitzer Prize for his *Life of William Osler*.

194

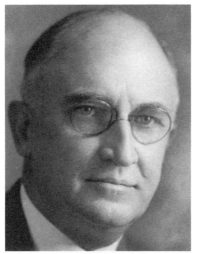

James S. McLester.

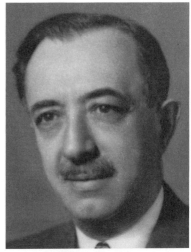

Israel S. Wechsler.

1927

Publication of the Cecil *Textbook of Medicine* (see Chapter 9), the McLester *Nutrition and Diet in Health and Disease,* and the Wechsler *Textbook of Clinical Neurology*—books each in their individual way the creative work of original minds and all destined to have long and influential lives.

Charles Mayo first successfully removes a pheochromocytoma. Wilder reports first pancreatic islet cell tumor producing hyperinsulinism. Noguchi shows causal relationship of *Bartonella bacilliformis* to verruga and Oroya fever. Tunnicliff introduces serum against measles. Bureau of Chemistry (United States Department of Agriculture) abolished.

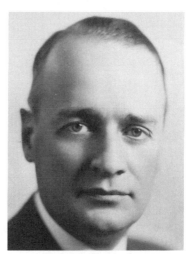

Frederick Christopher.

1929

Publication of the Christopher *Minor Surgery* (see Chapter 10). Seven years later Christopher would also publish with Saunders his equally durable *Textbook of Surgery.* Also in 1929 Sanford joins Todd in coauthorship of the *Clinical Diagnosis by Laboratory Methods* (see Chapter 7).

Smith demonstrates failure of growth and atrophy of endocrine glands following hypophysectomy. Fleming publishes his first paper on penicillin. Corner and Allen describe corpus luteum hormone. Berger constructs the electroencephalograph. Churchill performs first American pericardectomy

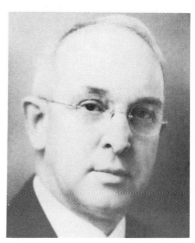

Arthur H. Sanford.

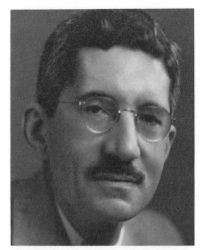

Harry Beckman.

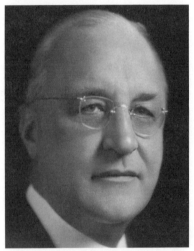

Evarts A. Graham.

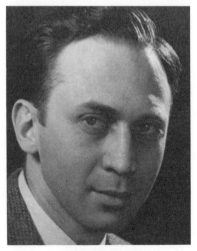

William Bloom.

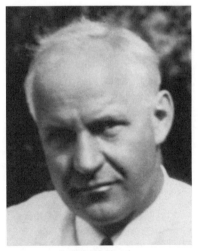

Arthur H. Curtis.

for constrictive pericarditis. Best and Murray report experimental use of heparin to prevent venous thrombosis.

1930

Publication of Beckman's *Treatment in General Practice*—probably the most widely used and beloved book for the general practitioner ever published. Beckman was a fine writer and a distinguished pharmacologist, and for many years he faithfully and carefully revised the *Treatment*; but as he got older, he found doing the book more burdensome than pleasurable, for what he had always really wanted to do was write a Textbook of Pharmacology. He tried twice in different formats. Each attempt produced a fine book of modest success, for Goodman and Gilman still stayed at the top, where it undoubtedly belonged (see Chapter 4). The year also saw publication of Evarts Graham's three-volume *Surgical Diagnosis*—a book eagerly anticipated and extensively sold; but it never did undergo revision, partly because surgical diagnosis was no longer seen as an independent entity separate from medical diagnosis. The Maximow and Bloom *A Textbook of Histology* was also published in 1930 (see Chapter 8), as was the Curtis *Textbook of Gynecology*—a text whose superb illustrations, meticulous attention to pathology and precise formal prose were to insure success for many editions. It would later be carefully revised by John W. Huffman, one of Curtis's many distinguished students. But eventually its full detail would make it unsuitable as a teaching text in a streamlined undergraduate medical curriculum.

Theiler develops immunization against yellow fever in animals. Wilson, MacLeod and Barker introduce the precordial lead. The electron microscope is developed. *American Standard Nomenclature* is completed.

1932

Publication of Feldman's *Neoplasms of Domesticated Animals*. By no means Saunders' first publication in veterinary science, it was an influential work of lasting value. Feldman was Director of the Division of Experimental Surgery and Pathology of the Mayo Foundation and his findings rested on an extraordinarily wide experience in animal pathology. The year also saw publication of the Trumper and Cantarow *Biochemistry in Internal Medicine*—a basic forward-thinking text carried on for many editions, the later issues the work of Cantarow alone. Still later he and Schepartz would do for Saunders a fundamental *Biochemistry*.

Urey describes heavy hydrogen. Lawrence develops the cyclotron. Cushing describes the disease

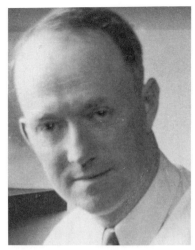

William F. Feldman.

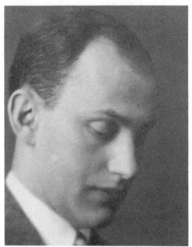

Max Trumper.

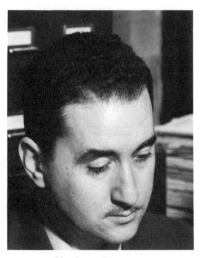

Abraham Cantarow.

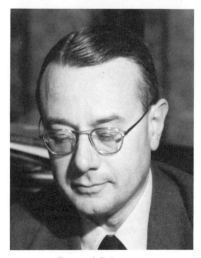

Bernard Schepartz.

that bears his name. Goldblatt produces experimental hypertension by renal artery stenosis. Domagk discovers Prontosil—the first sulfa drug. Later Domagk would be awarded the Nobel Prize for his epoch-making discovery—one Ehrlich had anticipated and one Jacobs and Heidelberger had narrowly missed in 1917 when they showed that sulfonamide-containing azo dyes exercise antibacterial activity—an observation that was somehow lost sight of in the turmoil of World War I.

1933

Publication of the four-volume Curtis *Gynecology and Obstetrics*—an exhaustive treatise not elsewhere mentioned in this account but one of great significance. Like the Abt *Pediatrics*, it established a kind of intellectual plateau in its specialty—a summation that made search of past findings and ideas no longer necessary.

Hamilton designs the manometer for measurement of intravascular pressure. Nobel Prize awarded to Morgan for his genetic studies.

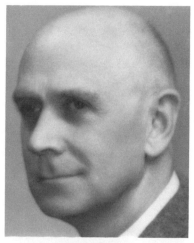

Alfred P. Noyes.

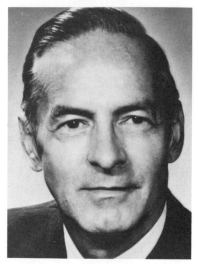

Lawrence C. Kolb.

1934

Publication of the Noyes *Modern Clinical Psychiatry*. Arthur Noyes was Superintendent of the Pennsylvania State Mental Hospital at Norristown; but his book, not one of institutional practice, was a balanced consideration of the theories and therapies of contemporary psychiatry. It became the leading textbook in its field and was carried on ably by Lawrence Kolb, Chairman of Psychiatry at the Columbia College of Physicians and Surgeons.

Henrik Dam discovers vitamin K after exhaustive studies into the mechanisms and causes of hemorrhagic tendency. Nobel Prize awarded to Whipple, Minot and Murphy for their discovery of use of liver in the treatment of pernicious anemia.

1936

Lawrence Saunders, son of the founder, is elected President of the W. B. Saunders Company. (See also Chapters 4, 12 and 15.) He had already demonstrated a keen sensitivity to the important issues of publishing and had played a major role in difficult negotiations with authors, especially those with Alexander Maximow; but in his earlier years with the company W. D. Watson and Ryland Greene continued to exercise a dominating influence on its affairs. It was only upon his election to its presidency that Lawrence Saunders was able to bring to bear his own strong influence on its policies and actions.

Publication of the Christopher *Textbook of Surgery* (see Chap. 10) and of Levine's *Clinical Heart Disease*, the latter one of the four or five finest texts in cardiology ever published but a highly personal work reflecting Levine's intense experience—a book that might someday be replaced but could never be revised by anyone else, no one having ever suggested revision of a major work of art. The year also saw publication of important titles in the Saunders dental list: Skinner's *Science of Dental Materials* and Thoma's *Oral Diagnosis.*

Bittner shows that mammary carcinoma of mice can be transmitted through the mother's milk to the offspring—the first demonstration of natural transmission of a tumor-inducing agent. Long and Bliss introduce sulfa drugs into the United States.

1937

Publication of Meredith Campbell's *Pediatric Urology* (he would later do for Saunders his splendid three-volume *Urology*) and of the Major *Physical Diagnosis* and the Tuft *Clinical Allergy*—all works of lasting clinical value.

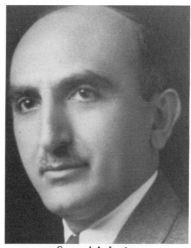

Samuel A. Levine.

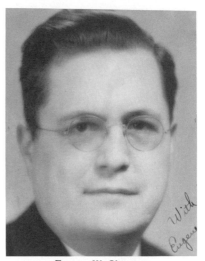

Eugene W. Skinner.

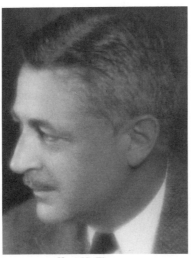

Kurt H. Thoma.

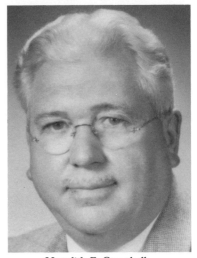

Meredith F. Campbell.

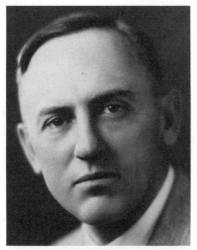

Ralph H. Major.

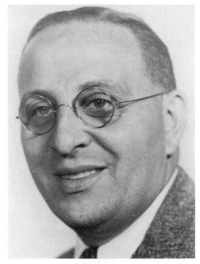

Louis Tuft.

Fantus establishes first blood bank. Chargaff and his associates begin their studies showing that there is a DNA molecule characteristic of each species of organism and that adenine and thymine are linked together in the DNA molecule—knowledge basic to the later deciphering of the structure of DNA.

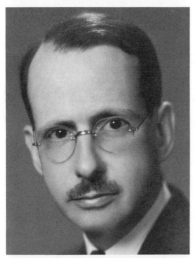

Sanford R. Gifford.

1938

Publication of Gifford's *Textbook of Ophthalmology,* to be revised in subsequent editions by Francis Heed Adler and later by Harold G. Scheie and Daniel M. Albert. The year also saw publication of a slim book of large influence—the Sturtevant and Beadle *Introduction to Genetics*—of the Cutler and Buschke *Cancer: Its Diagnosis and Treatment* and of the Barsky *Plastic Surgery.* In 1955 Barsky would agree to operate—in some instances with stunning success—on the "Hiroshima maidens," whose disfiguring injuries had been studiously neglected by the Japanese government and by Japanese surgeons, defensive perhaps about their own lack of expertise in reconstructive surgery. The complicated and difficult plan for treatment was organized by the humanitarian editor of *The Saturday Review,* Norman Cousins, who would also later become a Saunders author (*The Physician in Literature,* 1982—one of many fine books perceived as fascinating but not indispensable to the effective practice of medicine).

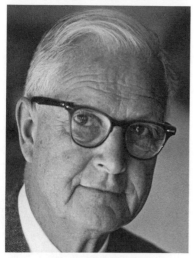

Francis Heed Adler.

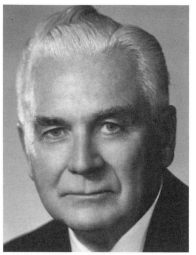

Harold G. Scheie.

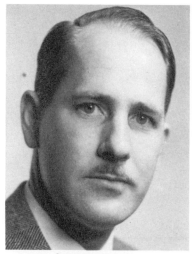

George W. Beadle.

In 1898 in Germany R. Tigerstedt and P. G. Bergman extracted from kidneys a substance they called renin that raised blood pressure in experimental animals. But their findings were never confirmed by the work of others until 1938, when Pickering and Prinzmetal rediscovered renin, leading eventually to the finding that it is an enzyme that causes release of a hypertensive substance in the plasma.

1940

Dwight Hotchkiss becomes Editor of the *Medical* and the *Surgical Clinics of North America*. Dwight had completely lost his hearing in military service during World War I but had become a skilled lip reader. Without a telephone, with no staff and with but a part-time secretary, he would for more than thirty years edit two of the most influential and successful of all medical periodicals. He could do this single-handedly partly because he kept his board of reviewers under his hat and partly because he knew no pause in his rounds of duty to correct knowledge clearly presented. In his spare moments he edited such important books as the Conn *Current Therapy* and never failed to give their authors the insight of his experience and wisdom.

Publication of Buckstein's *Clinical Roentgenology of the Alimentary Tract*—a richly illustrated encyclopedic work, but one that may have

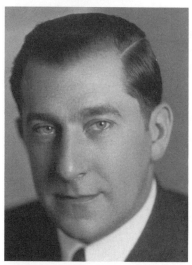

Max Cutler.

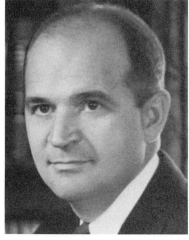

Waltman Walters.

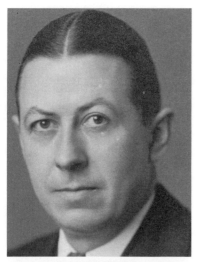

Albert M. Snell.

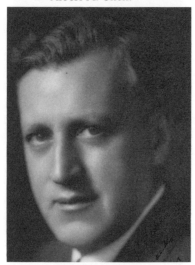

Russell M. Wilder.

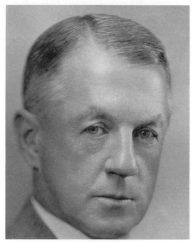

Frank H. Lahey.

missed out in its local sale, for Ryland Greene, pointing with authority to his bookshelves, said to the Philadelphia salesman, "Every radiologist in your territory should have this book." But the salesman thought he was pointing to Blumer's three-volume *Bedside Diagnosis*. One may still find a grizzled Philadelphia radiologist, perhaps missing a couple of fingers, who will tell you that forty years ago some crazy Saunders salesman insisted that he buy the still unopened volumes of *Bedside Diagnosis*. When Ryland Greene spoke, he expected his advices to be carried out. The year also saw publication of an important Mayo Clinic monograph, the Walters and Snell *Diseases of the Gallbladder and Bile Ducts* and of a much smaller but eventually more important monograph, Windle's *Physiology of the Fetus* that brought together many strands of thought into a single fabric; of Wilder's *Clinical Diabetes and Hyperinsulinism*; and of Emil Novak's *Gynecological and Obstetrical Pathology*.

Landsteiner and Wiener identify the Rhesus factor (agglutinogens) present on the membrane of red blood cells. Huggins describes effect of hormones in prostatic secretions. Gregg studies congenital malformations following German Measles. Hinshaw and Feldman show beneficial effect of Promin (synthesized in the Parke-Davis research laboratories) on experimental tuberculosis—the first antimicrobial substance proved unequivocally effective against experimental tuberculosis induced by the human-type tubercle bacillus. Link discovers dicumarol.

1941

Publication of the Graybiel and White *Electrocardiography in Practice*—for many years the standard against which electrocardiographic tracings were studied. Paul D. White's text on *Heart Disease* was a Macmillian publication; but the practical manual in electrocardiography escaped to Saunders. The year also saw publication of other fine Boston books: the Ladd and Gross *Abdominal Surgery of the Infant and Child* (see Chapter 11) and the first issue of the *Surgical Practice of the Lahey Clinic*. Frank Krusen's *Physical Medicine* was also published. Krusen headed up the

Mayo Clinic Section on Physical Medicine and his book became at once the bible of an emerging specialty.

Huggins describes estrogen therapy and orchiectomy for prostatic cancer. Hirst demonstrates influenza virus by agglutination of red blood cells. Coons perfects the identification of globulins by means of fluorescent labels. His technique—immunofluorescence—has become the means to elucidate interaction of antigen and antibody. First clinical trials of penicillin by Florey and his associates. Office of Scientific Research and Development organized.

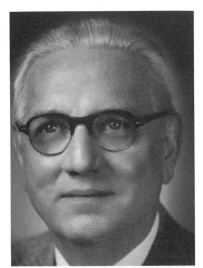

Frank H. Krusen.

The years of World War II— a time of strains and shortages; but medical education, practice, research and publishing were not unalterably affected by them. Saunders becomes official publisher for the National Research Council's War Manuals and supplies tens of thousands of books to the Medical Corps of the Armed Forces, to medical students in accelerated educational programs and to cadet nurses. Once again, business having outgrown its plant, additional space for warehousing and storage was acquired on Locust Street. One of the old houses purchased had been the home of Horace H. Furness during the years when he worked on his vast, scholarly and never completed *Variorum Shakespeare*. Especially during these years, despite world-wide material shortages, the volume of Saunders translations grew significantly.

1942 –1945

In 1943 Alexander M. Greene, son of Ryland Greene, becomes Vice President of the Saunders Company with sales and editorial responsibilities, the latter exercised under nominal direction from Editor Lloyd Potter. Greene had been deeply involved in the delicate negotiations creating a new and influential *Textbook of Pediatrics* under the editorship of Waldo E. Nelson (see Chapter 13). However, he never came to occupy at Saunders quite the spot he hoped to fill, and in 1948 he left to become President of Year Book Medical Publishers in Chicago, a post he filled with high distinction for twenty years, adding to his list a famous Saunders author, Harry Beckman, as compiler of the highly successful *Year Book of Drug Therapy*.

It was a busy publication time too. In 1942 Cutler's *The Hand*, Duncan's *Diseases of Metabolism* and Lundy's *Clinical Anesthesia* were among many important titles published. Also there appeared the first five of the *Military Manuals* authorized and sponsored by the Division of Medical Sciences of the National Research Council. All were well-conceived practical guides, but one that would have a long life of its own beyond its military purposes was

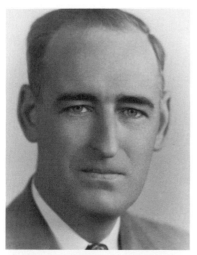

Garfield G. Duncan.

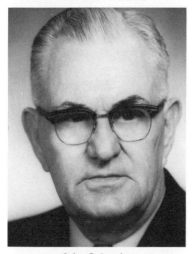

John S. Lundy.

the Pillsbury-Sulzberger-Livingood *Manual of Dermatology* (see Chapter 4). 1943 saw publication of the first volume of the Bockus *Gastroenterology*—a work of durable value whose contract of publication called for a single volume of six hundred pages. Its Fourth Edition was published in seven volumes in 1985 under the editorship of J. Edward Berk, Distinguished Professor of Medicine of the University of California at Irvine. It is dedicated affectionately to its original author and the mentor of so many of its writers: "creator and guiding genius of this work and the inspiration of this edition." A Foreword by Sir Frances Avery Jones evokes the memory of Harry Bockus as a truly international physician who helped put in place the foundations of modern gastroenterology. The year saw too publication of the Weiss and English *Psychosomatic Medicine*—the first thorough exploration of the interrelatedness of psyche and soma in the manifestations and natural history of disease. In 1944 appeared the Conant-Smith-Baker-Callaway *Manual of Clinical Mycology*—for many years the authoritative clinical guide to fungal infestations. In 1945 the Fourth Edition of the Mitchell-Nelson *Textbook of Pediatrics* (see Chapter 13) was published, and there appeared three important monographs that came out of medical military concerns in

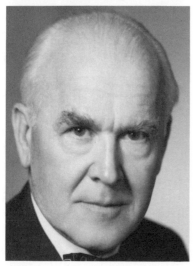

Henry L. Bockus.

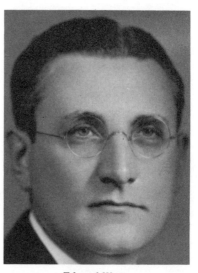

Edward Weiss.

which the Armed Forces Institute of Pathology and the National Research Council were involved. The Ash and Spitz *Pathology of Tropical Diseases,* the Haymaker and Woodhall *Peripheral Nerve Injuries* and the Mackie-Hunter-Worth *Manual of Tropical Medicine.* All were of great value, but of the three the *Manual of Tropical Medicine* has had the longest life. It has been carried on successively by George W. Hunter, William W. Frye, J. Clyde Swartzwelder and, in its current edition, by G. Thomas Strickland, Director of the International Center for Medical Research and Training (Lahore, Pakistan).

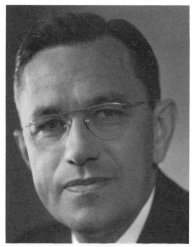

Waldo E. Nelson.

The war years saw the resources of science turned to military needs. The most remarkable of these achievements was the release and control of atomic energy in nuclear chain reaction. But startling advances were also made in the fundamental biosciences and in clinical research. Gilman and his coworkers describe the effect of nitrogen mustard on lymphomas. Earle demonstrates conversion of normal cells to cancer cells in tissue culture. Papanicolaou and Trout publish their *Methods of Exfoliative Cytology.* Waksman announces discovery of streptomycin. Adrenocorticotropic hormone (ACTH) is isolated from anterior pituitary gland. Avery, MacLeod and McCarty identify transforming factor in pneumococci as DNA (deoxyribonucleic acid)—work regarded by many as the single most significant bioscientific breakthrough of the twentieth century. Heilman and Kendall describe the beneficial effect of cortisone on experimental lymphosarcoma. Hinshaw and Feldman demonstrate effectiveness of streptomycin in experimental tuberculosis. Delbruck and Luria open up the new field of bacterial genetics. Synthesis of quinine achieved. Blalock and Taussig perform their first surgical procedure for the treatment of human cyanotic heart disease on a baby more than a year old who weighed only ten pounds, the infant not only surviving the operation but also thriving and gaining weight. Negarski performs first recorded resuscitation in a human after clinical death. Dam and Doisy receive the Nobel Prize (1943) for their work on vitamin K. Erlanger and Gasser receive the Nobel Prize (1944) for research on nerve fibers.

Foreign business expands rapidly after World War II, and Saunders organizes its first International Department under the direction of Regina Hassall, who vigorously pursues establishment of outlets for Saunders books all over the world (see Chapter 19). W. C. Shepard joins Saunders as its Art Director (see Chapter 6). But, more important, change is in the air. The tall, shiny brass cuspidors that had once stood beside the desks of most male Saunders employees are removed and now, possibly, may be purchased at Sotheby's for exorbitant prices. Women are no longer obliged to wear hats to and from work, and W. D. Watson has discontinued his hat-check surveillence. Dramatically, the hand-sewn book is abandoned after a cautious and judicious trial of machine-sewn books, which were thought unlikely to hang together for long. Swift advances come to office routines. A companywide intercommunication system is installed, calling for the full-time ineffectual services of a baffled and weary electrician named Charlie. The system's a push-button affair so that one may easily push the wrong button, allowing

1946

one's astonished boss to hear on his squawk box what an ignorant nincompoop he is. Even the accounting department feels the heady breeze of innovation and steel pens are discarded in favor of fountain pens or even newfangled ball points. Only one eyeshade persists. The interstory dumb waiter is demotorized in favor of more efficient hand operation. This may sound like a step backward, but it wasn't. Another forward step is taken—the red and green, two-wheeled pushcart, propelled by a fleet young man for swift local deliveries, is forsaken and its place taken by a jeep; but, hold, the evidence is not yet certain that deliveries were expedited thereby.

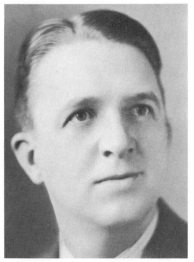

Edgar V. Allen.

Publication of one of the typically thorough Mayo Clinic monographs—the Allen-Barker-Hines *Peripheral Vascular Diseases*, a book that would long be an intellectual summation and synthesis of the new and vital in a developing field of internal medicine that would eventually move into surgery. The year also saw publication of the Daniels, Williams and Worthingham *Muscle Testing;* the revision of the Howell *Physiology* by John Fulton; the Masserman *Principles of Dynamic Psychiatry* (see Chapter 10); and the four-volume Hyman *Integrated Practice of Medicine*. The last was the single-handed work of a tempestuous internist from New York whose knowledge, friendship and capacities were all on a larger-than-life scale. It was published at an opportune time, and its success was immediate and far beyond the most sanguine expectations. Later Hyman would publish a fifth

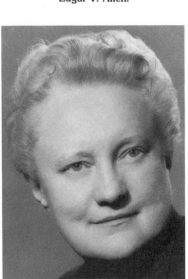

Catherine Worthingham.

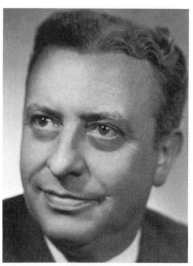

John F. Fulton.

Progress Volume with Saunders; but for reasons that are not entirely clear a revision of the whole book was never done, although updated material from it on diagnosis and on therapy would be published as independent volumes by the J. B. Lippincott Company.

Promin therapy proves effective against Hansen's disease. Penicillin is produced synthetically. The Nobel Prize is awarded to H. J. Muller for research on X-ray-produced mutations—work that extended the pioneering genetic studies of Thomas Hunt Morgan for which he had received the Nobel Prize in 1933. Passage of the Hill-Burton Act for construction of needed hospitals. Passage of the National Mental Health Act. Communicable Disease Center established in Atlanta.

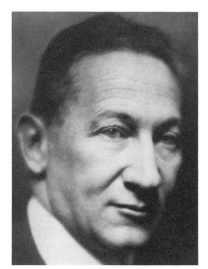

Harold T. Hyman.

Saunders buys the Partridge and Harris printing company, moving its somewhat aged presses to the plant at Sixteenth and Callowhill Streets. But the time was not far distant when thunderous letterpress equipment would be replaced by speedier, more compact offset presses. The transformation would be effectively and painlessly managed by Pressroom Superintendent John Hartman. J. F. Brown retires as Managing Director of the London office and is succeeded by William Carter (see Chapter 20).

1947

In 1947 Tyler Buchenau becomes Saunders College Editor, the most knowledgeable and perceptive of all editors in the field of college publishing. In the postwar years, when federal funds for education were beginning to seem unlimited and publishers indulged in indiscriminate programs and wild spending, Tyler was cautious and selective. He built a list of books, especially in biology, of outstanding excellence and distinguished authorship; but many of his authors were little interested in watered-down simplification of complex matters. Hence the Saunders College texts were widely respected but not quite so widely used.

Publication of the *History of the American Medical Association 1847 to 1947,* a volume of some twelve hundred pages put together somewhat haphazardly by JAMA Editor Morris Fishbein but containing archival material of great interest, especially that relating to Nathan Smith Davis, III, founder of the American Medical Association. Despite innumerable obstacles to the planned schedule, the book was miraculously published in time for the June AMA convention. It attracted a great

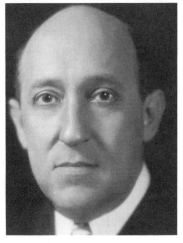

Morris Fishbein.

deal of attention, lavish festivities and favorable reviews; but association members did not beat a path to its door, and eventually some two thousand copies of the book were destroyed, although later evidence would suggest that this was done hastily. 1947 was also the first year in which the Saunders Company published more than fifty new books and revisions.

Parke-Davis announces discovery of Chloromycetin. Farber induces remissions of acute leukemia with folic-acid antagonists. Peter Bent Brigham Hospital begins work on the artificial kidney based on the earlier development of a prototype by Willem Kolff. Dalldorf uses suckling mice for virus inoculation—work that revolutionized research in the field of viral disease, including poliomyelitis and related human infections. Lederle announces discovery of Aureomycin. Bing catheterizes the coronary sinus. Nobel Prize awarded to Carl and Gerty Cori and to B. A. Houssay for their studies on metabolism of glycogen and sugar. Much of present knowledge of the relationship between the pituitary and carbohydrate metabolism springs from the work of Houssay and the Coris. Because the earlier investigations of Davidoff and Cushing were inconclusive, the crucial experiments of Houssay and his associate Biasotti provided altogether new insight into pituitary function.

1948

Publication of the Kinsey, Pomeroy and Martin *Sexual Behavior in the Human Male* (see Chapter 15). Although other medical books, e.g., the *Dorland Dictionary*, had had larger sales than the Kinsey report on the male, this was the first medical book ever to appear on best-seller lists.

Bailey performs first mitral commissurotomy. Vitamin B_{12} discovered—the liver substance that combats pernicious anemia and is, in its pure form, the most powerful medicinal agent ever identified. Soon Merck chemists announced that vitamin B_{12} could be obtained from a strain of *Streptomyces griseus*—the same species of mold that produces streptomycin—and early in 1949 Merck placed pure crystalline vitamin B_{12} on the market. Kendall and Hench describe the therapeutic properties of cortisone. Dalldorf and Sickles isolate Coxsackie virus.

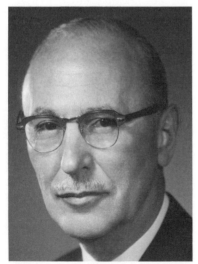

R. Philip Custer.

1949

Publication of the Allee-Emerson-Park-Park-Schmidt *Principles of Animal Ecology*. John Behnke, who had managed the Saunders College list before Tyler Buchenau, was a shrewd textbook man but also a partisan of the authoritative treatise; and *Principles of Animal Ecology* was one of the best. It put firmly in place the particular principles of a science Ernst Haeckel had defined eighty years before: "By ecology we mean the body of knowledge concerning the economy of nature—the investigation of the total relations of the animal both to its inorganic and to its organic environment." Saunders also published in 1949 a truly distinguished textbook in biology—the Romer *Vertebrate Body* (see Chapter 11). The year saw publication of two beautiful atlases from the Armed Forces Institute of Pathology that were to have a permanent influence in study of the morphology of disease, the Lyons and Woodhall *Atlas of Peripheral Nerve Injuries* and the Custer *Atlas of Blood and Bone Marrow.* The Friedberg *Diseases of the Heart* (see Chapter 16) and the first issue of the annual Conn *Current Therapy* (see Chapter 14) also were published.

Pauling and his coworkers describe the first molecular disease—sickle-cell anemia. Enders, Robbins and Weller cultivate poliovirus in human cells from tissues other than those of the nervous system. Zaimis and Paton introduce ganglionic blocking agents. Vaskil reports antihypertensive effect of rauwolfia. National Institute of Mental Health established.

1950

Publication of the Anson *Atlas of Human Anatomy*—much admired for its subtle depiction of anatomical variations but never competitive with the Grant Atlas as a teaching tool; the Sixth Edition of the Curtis *Textbook of Gynecology* with John W. Huffman as author; the Ogle *Researches in Binocular Vision*—a fine

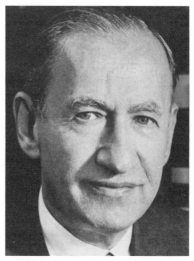

Charles K. Friedberg.

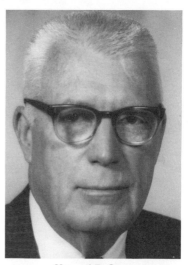

Howard F. Conn.

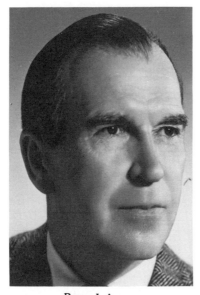

Barry J. Anson.

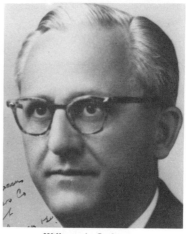

William A. Sodeman.

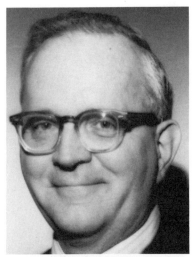

Claude A. Villee

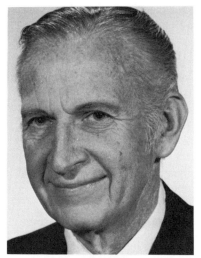

Robert H. Williams.

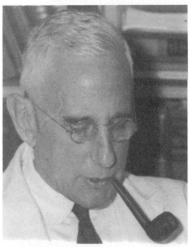

Robert F. Loeb.

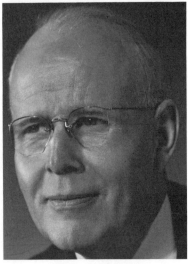

Walter C. Alvarez.

Mayo Clinic monograph; the Prosser *Comparative Animal Physiology*—the first thorough American text in comparative physiology; the Sodeman *Pathologic Physiology: Mechanisms of Disease*—its knowledgeable editor knowing the people to go to for what were then advanced ideas in internal medicine; the Villee *Biology; The Human Approach*—a text that, under the gentle guidance of editor Tyler Buchenau, would become America's leading textbook in biology; and of the Williams *Textbook of Endocrinology* (see Chapter 11).

Pfizer announces discovery of Terramycin. Nobel Prize awarded to Hench, Kendall and Reichstein for their studies in treatment of rheumatoid arthritis with cortisone and ACTH (adrenocorticotropic hormone).

1951

An IBM complete accounting and inventory-control system is installed in a daring and what proved to be disastrous flight of fancy.

Robert F. Loeb joins Russell L. Cecil as coeditor of the Eighth Edition of the *Textbook of Medicine* (see Chapter 9). Walter Alvarez publishes with Saunders his perceptive but curious work on *The Neuroses* (see Chapter 11). And the College Division publishes the Noller *Chemistry of Organic Compounds*—a text that took a daring new approach to the classification of organic compounds, in connection with which its author sent to the publisher a collect 192-page telegram listing last-minute changes in what had heretofore seemed an accurate and useful index. The year also saw publication of the Meschan *Atlas of Normal Radiographic Anatomy*, the first of many Meschan books beautifully illustrated and effectively conceived as teaching texts and clinical monographs in roentgenology; and of the first annual issue of the *Surgical Forum* from the American College of Surgeons. Eventually both the sponsoring society and the hard-pressed publisher would restore their equanimity after several years of stormy disagreement about what the *Forum* should be, how it was to be published and for whom it was intended (see Chapter 10).

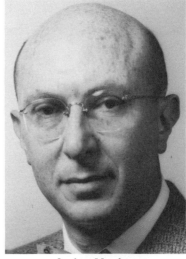

Isadore Meschan.

Gross demonstrates transmission of leukemia in mice. Hammon conducts trials of gamma globulin as prophylaxis against poliomyelitis. The effect of fluoride in prevention of dental caries is discovered.

1952

Publication of *Ophthalmic Pathology* from the American Academy of Ophthalmology and Otolaryngology—a stunning atlas-text initially the work of Jonas Friedenwald and continued in later editions under the editorship of Michael J. Hogan and of William H. Spencer.

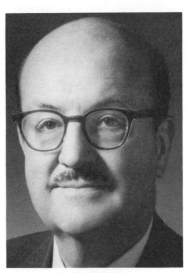

Michael J. Hogan.

Zoll introduces the first practical pacemaker and uses external cardiac stimulation in cardiac arrest. Hufnagel inserts first artificial heart valve. The first enzyme-deficiency disease is identified by the Coris. Bodian and Horstman demonstrate viremia in poliomyelitis. The discovery of isoniazid is announced. Bahnson removes an aneurysm of the arch of the aorta. The experiments of Hershey and Chase demonstrate that the genes must be DNA (deoxyribonucleic acid) and that DNA must carry the specifications for making new viruses. Hence DNA is the genetic material—the basis of life. Only now was the significance of the earlier investigations of Avery and his associates appreciated.

Publication of the Banks and Laufman *Atlas of Surgical Exposures of the Extremities*—a classic that would continue unrevised for more than thirty years as the definitive exposition of orthopedic incisional techniques. Originally Harold Laufman planned to do the drawings for the book from

1953

211

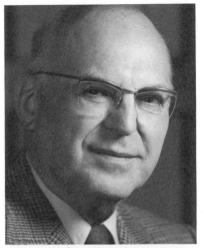

Sam W. Banks.

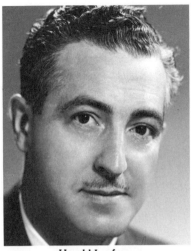

Harold Laufman.

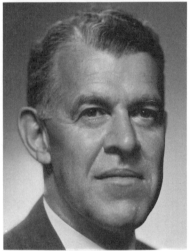

Richard B. Cattell.

photographs of dissections on cadavers; but in the end Jean McConnell did almost all the artwork, adding beauty to excellence of presentation. Five Boston books brought lustre to the year's list: The Cattell and Warren *Surgery of the Pancreas*, the Dunphy and Botsford *Physical Examination of the Surgical Patient*, the Glickman *Clinical Periodontology*, the Gross *Surgery of Infancy and Childhood* (see Chapter 10), and the Parsons and Ulfelder *Atlas of Pelvic Operations*. In the last Mildred Codding was to pelvic operative procedures what Jean McConnell was to orthopedic exposures. But Langdon Parsons, kindest and gentlest of

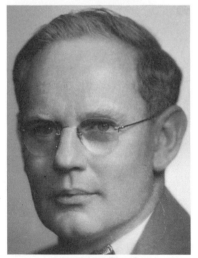

J. Englebert Dunphy.

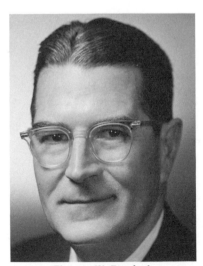

Thomas W. Botsford.

men, could never manage to express to his artist what he wanted in final revision of the drawings, so this unhappy task fell to Howard Ulfelder. Their book was the first medical title ever to make it in the annual book show of the American Institute of Graphic Arts. Lustre of a different sort was added in publication of the brief pioneering work on *Bacterial Genetics* by Werner Braun and of the Kinsey et al. *Sexual Behavior in the Human Female* (see Chapter 15).

Announcement by Watson, Crick and Wilkins of the double-helix configuration of DNA. Gibbon performs the first open-heart surgery by using an extracorporeal pump. The Nobel Prize awarded to Lipmann and Krebs for their studies of carbohydrate metabolism and coenzyme A.

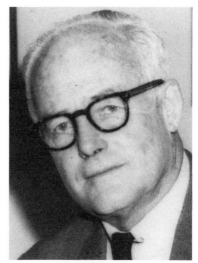

Langdon Parsons.

1954

John Dusseau elected Saunders Vice President and Editor-in-Chief and Robert Rowan Managing Editor. Bob Rowan, despite winning the Conn *Current Therapy* bet with Jack Lutz, had been appointed Advertising Director, becoming the best and often the most-behind-schedule copywriter in the business. He would later become Associate Medical Editor, then Vice President in charge of sales and thereafter Executive Vice President. To all these posts he brought a full knowledge of every aspect of publishing and a prevailing kindliness rare among executives and endearing him to many authors and friends of the Saunders Company. Now retired, his bald pate still gleams with the evidence of grace beneath it. (See also Chapters 10, 11, 14 and 15.) Bob was followed as Director of Advertising by George Brauckman, who also later succeeded him as Vice President in charge of sales. As talented as Bob and, some would say, more witty and less kindly, George had a managerial defect. He worked with such fierce devotion to every job he tackled that he had a barely concealed intolerance for the usual run of people who believe that six hours of work in a seven-hour work day is grounds for enlistment among the saints. George could never bring himself to expect or accept less than nine hours of work in a seven-hour work day.

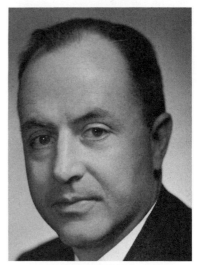

Harold Ulfelder.

Publication of the three-volume Campbell *Urology*—the definitive clinical monograph in its field to be carried on in later editions by J. Hartwell Harrison, who, like Meredith Campbell before him, dedicated his work "to those who may be helped by these volumes." The year also saw publication

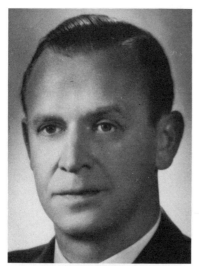

J. Hartwell Harrison.

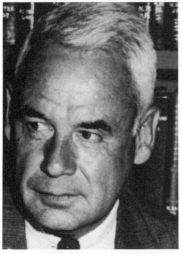

Richard T. Shackelford.

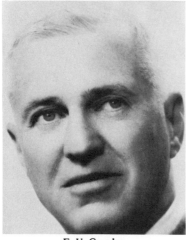

E. V. Cowdry.

of the Florey *Lectures in General Pathology.* Finally, the first issue of the *Pediatric Clinics of North America* came to publication—an addition to the *Medical Clinics* and *Surgical Clinics* undertaken with profound misgiving by some of the Saunders principals who thought that clinics, like the sexes, should be confined to two.

Farber describes effects of daunomycin in tumors. Sourkes reports antihypertensive effects of alpha-methyldopa. Howard and his associates report hypertension associated with impaired blood flow to the kidney to be dramatically improved by nephrectomy. Enders, Robbins and Weller receive the Nobel Prize for their work on tissue culture of poliomyelitis virus.

1955

Publication of Shackelford's revision (actually complete redoing) of the *Bickham-Callander Surgery of the Alimentary Tract* (see Chapter 12) and of Cowdry's *Cancer Cells*—a distinguished and valuable work greeted in America with admiration and slight interest; but its Russian translation had a phenomenal sale. Since no royalty therefrom could be taken out of the country, Cowdry traveled all over Russia on his accumulated royalty and returned home with huge tins of beluga caviar—the only thing tourists could then legally take out of Russia. His preface to the book sets out the problem and the goal of almost all scientific writing: "Available information on cancer cells increases much more rapidly than it can be even partially digested. Unless one immediately records what is thought to be really significant, it is displaced by the onrush of further data and forgotten. Writing this book is an instructive lesson of the need for bringing each line of evidence to some sort of conclusion before passing on to another aspect of cancer cells no matter how attractive. Winged fancy must not be permitted to roam unleashed." (See also Chapter 8.) The year included publication of the Masserman *Practice of Dynamic Psychiatry* (see Chapter 10) and of the Seventeenth Edition of the Howell *Textbook of Physiology* now under the scholarly editorship of John

Fulton, a man who enjoyed all good things, especially good writing and sound thought, and disdained pedestrian concerns. A basket lunch with him in his office at Yale was an epicure's delight, and his talk was as heady as the wine. His talk in 1950 included the flat statement that endocrine physiology was not important enough to be included in the textbook. He grudgingly changed his mind for this, the Seventeenth Edition. And the year ended with the publication of the Harvey and Bordley *Differential Diagnosis* (see Chapter 12) and of the Willier-Weiss-Hamburger *Analysis of Development*—a work of rich erudition and fundamental meaning that is still consulted for its germinal ideas.

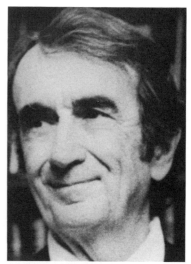

A. McGehee Harvey.

Salk introduces polio vaccine. Lawrence identifies transfer factor—a substance isolated from disrupted blood leukocytes that transfers delayed antigenic hypersensitivity from one individual to another. Conn describes syndrome of aldosteronism due to adrenal adenoma. DeBakey, Creech and Harris remove aortic aneurysm and replace with a homograft. Merrill, Hume, Miller and Thorn report their experience with renal transplantation in nine terminally ill patients. Four of the nine transplanted kidneys functioned, and two of the patients experienced marked relief of symptoms. The Nobel Prize in chemistry awarded to du Vigneaud and Theorell for their studies of chemical synthesis of oxytocin and of the oxygen transport system in living tissues.

1956

Lawrence Saunders is elected Chairman of the Board of Directors and Harry R. Most becomes President and General Manager of the Saunders Company. Lawrence Saunders, only son of Walter Burns Saunders, had come into the publishing house after graduation from the Wharton School of the University of Pennsylvania, thereafter serving as a Navy officer during World War I. The twenty years of his presidency had been a period of dramatic growth; but he always insisted that the business be conducted with the same attention to honesty, dignity and personalized service that had characterized the house when it was smaller. During those twenty years it became generally recognized as the largest and most important medical publishing house in the world. (See also Chapters 4, 12 and 15.)

Harry R. Most, Lawrence's successor and the first president of Saunders not a family member, was graduated *cum laude* from Wesleyan University in 1934 and joined Saunders in 1937 shortly after his admission to the Pennsylvania bar. Keeping a publishing ship on an even keel requires an aptitude greater than agreeable persuasiveness, and Harry had it. In a small family-owned business the interests of owners and employees may not always coincide; but Harry was a masterful tactician in the fine art of bringing diverse interests into approximation. He also knew how to restrain grandiose ideas without recourse to the power of veto. He did it by instituting pauses, and there is nothing more fatal to grandiosity than slow deliberation. His

215

decisions were characterized by the wisdom of experience rather than by arbitrary forcefulness. He is now actually retired, following meteoric publishing flights after his pseudoretirement from Saunders, and devotes himself to farm, horses and dogs. (See also Chapters 4, 15 and 20.)

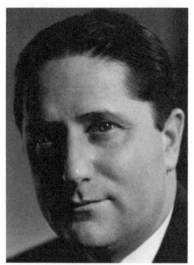

Loyal Davis.

Publication of the Christopher *Textbook of Surgery* in its Sixth Edition edited by Loyal Davis (see Chapter 10); of the Guyton *Textbook of Medical Physiology* (see Chapter 17); of the Haagensen *Diseases of the Breast*—the definitive study of breast disease based on long-term surgical experience of exquisite skill, solid pathology and scrupulous statistical analysis; of the Hinshaw and Garland *Diseases of the Chest*—Hinshaw a superb clinician who carried out early investigations of isoniazid and streptomycin in the therapy of tuberculosis contemporaneously with McDermott and Muschenheim, Garland a roentgenologist who appreciated that radiologic examination is the study of living gross pathology and, when used unnecessarily, may be harmful; and of the beautiful Pillsbury-Shelley-Kligman *Dermatology*, to be carried on effectively in later editions by Sam

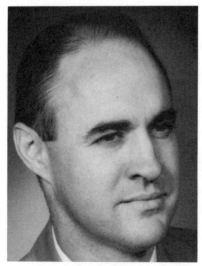

Arthur C. Guyton.

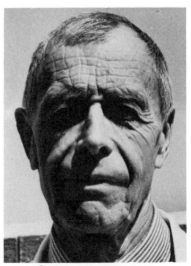

Cushman D. Haagensen.

Moschella and Harry Hurley (see Chapter 11). The year also saw publication of the *Handbook of Biological Data*, edited by William S. Spector and sponsored by the National Academy of Sciences and the National Research Council. A vast putting-together of quantitative data, it proposed to do what similar tabular manuals had achieved in physics and engineering, and it enlisted the contributions of more than four thousand scientists and the advice and counsel of an additional thirteen thousand. Other similar volumes from the NAS-NRC were to follow—of them the *Handbook of Respiration* the most valuable. All were meticulous compilations; but all suffered from the disadvantage that the biosciences are not readily compressible into tables.

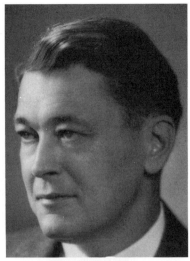

Donald M. Pillsbury.

Tigo and Levan arrive at the true number of diploid chromosomes in man—forty-eight. Zoll introduces external defibrillator. Nobel Prize awarded to Forssmann, Cournand and Richards for cardiac catheterization. James A. Shannon is appointed Director of the National Institutes of Health. Shannon had made significant studies in renal physiology and his investigations of malaria during World War II had won him the Presidential Order of Merit. Working with Congressman John Fogarty, Senator Lister Hill and Secretary Marion Folsom, he would insure support for and give intelligent direction to the NIH.

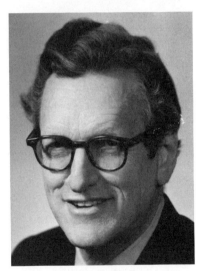

Walter B. Shelley.

A. Paul Burton becomes Saunders Executive Vice President, having previously been Sales Manager and later Vice President in charge of sales. A graduate of Rutgers University, Paul had also participated in the Advanced Management Program at Harvard School of Business Administration; but a more unlikely MBA could not readily be imagined, for his shrewd business judgments were essentially intuitive. A superb salesman, he became a superb manager of salesmen, because he knew the secret of good management: Never ask anyone to do what you can't do or haven't done yourself. A man of forthright opinions, he commanded a persuasiveness sometimes more compelling than the reasons behind it; but in all games of chance his persuasiveness was unalloyed. Every Saunders subscription salesman believed he had in Paul a steadfast friend and an ally at a foreign court in which intrigue and subtle machinations were daily directed against the well-being of those unappreciated workers who bring in the business.

1957

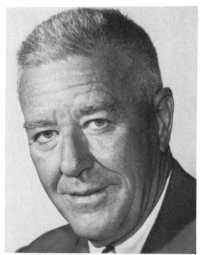

John H. Mulholland.

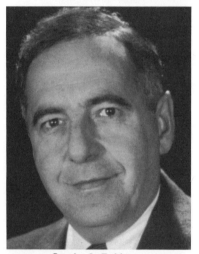

Stanley L. Robbins.

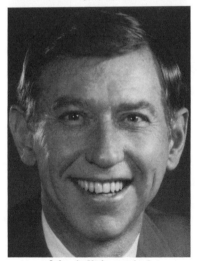

John A. Kirkpatrick, Jr.

Publication of the first issue of the *Dental Clinics of North America*. The new Clinics were managed by newly appointed Dental Editor Bob Wright, who would bring to books in dental and veterinary medicine and later in nursing a keen insight into what makes effective writing and teaching. The year saw too publication of the Dripps-Eckenhoff-Vandam *Introduction to Anesthesia*, the Mulholland-Ellison-Friesen *Current Surgical Management*, the Nadas *Pediatric Cardiology* ("I wish to thank my secretary for her efficiency in holding together the cardiology department during the trying period in which this book was written") and of the Robbins *Textbook of Pathology* (see Chapter 17).

Ingraham discovers specific amino acid change in sickle-cell hemoglobin. The Sabin oral poliomyelitis vaccine tested in Russia. Freis and Hollander observe antihypertensive effect of thiazide derivatives. Witebsky sets out "Postulates for Autoimmune Disease," which have been compared with Koch's "Postulates for Infectious Disease." When these postulates were proposed, no experimental animal was known to exhibit spontaneously any disease similar to human autoimmune disease; but since then strains of New Zealand mice have exhibited spontaneously occurring acquired hemolytic anemia.

1958

Publication of the Roberts *Difficult Diagnosis*—a synthesis of the most advanced medical ideas relating to diagnosis obscured by uncertain and conflicting findings. A work built on Harvey's observation in 1657 that "Nature is nowhere accustomed more openly to display her secret mysteries than in cases where she shows traces of her workings apart from the beaten path." Also a book of immense success but never revised by its author, partly because to him the challenge of writing lay in the new, not in redoing the old. The year also saw publication of the Aegerter and Kirkpatrick *Orthopedic Diseases*—a text uniting expert pathology with elegant roentgenology; of the Shafer-Hine-Levy *Textbook of Oral Pathology*— the Robbins of dental science; and of the Hebb *Textbook of Psychology*—no nonsense about how to get on with your boss.

First use of closed-chest cardiac massage combined with mouth-to-mouth respiration for cardiac resuscitation. Nobel Prize awarded to Beadle, Tatum and Lederberg for their genetic studies.

1959

Publication of the Guyton *Function of the Human Body* (see Chapter 17), of the Moore *Metabolic Care of the Surgical Patient* (see Chapter 11), of the Shambaugh *Surgery of the Ear*, and of the DePalma *Management of Fractures and Dislocations*—the most vividly graphic of all surgical guides to technique.

Ford and Jacobs discover role of Y chromosome in sex determination in humans. Ciba introduces guanethidine—an adrenergic blocking agent—for treatment of hypertension. Avery and Mead discover surfactant deficiency in lungs of premature infants. Ochoa and Kornberg share the Nobel Prize for work on enzyme synthesis of RNA and DNA.

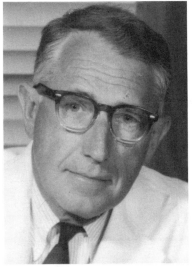

Francis D. Moore.

1960

In 1938 W. D. Watson had written a brief history of the Saunders Company distinguished by a curious parade of office boys and clerks, over whose performance W. D. kept vigilant watch, who had been dismissed for incompetence but later became presidents or chief executive officers of large corporations. Clearly, Watson could no more foresee the future than the rest of us; and he had this to say about advertising: "After Mr.

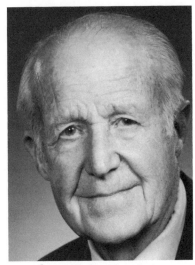

George E. Shambaugh, Jr.

Greene took charge of advertising, we were soon taking space in 88 journals throughout the United States and foreign countries. Our policy in the very beginning was not to take space in any journal unless we could get 'front cover.' This policy has never been changed and we, even now, see no reason for changing it." In 1960 with some reluctance but admission of its inevitability Saunders abandoned its front-cover position on the *Journal of the American Medical Association*. An editorial in the April 16th issue of the *Journal* recalls the privileged past:

> Scarcely a physician in practice remembers a time when, as he glanced down the cover of each issue of *The Journal*, he did not see a description of a new book from the W. B. Saunders Company. The Saunders box on the cover of this issue is unique. It contains a farewell message after 60 years and after more than 3,000 consecutive appearances. The position will be relinquished so

that we may present a more attractive face to our readers. Although this small window through which the progress of medical publishing has been evident is now gone, it is not forgotten. A medical landmark does not vanish without some nostalgia—and so it is with us.

Some of us may remember when Saunders had an obvious half-page on *The Journal*. This brought to the attention of the practicing physician such excellent tomes as Labat's "Anesthesia," Abt's "Pediatrics," Beckman's "Treatment," and Bickham's "Operative Surgery." Each of the 23 editions of Dorland's Illustrated Medical Dictionary was announed on the front of *The Journal*.

Medical publishing is the handmaiden of medical education, in spite of other mediums that may claim this honor. Both have marched forward together, and many of the titles of Saunders' books which have appeared on the front cover constitute a composite of America's best medical writing for more than a half-century. The first announcements of the publication of the following excellent volumes appeared on the cover of *The Journal*. Arey's "Developmental Anatomy," DeLee's "Principles and Practice of Obstetrics," Ewing's "Neoplastic Diseases," Garrison's "History of Medicine," Jordan's "Bacteriology," Maximow's and Bloom's "Histology," Ranson's "Neuro-anatomy," and Sollman's "Pharmacology." This was as much a matter of pride to us as it was for the House of Saunders, because a prime concern of the American Medical Association has been the sound as well as imaginative advancement of medical education. There is little doubt that the titles and authors of these books would have done honor and added prestige to the front cover of any medical journal. They were books that looked forward and extended the frontiers of medical knowledge. Among them were books that took courage to write and courage to publish.

Through all these years, the front cover notices have been calm and unhurried. No extravagant claim, except the occasional intimation of universal interest in a work of highly specialized knowledge, has betrayed fundamental faith in a worthy product. We hope to continue to see the Saunders book announcements on the inside pages of *The Journal* for many years to come.

This, then, is a farewell message to an old friend in a tweed jacket. This friendship was never more manifest than at the time that Saunders agreed to relinquish this desirable spot. The conference that led to this momentous decision lasted less than two hours.

Giving up the front cover was done wryly but graciously. The cover will be permitted a little more of that most valued of earthly possessions—elbow room. Possibly we should confess sympathy for Thoreau, who preferred to sit on a pumpkin and have it alone than to be crowded on a velvet cushion.

At this time, too, Sherman E. Perkins, grandson of Walter B. Saunders, became Secretary of the company and member of its Board of Directors. A graduate of the University of Pennsylvania and a paratrooper on combat missions in the Pacific during World War II, he carried on a family tradition of friendliness and interest in people. Since 1953 he had been Sales Manager in charge of subscription sales; and, although he was not himself an adept salesman, he had a fine-honed sympathetic understanding of sales people. They often work with little direct contact with the home-office base and sometimes cover territories far too extensive for frequent trips home. Perk knew their problems and their defensive attitudes; and all the subscription salesmen felt they had in him an honest friend at the office who was not trying furtively to reduce either their territories or their commissions. Later, Perk would be named a Saunders Vice President; but this appointment little changed his responsibilities, and he continued to travel at least 50,000 miles a year visiting sales personnel and attending medical meetings. But however friendly and cheerful Perk is, what he really loves is plants. With acquisition of the company by Columbia Broadcasting System, Perk felt that an era of good will and mild indulgence in informality might be passing. He therefore resigned to take up ranching and attend to the two thousand azaleas he had grown from cuttings. In his many years with Saunders he had never carried a watch or a grudge, steadfastly keeping appointments and friends.

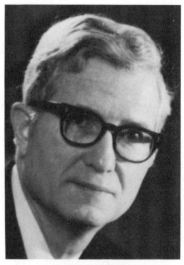

James D. Hardy.

Publication of the American College of Surgeons *Management of Fractures and Soft Tissue Injuries*, of the Artz and Hardy *Complications in Surgery and Their Management*, of the Balinsky *Introduction to Embryology*, of the Leonard *Orthopedic Surgery of the Dog and Cat*, of the Poppen *Atlas of Neurosurgical Techniques* (see Chapter 11), of the Schaffer *Diseases of the Newborn* and of the Eighteenth Edition of the *Howell-Fulton Textbook of Physiology*, edited by Theodore C. Ruch, Chairman of the Department of Physiology and Biophysics at the University of Washington and author of *Diseases of Laboratory Primates*, a fascinating account of somewhat restricted interest. Ruch brought to the textbook a heightened sense of the importance of biophysics to future physiologic investigation and teaching, a keen perception of the necessity for correlation in the neurosciences, and a more rounded view of physiology than that of Fulton, who rather thought neurophysiology the only proper study of function. The year

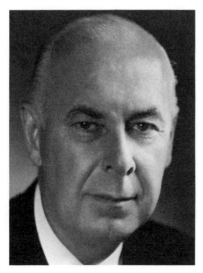

James Poppen.

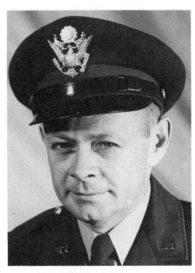

Curtis P. Artz.

221

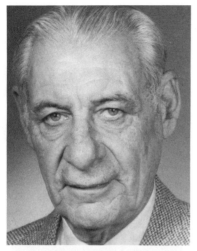

Alexander J. Schaffer.

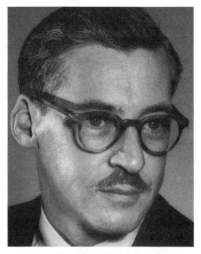

Theodore C. Ruch.

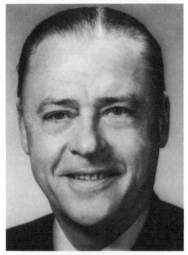

Ernest Gardner.

also saw publication of Saunders' first text-book in gross anatomy—the Gardner-Gray-O'Rahilly *Anatomy*. Regionally organized and illustrated in sharply contrasting line draw-ings by Caspar Henselman, it was a depar-ture from tradition that elicited lavish admi-ration from derring-do young anatomists and disdain from some older fundamentalists. But it fit nicely into changing patterns of medical education, and youth carried the day. Henselman's severely black figures were later compromised in the interest of amelio-rating outright dislike. The year ended with publication of the Felson *Fundamentals of*

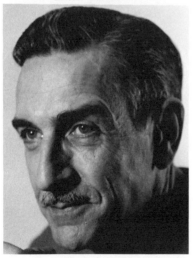

Donald J. Gray.

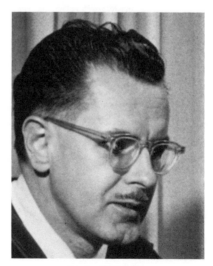

Ronan O'Rahilly.

Chest Roentgenology by an author dedicated, lucid, witty and exacting.

Farber describes effect of daunomycin on Wilms' tumor. Barski delineates techniques of cell hybridization. Choh Hao Li and his group synthesize a peptide composed of the first 19 amino acids of ACTH (adrenocorticotropic hormone) and demonstrate that it possesses all the biological properties of the natural hormone. Berson and Yalow describe technique for radioimmunoassay of hormones. Laragh discovers that angiotensin stimulates secretion of aldosterone. Laser (light amplification by stimulated emission of radiation) is introduced—a device for creation, amplification and transmission of a narrow, intense beam of coherent light.

1961

The new printing and warehousing facility in Cherry Hill, New Jersey, is now in full swing, and additional offset presses are being installed that will print precisely such delicate electronmicrographs as those of the Fawcett *Cell*. The home office, too, is renovated and even air-conditioned.

Publication of the Cherniack and Cherniack *Respiration in Health and Disease*—one of several Canadian texts of enormous success and teaching value (see Chapter 17); of the Graber *Orthodontics*—an outstanding text in the growing dental list; of the three-volume *Atlas of Acquired Diseases of the Heart and Great Vessels*—a visually superb study of cardiac pathology from Jesse Edwards of the Mayo Clinic; and of the first issue of *The Journal of Surgical Research* under the editorship of Gardner Child—a daring journal venture but only partially successful, because few surgeons are interested in the whole field of surgical research. The year also saw publication of the Marlow and Sellew *Textbook of Pediatric Nursing*. This was called a revision of the Sellew but was a complete rewriting by Dorothy Marlow, the first of many editions under her authorship of the leading text in its field.

Gorman, Frida and Pollack describe use of gamma globulin in prevention of hemolytic disease of the newborn. Schally and Guillemin separately identify

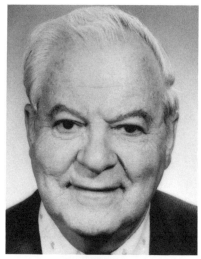

Benjamin Felson.

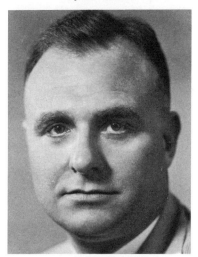

Jesse E. Edwards.

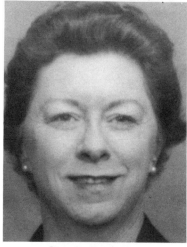

Dorothy R. Marlow.

223

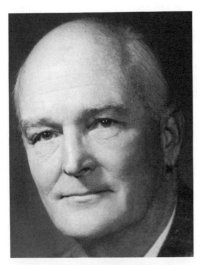

John H. Gibbon, Jr.

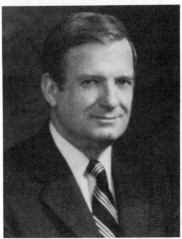

David C. Sabiston, Jr.

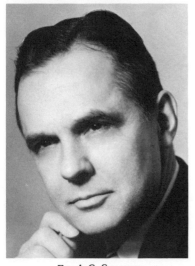

Frank C. Spencer.

hypothalamic releasing factors. Good and Miller show that thymectomy in the newborn inhibits development of the immune system. U.S. Public Health Service licenses Sabin's oral poliomyelitis vaccine.

1962

Veterinary books become an increasingly important segment of Saunders publishing. Such titles as Miller's *Anatomy of the Dog* by Evans and Christensen, the Kirk *Current Veterinary Therapy*, Leonard's *Orthopedic Surgery of the Dog and Cat*, and the Ettinger *Veterinary Internal Medicine* will make Saunders America's leading veterinary publisher. The year saw publication of the Engel *Psychological Development in Health and Disease*—a dynamic introduction to modern principles of psychology as they apply to the understanding of disease; of the great Gibbon *Surgery of the Chest*, to be carried on in later editions by David Sabiston (see Chapter 10) and Frank Spencer; of the Parsons and Sommers *Gynecology*, and of the Reid *Textbook of Obstetrics* (see Chapter 11), the two specialties united that year in the Huffman *Gynecology and Obstetrics*—an elegantly illustrated and written book that appeared ahead of its time, although well-worn and well-thumbed copies are still in constant use in many medical-school libraries. Huffman would later do for Saunders his much more successful *The Gynecology of Childhood and Adolescence*—a book nearer to his experience and interests than the combined text. The Thirteenth Edition of the *Todd-Sanford Clinical Diagnosis by Laboratory Methods*, with Israel Davidsohn as editor, appears (see Chapter 7). The College Division published Welty's *The Life of Birds*—the most fundamentally scientific of all American texts in ornithology.

Trentin and his coworkers demonstrate that a human virus has oncogenic potential in animals. Lown demonstrates electrical conversion in treatment of cardiac arrhythmias. Watson, Crick and Wilson awarded the Nobel Prize for their work in constructing the double-helix model of the DNA molecule in which the known elements of the molecule (sugar, phosphate and the four nucleotide bases) fit together in a functional unit. The National Vaccination Assistance Act is passed.

1963

Saunders' 75th anniversary is celebrated by awarding two writing fellowships to investigators doing significant work in biomedicine and needing time away from the pressures of daily responsibilities in order to think and write. A distinguished selection committee of twenty members headed by Robert F. Loeb, assisted in final decisions by René J. Dubos, Henry Allen Moe and Robert S. Morison, awarded the fellowships at a meeting of the American Philosophical Society to Herman M. Kalckar and Paul B. Beeson. For Saunders folk a splendid dinner marked the occasion and for it the Saunders Speedee Service Cart (see year 1946) was restored to usefulness.

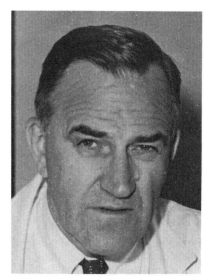

Duncan E. Reid.

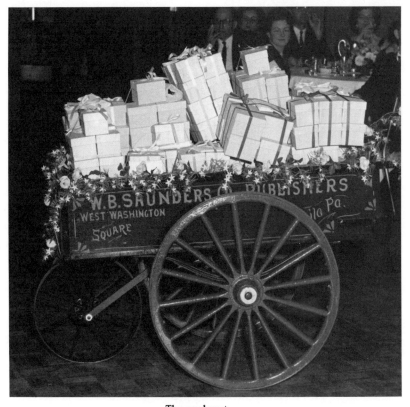

The pushcart.

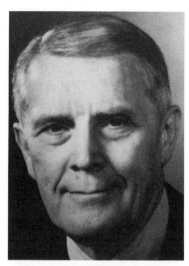

Paul B. Beeson.

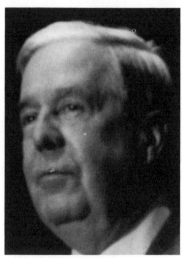

Walsh McDermott.

While the dinner was being held the press-room night shift was printing the first issue of the *Radiologic Clinics of North America*—the first truly special Clinics on the Saunders list. And a new editorial department came into being charged with creating Skinnerian programmed texts. Its first try was a nail-hitter—Christensen's *Ph and Dissociation*, which would endure long past the heyday of Skinner's principles of learning. A phenomenon of the program was the Felson-Weinstein-Spitz *Principles of Chest Roentgenology*, still selling briskly in its original form twenty-some years later and long ago having passed the 100,000-copy sales mark. Similarly, its German translation is also still selling vigorously—in total copies sold far surpassing the record of any other Saunders book in German and indeed that of almost all indigenous German medical titles.

Publication of the Warren *Surgery* (see Chapter 11), and of the Eleventh Edition of the Cecil *Medicine* under the editorship of Paul Beeson and Walsh McDermott. (See also Chapter 9.)

Johnson and his associates show the effect of vincristine in leukemia. Blumberg describes Australia antigen and relates it to hepatitis B. Community Mental Health Center Act passed by Congress.

1964   Lawrence Saunders is honored on the fiftieth anniversary of his service to the Saunders Company by foundation of an annual Art Fellowship at the Johns Hopkins University School of Medicine (see also Chapter 12). Tributes from all over the world come to him on his occasion. Of these the warm greeting from Cushman D. Haagensen is quoted here:

> Dear Larry,
> My congratulations on the fiftieth anniversary of your leadership of Saunders.
>
> During the many years of my own association with you I have looked upon you as a beloved "Chief"—as the head of another academic department of my life. This is in fact what you are—a Professor of Medicine without portfolio in the truest sense—for with your books you teach medicine to students and physicians everywhere. And the printed word is surely the most potent way of teaching. The superiority of American medicine is closely related to the

superiority of American textbooks of medicine which you have done so much to achieve. With your leadership Saunders has not only produced the best medical texts, but you have generously made them available all around the world.

As a "Chief" you have been superb. You have given those who write for you the patient encouragement which brings out the best in them; and with your expert technical staff of editors, illustrators, and printers you have made writing easy.

I can truly say that as I look back, the writing I have done for you has been the most pleasant, the most satisfactory, and I hope, the most useful part of my life.

Hail to the Chief! May you now, at your 50th anniversary, have all the blessings that you so richly deserve.

From a devoted friend.

Carolinen

The fellowship too attracted much favorable notice, and an editorial in the *New England Journal of Medicine* summed up nicely its purpose and hoped-for effect:

ART OF MEDICINE

Among the many paramedical pursuits, most of which are usually considered sciences, the field of medical art has become increasingly important. In the modern context communication is in many of its aspects a highly sophisticated science. However, the presentation of medical data in journals and at conferences and meetings also involves the art of writing, the art of speaking and the art of illustration.

To encourage the career of the medical artist, the W. B. Saunders Company has endowed an annual art fellowship at Johns Hopkins University School of Medicine. The endowment is in honor of Lawrence Saunders, chairman of the board and son of the founder. The fellowship will provide tuition fee for one student each year in the University's Department of Medical Art.

It is hoped that the fruits of Saunders's generosity will be seen on the pages of the *Journal* in the future.

Publication of Avery's *The Lung and Its Disorders in the Newborn Infant*—the first and an outstanding issue in the series Major Problems in Clinical Pediatrics under the editorship of Alexander Schaffer. Mary Ellen Avery, after leaving Johns Hopkins to become Chairman of the Department of Pediatrics at McGill University and later at Harvard, would take on the authorship of Schaffer's *Diseases of the Newborn*. The year also saw publication of the elegant Bates and Christie *Respiratory Function in Disease* (see Chapter 17), of the daring Starzl *Experience in Renal Transplantation*, of the altogether new Emmett

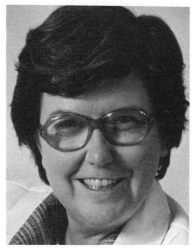

Mary Ellen Avery.

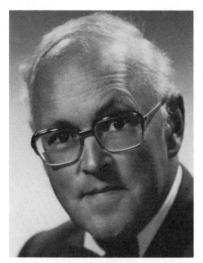

David V. Bates.

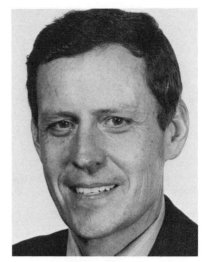

Thomas E. Starzl.

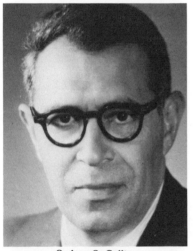

Sydney S. Gellis.

Clinical Urography in two volumes, of the first issue of Gellis and Kagan *Current Pediatric Therapy* and of the great Converse *Reconstructive Plastic Surgery*. The last was intended to be a rather modest one-volume survey of an emerging field of surgery and surgical investigation, reconstructive surgeons having had long experience in the possibilities and problems of transplantation. But John Marquis Converse—in a life frantically busy in surgical research, administration, surgical practice, fine writing and the enjoyment of all good things from Picasso to Zermatt—was

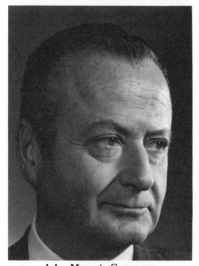

John Marquis Converse.

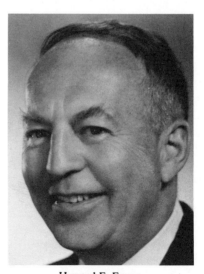

Howard E. Evans.

never one to do things by halves. Like so many well-intentioned plans, this one profited by going astray and resulting in five volumes of generous format and detailed surgical insight. On the other hand, the Miller-Christensen-Evans *Anatomy of the Dog*, a work of similar dedication and erudition completed by Howard Evans after Mac Miller's death, turned out to be precisely what it was intended to be—a one-volume superbly illustrated and meticulously accurate depiction of canine anatomy valuable to veterinary science and to surgical research the world over.

Bloch and Lynen receive the Nobel Prize for their work on the mechanism and regulation of cholesterol and fatty-acid metabolism. National Library of Medicine introduces its computer-based system for analysis, storage and retrieval of medical literature—MEDLARS.

1965

By now Saunders Linofilm composition is in solid working order and proves to be beautifully adapted to the new list in mathematics and physics inaugurated by Abian's *The Theory of Sets and Transfinite Arithmetic* and the Stevenson and Whitehead monograph series Studies in Physics and Chemistry. Publication of the Edwards-Carey-Neufeld-Lester *Congenital Heart Disease*—a complement to the Edwards *Atlas of Acquired Diseases of the Heart and Great Vessels*, of the Ingelfinger, Relman and Finland *Controversy in Internal Medicine* (see Chapter 11) and of the Krusen-Kottke-Ellwood *Handbook of Physical Medicine and Rehabilitation*—a successor to the original Krusen *Physical Medicine* with its character of explicit direction derived from careful analysis of long experience. The Nursing Department publishes the Jacob and Francone *Structure and Function in Man*—a beautifully illustrated anatomy-physiology text that would long dominate the teaching of anatomy to nurses and paramedical personnel.

Proinsulin discovered by Steiner and Oyer. Introduction of immunization against measles based on the long-continued viral studies of Enders and Peebles. Congress passes the Medicare, Medicaid and Higher Education Acts.

1966

The *Nursing Clinics of North America* under the office editorship of Helen Dietz is launched and is an immediate success. Publication of *Emergency Care of the Sick and Injured*, sponsored by the American College of Surgeons and edited by Robert H. Kennedy; and of Fawcett's *The Cell* (see Chapter 8). An important brief book off the beaten track of widely used popular texts was the Thompson and Thompson *Genetics in Medicine*—the husband-wife creation of a fine teaching text for courses that scarcely yet existed but one satisfying a learning need already keenly felt. A text in more classic tradition was the brief Leeson and Leeson *Histology*—a thoughtfully

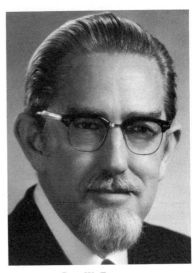

Don W. Fawcett.

229

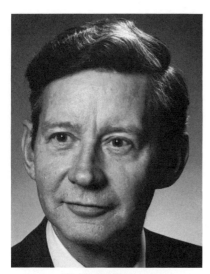

Thomas S. Leeson.

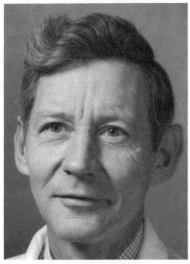

C. Roland Leeson.

conceived instrument of learning whose authors, who had studied in England and taught in Canada, thought sound teaching in medical science to be important but need not be exhaustive. The year also saw publication of the First Edition of Masterton and Slowinski *Chemical Principles*, whose manuscript had been under contract to a distinguished publisher who had declined to publish. In later editions, under the skillful editorial guidance of John Vondeling, the book would become the leading text in general chemistry in the world and its authors would write for Saunders another half dozen splendidly successful texts in chemistry. A natural-born teacher-editor, Howard Conn (see Chapter 14), added a new important serial publication to the Saunders medical list—the Conn-Clohecy-Conn *Current Diagnosis*: "Our principal aim is to assist the physician to cope with one of the most difficult and yet most common of all problems in medicine—the patient with atypical symptoms, with misleading signs, with a clinical picture produced by a combination of diseases."

Parkman and Meyer develop rubella vaccine. Ishizaka describes gamma E immunoglobulin (IgE) and its association with allergic states. Huggins and Rous receive the Nobel Prize for their momentous contributions to cancer research. When Rous left Hopkins to join the staff of the Rockefeller Institute, his mentor, William Welch, said to him, "Whatever you do, do not commit yourself to the cancer problem."

1967   A long-standing distribution arrangement with McAinsh & Company in Canada is terminated, and a wholly owned Saunders subsidiary, W. B. Saunders Company Canada, Ltd., is established with offices in Toronto and A. J. Cornwall as manager (see also Chapter 20).

Publication of the Federman *Abnormal Sexual Development*—a brilliant and beautifully written book but sufficiently complex in its scientific explanations to scare off some readers. Dan Federman would later play an important role in development of the *Scientific American Medicine* (see Chapter 9). The year also saw publication of the *Manual of Preoperative and Postoperative Care*, sponsored by the American College of Surgeons and edited by a triumvirate of excellence—Henry T. Randall, James D. Hardy and Francis D. Moore; and of the Fomon *Infant Nutrition*—a book of thoughtful balance whose immediate sale was disappointing but eventually encouraging. The year saw too publication of the first issue of *Pharmacology for Physicians*, edited by Walter Modell.

Favaloro performs the first coronary artery bypass utilizing a vein. Nobel Prize awarded to Hartline, Wald and Granit for their discoveries concerning primary chemical and physiolgical processes of vision.

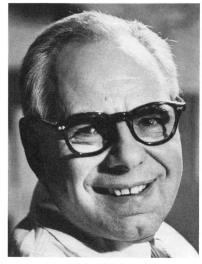

Walter Modell.

1968

The death of Lawrence Saunders ends a lifetime of service not only to the Saunders Company but to the idea of intelligent dissemination of knowledge. It is shortly followed by acquisition of the company by CBS Inc., ending eighty years of independent operation and ownership by the Saunders family.

Celebration of Sam Mink's fiftieth anniversary with Saunders. Sam came to work for Saunders as an office boy at the age of fourteen. Not abundantly educated, Sam knew more about the human heart than most cardiologists and more about the mind of man than many psychologists. He also knew better than most radiologists how printed roentgenograms should look; but one or two holdouts might dispute this, although not with conviction. In any event, he sized up pictures and everything else with easy accuracy; but his real art was conciliation. When all else had failed to calm some irate author, Sam was dispatched to pour oil on him. A writer who had been eagerly and impatiently awaiting first proof of his book for eighteen weeks could somehow be convinced by Sam that actually only six weeks had gone by and that the other twelve were some kind of easily imaginable aberration on the part of an understandably anxious person. Sam was also Mr. Malaprop. "Lead the way," he'd say, "and we'll precede."

Publication of the Shackelford *Diagnosis of Surgical Disease*—a successor to the famous Graham *Surgical Diagnosis*; of the Wagner *Principles of Nuclear Medicine*—the first thorough text in an emerging new technical field of medicine; and of the first issue of the *Otolaryngologic Clinics of North America*.

Gertrude and Werner Henle relate Epstein-Barr virus to infectious mononucleosis. Cotzias introduces L-dopa treatment of Parkinson's disease. Nirenberg, Khorana and Holley receive the Nobel Prize for their work on the genetic code.

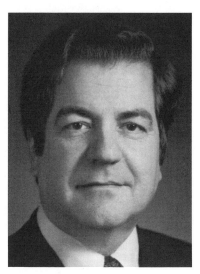

Henry N. Wagner, Jr.

1969   Eugene Hoguet becomes Vice President in charge of production. Gene began his career with Saunders in 1940 as office boy in the Production Department. From the very outset he proved himself extraordinarily capable—never too busy to answer a question, never unable to inform an author of the exact status of his manuscript. (See also Chapter 15.) Upon his retirement in 1982 testimonials from writers, friends and colleagues poured into the Saunders Company. Here is part of one from George Brauckman:

> Congratulations on your retirement from Saunders after 40 years of fire-breathing and dedicated service. You were one of the company's sturdiest pillars during those growing, changing and exciting years.
>
> You were a non-stop dynamo, interested and involved in every little detail that made up the whole of a great publishing house. Your honesty was almost embarrassing to the rest of us. I guess I remember most your quickness to anger at deceit or unfairness. The color would start at your collar and flame up your face and ears to blend with your red hair (in the days when you had considerably more). We always knew where you stood.
>
> I remember vividly my first day at Saunders in 1949, when you were production manager and I was hired as your assistant; we worked on the decrepit drafty first floor of 711 Locust Street. You, Sam Mink, George Laurie and a stenographer were the entire production department. Manuscripts, galleys, page proofs, and type pages littered the room. You called me to your desk and patiently explained the details of the job: the politics at the compositor, Westcott & Thomson; the importance of being respectful to W. D. Watson and Jack Lutz; not to hang around with the girls in the accounting department; and how glad you were to have me aboard. I thought you were a great boss.

Gene spent his working life fighting the never-ending and never-altogether-won battles of schedule, quality and cost. He did not know how to give an important task anything but all his splendid resource.

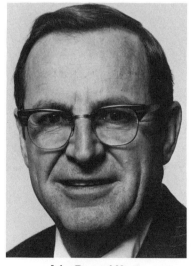

John Bernard Henry.

A warehouse and office designed to serve bookstore accounts in the western United States is opened in Mountain View, California, as part of a major change in book distribution arrangements. The contracts under which book wholesalers had distributed medical, dental, veterinary and allied health books were terminated—only nursing books were excepted. Like many sweeping changes, this one proved to be a not altogether unmixed blessing.

John Bernard Henry becomes coeditor with Israel Davidsohn of the Fourteenth Edition of the Todd-Sanford *Clinical Diagnosis by Laboratory Methods* (see also Chapter 7).

Philip K. Bondy of Yale assumes editorship of the Duncan *Diseases of Metabolism*—in later editions joined by Leon E. Rosenberg as coeditor of the book retitled *Metabolic Control and Disease* to indicate a shift in emphasis toward the mechanisms by which metabolic reactions are controlled and modulated. A more special volume of similar nature also appeared—the Gardner *Endocrine and Genetic Diseases of Childhood*. The Kirk and Bistner *Handbook of Veterinary Procedures and Emergency Treatment* adds a new dimension of instant success to an already lively list, and the Scheie and Albert revision of the Adler-Gifford *Textbook of Ophthalmology* meets a similar cordial reception.

Man walks on the moon and interstellar space suddenly seems part of our travel world. Good and his coworkers describe homograft treatment of thymic agenesis. Guillemin synthesizes the thyrotropin-releasing hormone of the hypothalamus. Delbruck, Luria and Hershey receive the Nobel Prize for their work on bacteriophage and viral genetics.

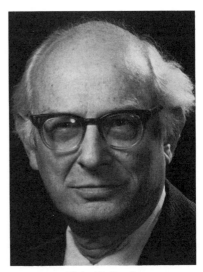

Philip K. Bondy.

William R. Carter, Manager of the Saunders London Company, retires and his post is taken by Michael Jackson, who had served for some years in the Philadelphia office as Associate Medical Editor—a post he richly enjoyed, but return to England was attractive to him. CBS International Publishing acquires the outstanding Mexican scientific publishing house Nueva Editorial Interamericana, S. A. (NEISA) with branch offices in Argentina, Brazil, Colombia, Ecuador, Peru, Venezuela, Uruguay and Spain. As an independent publisher, NEISA had long had a cordial relationship with Saunders as translator and distributor of its books; the acquisition strengthened these ties and opened up new market possibilities.

1970

Publication of the superbly illustrated Braverman *Skin Signs of Systemic Disease*—a seemingly special work that would also be used as a teaching text in dermatology. The year also saw publication of the magnificent Fraser and Paré two-volume *Diseases of the Chest*—one of those books whose fine quality was at once recognized and whose Second Edition in four volumes would take its place among the classics of medical literature; and of the McGilvery *Biochemistry: A Functional Approach*—a new and daring look at the fundamentals of biochemistry. The first of a series of brief volumes written and edited by Lucy Squire also appeared. This first volume—Squire, Colaiace and Strutynsky *Exercises in Diagnostic Radiology: The Chest*—set the tone

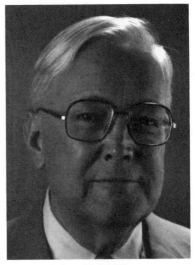

Robert W. McGilvery.

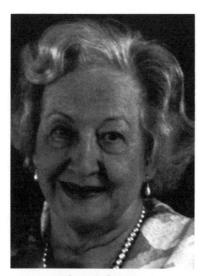

Lucy F. Squire.

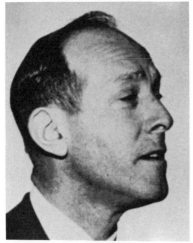

Richard H. Marshak.

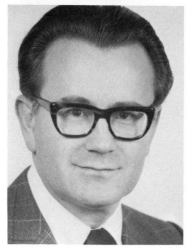

Norbert W. Tietz.

and character of excellence that would distinguish all the series titles. 1970 also saw publication of the Marshak and Lindner *Radiology of the Small Intestine*—a book eagerly awaited by all those interested in roentgenology of the gastrointestinal tract—of the immediately successful Tietz *Fundamentals of Clinical Chemistry;* of the first issue of *Human Pathology*—a vehicle for new thought and new ideas, but not all of them originating from experience with humans—and of the first issue of the *Orthopedic Clinics of North America*—a book-journal in direct competition with other similar publications but one that would achieve great success and influence—and of the Evans and Cruickshank *Epithelial Tumours of the Salivary Glands,* the first and an excellent title in the series Major Problems in Pathology under the editorship of James L. Bennington. Bennington would later direct compilation of the *Saunders Encyclopedia and Dictionary of Laboratory Medicine and Technology*—a reference source of incomparable value.

Khorana synthesizes the first artificial gene. Discovery of reverse transcriptase by Temin and Mizutani brings molecular virology to the forefront of cancer research. The first cardiac pacemaker is implanted. Axelrod, Katz and von Euler receive the Nobel Prize for work on humoral transmission in nerves.

1971

Saunders goes on a popular work schedule of a four-and-a-half-day week. Its effects are unknown except for general employee satisfaction.

Publication of the Hogan-Alvarado-Weddell *Histology of the Human Eye*—one of the most beautifully illustrated books in a field in which elegant illustration is both customary and mandatory; and of the Hardy *Critical Surgical Illness*—a book summarizing the sudden new array of concepts and techniques applicable to the care of the critically ill surgical patient, especially those experiencing metabolic imbalances. The first issue of the *Veterinary Clinics of North America* also appears in 1971, and Saunders launches the first of its audio-tape series with *Pediatric Conferences with Sydney Gellis.*

234

The structure of the gonadotropin-releasing factor is determined. Sutherland receives the Nobel Prize for discovery of cyclic adenosine monophosphate (cAMP).

The London Company begins its indigenous publishing program and brings out within the year the first issues of three new international Clinics: *Gastroenterology, Endocrinology and Metabolism,* and *Hematology.*

1972

Harry R. Most becomes Acting President of the CBS Education and Publishing Group and, later, President of the Macmillan Book Company; and Theodore vanden Beemt, Executive Vice President, becomes the new Saunders President. A certified public accountant who knew that figures are not the main point of life or even of publishing, Ted never allowed his extensive background in finance to dominate his thinking as president. He properly regarded writing as a mysterious process whose motivations and very content are difficult to analyze or even account for. He enjoyed dealing with authors and felt of editorial gaffes that he should let sleeping dogs lie. In fine, a vigilant but sympathetic chief executive who did make one foray into the cloud-shrouded editorial world. He insisted that Saunders publish a gadgety book called *The Doctor's Easaccount System.* Any editors reading here will be pleased to learn that it sold fewer copies than any other book Saunders published—indeed, for all anybody knows, fewer than any book anybody has published. Under his presidency the Linofilm Department added a PDP-8 computer to achieve a high level of both sophistication and versatility in film composition. Perhaps because Ted vanden Beemt understood computers, computerized composition fell into none of those traps that betrayed the earlier electronic accounting venture.

Over many years Saunders and other publishers had tried without noticeable success to produce an encyclopedia-dictionary in nursing to compete with the F. A. Davis *Taber's Cyclopedic Dictionary of Medicine*; and in 1972 Saunders did it with the Miller and Keane *Encyclopedia and Dictionary of Medicine and Nursing* (see also Chapter 18). The year also saw publication of the first of the brief and brilliant Shelley *Consultations in Dermatology*—perhaps not quite as widely sold as it should have been, because many physician book-buyers still equate wisdom with weight (but the wise and elegant *Advanced Dermatologic Therapy* he would later write with his wife Dorinda would become an immediate success); and of the Tachdjian two-volume *Pediatric Orthopedics* (see Chapter 11). Dave Sabiston becomes editor of the *Davis-Christopher Textbook of Surgery* (see Chapter 10) and Saunders publishes *Early Care of the Injured Patient* from the Committee on Trauma of the American College of Surgeons.

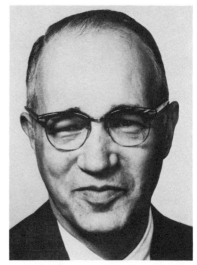

Benjamin F. Miller.

235

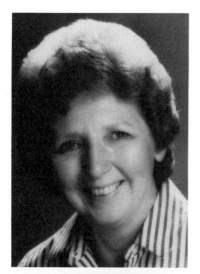

Claire B. Keane.

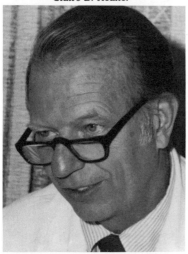

Robert A. Chase.

Guillemin isolates somatostatin, suggesting the possible role of growth hormone in the pathophysiology of diabetes. The Nobel Prize in Chemistry is awarded to Anfinsen, Moore and Stein for their studies on ribonuclease.

1973

Publication of the Chase *Atlas of Hand Surgery*—beautifully illustrated by Daisy Stilwell and having its origin as part of a plan for a much larger work that, perhaps wisely, was never completed; of the Sloane *Medical Word Book*—Saunders' first entry, and a good one, into the growing and increasingly professional field of medical transcription; of the Conn-Rakel-Johnson *Family Practice*—a comprehensive exposition of both the principles and practice of a new specialty in medicine that would help restore dignity and usefulness to general practice; of the Linton *Atlas of Vascular Surgery*—a magnificently illustrated depiction of the fine details of blood-vessel surgery; of the three-volume Youmans *Neurological Surgery*—the kind of complete and expert monograph that Ryland Greene, as editor and publisher, would have greatly admired; of the Hill *Outpatient Surgery*—a sophisticated succesor to the Christopher *Minor Surgery*; of the Warwick and Williams Thirty-fifth Edition of *Gray's Anatomy* (see

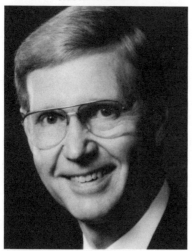

Robert E. Rakel.

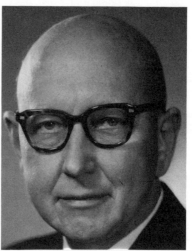

Robert R. Linton.

236

Chapter 20) and of Moore's *The Developing Human*—a modern brief treatment of development that would again give Saunders the leading textbook in embryology, the Arey having grown too detailed for the less rigorous science of the preclinical years of medical education.

Chang and Cohen and Bayer and Heiling construct molecules that combine genetic information from two somas. Their work with that of other molecular biologists further opens the prospect through gene manipulation of constructing bacterial cells that can synthesize a variety of biologically produced substances and of introducing genetic information into plant or animal cells.

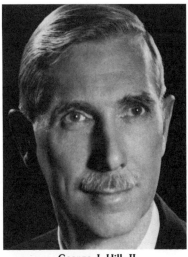

George J. Hill, II.

1974

John J. Hanley is named Vice President and Editor in Health Sciences, succeeding John Dusseau, and Albert E. Meier is appointed Vice President and Editor for Serial Publications. The future looks bright, and 65,000 square feet of warehouse space are added to the Cherry Hill plant.

Publication of the Nathan and Oski *Hematology of Infancy and Childhood*—the definitive collaborative work of brilliant investigators and clinicians with a lovely introductory "Pediatric Hematology in Historical Perspective" by Wolf Zuelzer. The year also saw publica-

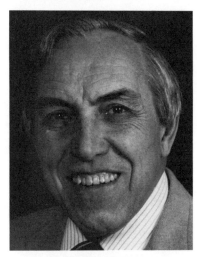

Keith L. Moore.

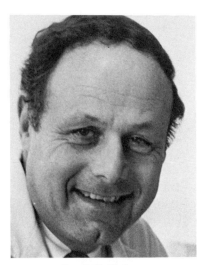

David G. Nathan.

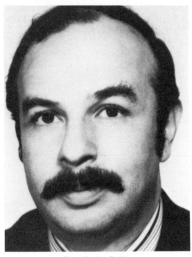

Frank A. Oski.

tion of the Luckmann and Sorensen *Medical-Surgical Nursing: A Psychophys-iologic Approach*—the culmination of years of unremitting work by its authors and of patient counsel and support from Nursing Editor Bob Wright and his later successor in that post, Helen Dietz, authors and editors together creating what is possibly the most widely used nursing textbook ever published. The Twenty-fifth Edition of *Dorland's Illustrated Medical Dictionary* is composed by computer and the entire entry file converted to magnetic tape, in an attempt to replace thousands of boxes of cards that had stubbornly refused to stay in proper order or to be uniformly legible.

The Nobel Prize is awarded to Claude, deDuve and Palade for their pioneering work in cell biology. Congress passes the National Health Planning and Resources Development Act.

1975

The Saunders medical, dental, veterinary and nursing departments are at their peak levels of performance; and the college lists in biology, chemistry, physics, mathematics, psychology and physical education are both solid and promising. Saunders is recognized as the leading publisher of the world in health sciences—a position it had long held but one it continued to enjoy only because of its willingness to break old molds but abide by a steadfast belief in excellence. W. D. Watson began his little history of the Saunders Company with a homely but pointed sentence: "Anyone would be proud to be associated with a business that has come from the very bottom of an industry to the very top."

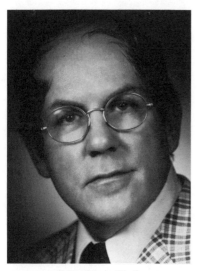

Peter James Dyck.

Publication of the Dyck, Thomas and Lambert two-volume *Peripheral Neuropathy*—one of the many splendid clinical monographs from the Mayo Clinic; of the two-volume Ettinger *Textbook of Veterinary Internal Medicine*—to become a standard reference in veterinary education and in the practice of small-animal veterinary medicine; and of the Rothman and Simeone *The Spine* in two volumes—the work of an orthopedic surgeon and a neurosurgeon with profound understanding of the importance of each specialty to the other.

238

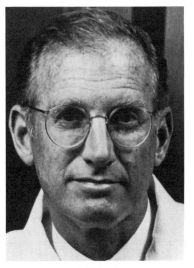

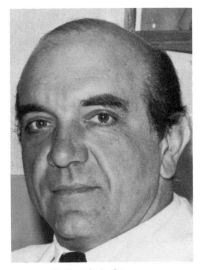

Richard H. Rothman.   Frederick A. Simeone.

Cohn and Hirsch at the Rockefeller Institute show that the granules of white blood cells are true lysosomes. The Nobel Prize is awarded to Dulbecco, Baltimore and Temin for their research studies relating to the pathogenesis of cancer.

Celebration of the bicentennial (see also Chapter 12) of a nation that spends a greater portion of its gross national product on health care and on medical research than that of any other country. It also publishes more journals and books (including, one might say, this one) devoted to these subjects than those of any other four nations.

1976

Meantime the researches of science pursue even smaller particles. Genetics did not rest until it had hypothesized a submicroscopic world of hydrogen bonds linking atoms in the structure of the double helix. But when the life sciences are reduced to study of the motion of electrons, we are left to stare at spinning electrons. Medicine reminds us that science has goals linked to the human condition.

> It is often pointed out that research in the basic sciences provides the base of new knowledge essential for the development of the applied sciences, including medicine. We are less frequently reminded that the reverse can also occur. Research directed against a specific medical problem has resulted in contributions to fundamental biological knowledge. The most dramatic example of this is the discovery that deoxyribonucleic acid (DNA) is the substance that transmits genetic information. From the initial discovery of the phenomenon known as "the transformation of pneumococcal types" until the identification of the transforming substance as DNA, all of the researchers were medical bacteriologists primarily interested in the cause and control of human pneumonia.
>
> Maclyn McCarty: *The Transforming Principle*

PART IV

THE PRESENT

21

A Decade of Change

By Albert E. Meier

In America's bicentennial year the Saunders catalog featured a striking cover illustration of Independence Hall and listed 776 active titles. Just above half were medical books; but 260 titles plus their associated lab manuals and study guides comprised the Saunders college textbook list at that time. The college publishing program was a vigorous one, traditionally strong in biology and chemistry but expanding into such disciplines as business and police science.

1976

In addition to the medical and college lists the 1976 catalog showed 75 active nursing titles, 47 in dentistry, and 21 in veterinary medicine, all important if necessarily smaller lists than in medicine. And all of these titles so far enumerated were free-standing books published from West Washington Square. Saunders also sold books published by its London affiliate, translations and coeditions of books originating at outstanding European houses, and the "Clinics," of which there were then 20 series (five from London, the rest published in Philadelphia).

Worthy of note was the company's increasing involvement with audiovisual titles, either as supplements to books or as independent projects. An early and successful venture was a set of slides used for teaching positioning to radiologic technologists. Made from the illustrations in *Radiographic Positioning and Related Anatomy* by Isadore Meschan, the slides enabled instructors to emphasize key points while students could later refer to the same pictures in their own copies of the textbook. A similar approach was used in connection with several other books in the early 1970s and indeed continues today.

More of an innovation perhaps and clearly a response to demand were the audiovisual titles designed for self-study. In that era a perceived shortage of teaching time, especially on the individual student level, was a problem throughout health science education. Anatomy, embryology, and pathology lent themselves particularly well to coordinated filmstrips and audio tapes

243

(no personal computers back then). In 1976 Saunders offered no fewer than 58 separate audiovisual programs of one kind or another, including experimental ventures in patient education.

To be sure medical books were the Saunders mainstay. In celebration of our nation's bicentennial Saunders offered *Two Centuries of American Medicine*, written by James Bordley, III, of the Mary Imogene Bassett Hospital, Cooperstown, and A. McGehee Harvey of Johns Hopkins University. *Two Centuries* wasn't quite published on the Fourth of July, but it *was* appropriately priced at $19.76.

In their preface these two distinguished clinician-authors, collaborators as well on an earlier Saunders textbook of *Differential Diagnosis*, pointed to the enormous role of the federal government in American medicine:

> After World War II, massive financial support for medical research came from the federal government. The atomic bomb had been developed by unlimited funding of nuclear research, and the belief became prevalent that in order to conquer the remaining great killer-diseases, such as cancer, cardiovascular disease, and kidney disease, it was necessary only to allocate huge sums to medical research. So much emphasis and so much money were devoted to research that medical education and medical care were relatively neglected at a time when both of these attributes of medicine were increasing almost prohibitively in cost. As a result of the concentration upon research, much new and valuable knowledge was acquired, and new forms of therapy were devised, but as the second century reached its end, the major killer-diseases were still unconquered. In the last decade of the nation's second century, the federal government shifted its principal emphasis, in the domain of medicine, from support of research to support of the planning and delivery of health services. A nagging residual question that can only be answered by future experience is whether medical care of the high quality made possible by a century of extraordinary progress in medical science can be delivered to the entire population at a level of funding, whether by taxation or insurance, that the public can afford and will tolerate.

The question still nags. Changing governmental priorities and the continuing high cost of medical care have altered the practice of medicine and force continuing reassessment of publishing goals and strategies. It was in 1976, too, that CBS put in place a new senior management team at Saunders as part of an effort to direct some of the company's attention toward new businesses. Extensive (and expensive) groundwork was laid, for example, in the area of medical books for the general public. These endeavors, it seems, were distracting at a time when the basic business faced an uncertain, but certainly changing, environment.

Among the new medical books published in 1976, three deserve mention as examples of a broad range. There was as yet no list identified as directed to the allied health professions; but such a list would soon be formed out of the medical textbook program, and one of its foundation stones was *The Language of Medicine* by Davi-Ellen Chabner. An understanding of medical terminology is basic to the further education of medical technologists, office assistants, radiologic technologists and all the other professionals who participate in today's health care. Though larger and more expensive than

244

some competing texts, *The Language of Medicine* was readily accepted. Sales increased in every year that the first edition was in print, establishing a pattern that has since been seen with other successful titles in the allied health disciplines.

As specialization sharpened the focus of most practicing physicians, publication of clinical references in narrower fields than formerly became not only possible but vital. Such works shared with the more general ones certain requirements for success: first, the happy combination of eminent authors, authoritative contributors, and a genuinely significant topic; and second, the ability of busy authors to actually carry out the task set for themselves in minimal time. Largely memories now are the painstakingly composed distillations of a life's work that in earlier times constituted many of the landmarks of publishing in medical subspecialties. Today's sophisticated readers demand currency; published reviews consistently cite the dates of the most recent references. Authors and publishers alike adhere as best they can to ever faster schedules.

Two examples will be chosen from 1976, in quite different areas. *Infectious Diseases of the Fetus and Newborn Infant* was edited by Jack S. Remington, a Stanford internist, and Jerome O. Klein, a Harvard pediatrician. Fellows together at the Thorndike Memorial Laboratory (Harvard Medical Unit, Boston City Hospital) in the early 1960s, these distinguished scientists sustained a joint interest in the subject of infections of the fetus and newborn infant and their long-term effects. Their work and that of their contributing writers proved to have wide appeal in the specialties of neonatology and infectious disease—disciplines that had scarcely existed a decade earlier.

With publication of *The Kidney* renal medicine was added to gastroenterology as subspecialties of internal medicine covered by substantial Saunders reference books based solidly in pathophysiology. Barry M. Brenner and Floyd C. Rector, Jr., both at the University of California, San Francisco, School of Medicine when the plans for the book were made and when the first edition appeared, have both made significant contributions to the understanding of kidney function. Their inspiration, and the charge they gave to their contributors, was to analyze disorders of whole kidney function in terms of alterations of function at the nephron and cellular levels. Called by one reviewer "a clinical house built of basic science bricks," *The Kidney* became as soon as it was published the standard reference work in nephrology.

Saunders had previously published a two-volume nephrology edited by Jean Hamburger of Paris and translated from French. The need for a contemporary work of American origin was apparent, and the Saunders editor had gotten as far as a preliminary plan and a list of potential authors. Marvin Sleisenger telephoned from San Francisco to say that his colleague Barry Brenner was thinking about undertaking a major book on the kidney and that if it went forward it would without any doubt be an excellent work. Was Saunders interested?

As it happened the Saunders editor was scheduled to spend most of the following week in San Francisco, and a meeting with Dr. Brenner was soon arranged. The trip was already crowded with appointments and was in connection with a national medical meeting, so that the initial discussion of *The Kidney* took place over pots of coffee late one evening in the editor's room at the San Francisco Hilton. A fruitful discussion it was, too; the editor's outline was quickly discarded, to be replaced in time by the plan that had much to do with making the book the success that it was.

1977 The never-ending watch for emerging medical disciplines susceptible of being defined in comprehensive reference works has certainly given the Saunders list a fair number of extra-base hits but also a few slow rollers that never get out of the infield. In the spring of 1977, after years of preparation, Saunders published to critical acclaim a three-volume 1700-page book on *Forensic Medicine*. Conceived and begun by Cesare Tedeschi of Boston University and the Framingham Union Hospital, the work was completed after his death by his son Luke and William G. Eckert.

Defining their subject as concerning "the causes of death, identity of the living and dead, results of injuries of all kinds, effects of violent crimes and unnatural offenses, and the nature of toxic or lethal agents," the authors and the international experts in medicine and law who contributed richly detailed chapters anticipated that *Forensic Medicine* would attract the lawyer who "wants to know how far medical science can go" and the physician who "must be acquainted with the legal theories pertinent to trauma and hazards." Perhaps, indeed, it did; but in that case there were not all that many such people. The first printing, somewhat under half the estimated total sale, remained in stock for many years. Plans for an annual or biennial supplement were shelved.

Elegantly written, comprehensive, and attractively produced, *Forensic Medicine* even won awards, and indeed it gathered between its covers medical expertise and legal precedent unique in the literature of the two professions. But the best that can be said for its commercial success is that it failed to earn a return on the considerable investment.

An important development in surgery during the early 1970s was the move toward separation of vascular surgery as a subspecialty, consisting mainly of reconstructive procedures for occlusive disease of the arteries. Skilled surgeons who dedicated themselves to vascular problems had not been rare. Saunders had published Robert R. Linton's *Atlas of Vascular Surgery* in 1973. The development of noninvasive diagnostic techniques together with surgical advances had subsequently combined to remove peripheral vascular disease from the realm of internal medicine almost completely.

In 1977, well before vascular surgery had its own certifying examination, Saunders published *Vascular Surgery*, edited by Robert B. Rutherford of the University of Colorado and a group of associates. These editors provided an apt description of how new surgical and medical specialties come into being: "Vascular surgery," they wrote, "has emerged as a specialty at least to the extent that it now represents an identifiably separate area of special interest within surgery and one that is of sufficient scope and complexity to occupy all or most of the time and interest of an increasing number of surgeons. It is not improbable that in the future, *major* elective vascular surgical procedures will be performed only by those with proper formal training and extensive personal experiences in this field. Whether this training consists of a separate distinct experience during a general surgical residency or a postgraduate vascular fellowship, and whether these qualifications are eventually formalized by board certification or bestowed by a certificate of competence, are, for the moment, immaterial. At the very least, it seems clear that the vascular surgical experience in general surgical residencies should no longer be random and diffuse but concentrated and closely supervised, so that those who elect to pursue vascular surgery as a major professional interest may be assured an adequate opportunity to gain competence. Equally clear is the need for continuing experience so that competence can be maintained."

To take advantage of the emergence of new disciplines is the task of the innovative medical publisher, the house that would rather lead than follow. To define the content and scope of a reference book, on the other hand, is the task of the author. Conceived and put under contract at 800 pages, the Rutherford *Vascular Surgery* came in at over 1400 pages. Its sales exceeded its publisher's expectations.

1978

The path toward publication of the Langman-Woerdeman *Atlas of Medical Anatomy* began with a telephone call from Jan Langman to the Saunders editor shortly before Christmas 1973. Professor and chairman of the Department of Anatomy at Charlottesville, Dr. Langman was a renowned teacher and author of a best-selling embryology textbook published not by Saunders but by Williams & Wilkins in Baltimore. The embryology text, in its first (1963) edition, had been translated into eight languages, possibly a record for a medical textbook, and both book and author were known all over the world.

Professor Langman had been born in Holland and was educated there, and he was well acquainted with Martin W. Woerdeman. Nearly 80 at the time of that first telephone call, Professor Woerdeman had undertaken preparation of an anatomy atlas back in the late 1930s. Preparation and labeling of some two thousand drawings by a team of illustrators was interrupted by World War II, when the completed plates had to be securely hidden in a safe place outside Amsterdam. The Woerdeman atlas was published finally in 1948, entirely in black and white and profusely labeled in Latin.

The new atlas was projected to involve about half of the Woerdeman plates with color overlays added, much of the labeling deleted, the remaining labels changed to English and, most significantly, clinically oriented text material was to be added so that medical students would be able to see how the anatomy was to be used in their subsequent education and in practice.

Compared with preparation of an altogether new atlas, here was an opportunity to secure a major work at reasonable cost and in a reasonable amount of time. The aim was to challenge, possibly even to dislodge, the most popular of all anatomy atlases, prepared by J. C. Boileau Grant of the University of Toronto and first published by Williams & Wilkins in 1943. The chance had to be taken; the opportunity was too good to pass up.

Still, the cost would not be small, and the risk was considerable. From the start the plan was to secure commitments to translate the work from leading medical publishers in many countries. Dr. Langman's reputation and the existing successful translations of his embryology book were expected to pave the way to these arrangements. Saunders would then be able to make a substantial initial printing of the illustrations only and make the printed sheets available to translating publishers, thus reducing the cost per copy for all the parties.

When the first sections of the atlas were put into production it was with the highest of hopes and the greatest of expectations, but not without a nagging worry that the project was more difficult than had been anticipated. Though many labels were being deleted, many remained, and the task of positioning these on reproductions of the plates, already reduced to their final dimensions, was a tedious one. Leader lines, which connect the labels to the indicated structures, had been included within the original art; removing the now unwanted ones took time and great effort. Meanwhile, in Charlottesville, Professor Langman superintended the preparation of color overlays, a process itself confounded by the nature of the original art, for an added color looked different with variations in the gray tone beneath.

Type was set and pasted-up page dummies were prepared, but new complications arose. Sometimes there was too much text, so that a page was overcrowded even with the illustrations reduced. Sometimes there was not enough. Many drawings were clearly too small for teaching effectiveness, meaning that new labels had to be set and put in place to accompany the revised, larger reproductions. Illustrations that logically belonged together, so that they could be compared, stubbornly refused to fit in spite of a generous page size.

Art director, illustration coordinator and book designer persisted. There were conferences, lengthy memos, trips to Charlottesville and innumerable telephone calls. Illustrations were added and deleted, reduced and enlarged, labeled and re-labeled. Color overlays were done and re-done. Time was passing, and costs were mounting.

Page proof of the first section, on the thorax, was ready in January 1977, when for the first time more than just a few people were able to see how the long-awaited atlas was shaping up. "I'm not terribly impressed," said a note from one of Saunders' sales principals. "The main criticism from my colleagues concerns the small size of the drawings," wrote Dr. Langman. "Sorry we cannot take over German edition," cabled Thieme from Stuttgart; "the illustrations were published (in a German edition) 20 years ago with little success."

If these were storm warnings, they went unheeded, the hard-working crew proceeding under full sail. Publication in April 1978 was with great fanfare including a reception at the Anatomists' meeting in Vancouver. An exuberant first printing and boundless editorial enthusiasm ("one of our most important medical books for the remainder of this century") helped to establish the selling price at an attractively competitive level.

Professor Langman went off to Berlin on sabbatical leave not long thereafter, and waited anxiously for the good news that was not to come. Shipments of the atlas that first summer were disappointing; teachers did not think the small pictures would make the book useful in the dissecting room, and in time, when the students were queried on this point, they agreed. Teacher and student alike gave high marks to the newly written and stimulating text; but in this as in any atlas the words could not save the pictures. Even the committed translations mostly failed to materialize.

Thus the Langman-Woerdeman joined the line of atlases that had tried but failed to dethrone Grant's, still on top today after so many years. It took a trade paperback edition a few years later to finally exhaust the storehouse of printed sheets. Years after that a proposed revision by new authors (Dr. Langman having died) was, wisely, abandoned.

Happier publishing stories of 1978 included the thirtieth annual *Current Therapy* volume, its appeal like that of *Grant's Atlas* undimmed by time and by the sweeping changes in medical education and medical practice over the years. In that year too Saunders published *Principles and Practice of Emergency Medicine,* edited by George Schwartz, Peter Safar, John Stone, Patrick Storey and David Wagner. Capitalizing again on the need of a nascent medical specialty to establish its boundaries and define its territory, the two-volume work stood alone in the field for some time. It enjoyed an enthusiastic critical reception and had spectacular and sustained success in the marketplace.

Spectacular too in its own way was the beginning of an ongoing venture that came after some discussion to be titled simply the Saunders Blue Book Series. Pocket-sized (at least in the beginning) and spiral-bound, each Blue Book was a concise compendium, sometimes in outline form, of a specific subject area. The first offering dealt with *Emergency Medical Therapeutics* and was priced at $9.95. It had been conceived and was largely written by Mickey S. Eisenberg of Seattle, whose enthusiasm and energy for the project were soon put to further good use when he became consulting editor for the series.

Linked by their common purpose and by an overall similarity in format and design, the Blue Books benefited by being members of an identifiable family and later by special bookstore promotion that included a free-standing rack designed specifically to accommodate them. The list expanded quickly and eventually stood at 30 titles, ranging from *Admitting Orders* to *Pharmacologic Therapeutics.*

1979   In 1979 the Saunders medical publishing staff devoted most of its time and effort to a number of new titles that appeared in succeeding years, some breaking new ground and others representing logical extensions of formulas that had worked well in the past. In addition revisions of "Cecil" and of "Nelson" were published, and in each there was a strong new editorial voice, as James B. Wyngaarden, then chairman of medicine at Duke, joined Paul Beeson and Walsh McDermott in "Cecil" and Richard E. Behrman, chairman of pediatrics at Case Western Reserve, came into "Nelson." But in terms of altogether new books, 1979 was principally a year of attention to the nursing list and to allied health, now identified as a separate publishing discipline.

Whatever publishing news there was in that year was overshadowed for many Saunders people by the corporate decision to consolidate its college publishing activities. The entire Saunders college operation, which had overlapped with that of Holt, Rinehart & Winston in a few subject areas, was placed under Holt's direction.

This change followed by about a year another switch in Saunders management. In its first 88 years Saunders had four presidents, and its progress throughout those years was evolutionary. But in the last 12 years under CBS there were also four presidents. Each brought to the office (or was given) a somewhat different set of expectations. At the same time, each has needed to respond to direction given by senior managers in New York, which has undergone changes of its own.

Separation of the college publishing business removed sales dollars from Saunders while leaving behind essentially all of the assets invested in the business. College textbooks, with their long press runs and two-color requirements, necessitated certain types of printing equipment which could not be as efficiently utilized once the college work was taken away. Promotion of basic science textbooks from the medical list into undergraduate departments was not feasible without the flow of new books and new editions in biology and chemistry that had made up the bulk of the work of the textbook representatives. Thus the repercussions of the divorce had long-term effects that may not have been fully realized even today.

1980   The seed that had been planted when Eugene Braunwald was invited to undertake a new reference book in cardiology bore fruit in May 1980, when the first edition of *Heart Disease: A Textbook of Cardiovascular Medicine* was published. Already one of the busiest people in American medicine, Dr. Braunwald had found the time and energy to participate in the writing of close to half its chapters—this in a two-volume work of over 1900 large pages.

Reviewers were impressed and enthusiastic, one calling *Heart Disease* "the gold standard" against which future books in cardiology would have to be measured. Sales were gratifyingly substantial; but even though the book enjoyed a wide sale, its record underscored the need for a medical publisher never to lose sight of the changing marketplace. When the second edition

250

was in active preparation the Saunders editor observed to Dr. Braunwald that the first edition had probably outsold any other contemporary work in its field but had not come up to the third edition of Friedberg's *Diseases of the Heart*, published 14 years earlier. "Why not?" was Dr. Braunwald's reasonable question. "Because there are so many more cardiologists now," said the editor. In the 1960s generalists still purchased books like these; in the 1980s they do not.

As the medical specialties grow in the power of their theories about normal and disordered physiology and in their ability to diagnose and to treat, they grow as well in numbers, until, imperceptibly or suddenly, new subdisciplines begin to form, because no one can master the expanding range of essential knowledge. Even as the publisher strives to take advantage of increasing medical specialization, he is aware that the potential audience for each of his titles is shrinking. Smaller print runs cause increased prices, which logically must work to further limit sales. The business problem thus posed had become apparent earlier; but as the 1980s began it was an overriding concern.

The pages of this history are full of examples of books whose gestation took not months but years. Faithfully carrying through commitments made in years past, when times were different, is common enough in publishing; but perhaps uniquely in medical and scientific publishing not only the material but also the audience may have changed significantly between signing the contract and publishing the book. Guessing about the future is not a productive enterprise. Rather hold fast to faith in the knowledge and experience of the author, who even more than the publisher wants to do a useful and not a useless book.

Five years was the development time for *Clinical Pediatric Dermatology* by Sidney Hurwitz, published by Saunders in 1981. Dr. Hurwitz had devoted the early years of his medical career to a general pediatric practice in New Haven before he took a residency in dermatology at Yale and then concentrated his private practice on disorders of the skin in children. As a private practitioner Dr. Hurwitz brought to the book both extensive experience and evident enthusiasm, but like most authors in private practice he had a limited amount of time and resources to dedicate to the project. The Saunders editor viewed these limitations as minor, for what was wanted (and specified in the contract) was a small book that was directed to pediatricians and that could be sold for $20.

1981

There was little or no competition for such a work, even though the number of pediatricians was large and even though a sizable proportion of their patients come to them with skin problems. Saunders had traditionally offered a wide range of titles in pediatrics and almost always had success in selling them. The proposed dermatology book was to be another pearl on the string.

As Dr. Hurwitz slowly assembled his material and wrote his chapters, late at night and entirely by himself, the nature of his book began to change in a way that, at one stage, made his editor uneasy. In the first place it was clear that the finished work would be not only much longer but also much more comprehensive than had been anticipated, for there was a good deal of descriptive material on, for example, the histologic diagnosis of skin lesions, not contemplated in the original plan and not perhaps essential to the generalist pediatrician. Moreover, and more worrisome, Dr. Hurwitz had reached the firm conclusion that the clinical illustrations would have to be reproduced in color. So certain was he that color was not only desirable but necessary that he offered to subvent the cost of the color separations.

Still clinging to the notion of a practical and inexpensive book for pediatricians, perhaps unwilling to take into account the fact that dermatologists constituted a good market too, the editor took an unusual next step. Clinical books for practicing physicians, as opposed to textbooks for medical students, have been only rarely sent out for review prior to publication. But most of the manuscript chapters of the pediatric dermatology were shown to other authorities in the field. The editor supposed that the reviewers would confirm his fears, while the author embraced the idea of reviews in the hope that the reviewers might offer valuable suggestions and guidance.

In the event the comments were surprisingly uniform. The book must be published just as it was, they said, for the need was great and the material appropriate. And of course the illustrations must be in color. The proferred subsidy allowed the project to make economic sense, at least on paper, while Dr. Hurwitz was so buoyed by the favorable opinions of his peers that he redoubled his efforts to complete the work.

Book and audience had indeed changed with time, but both in the same direction. Pediatricians and dermatologists alike welcomed *Clinical Pediatric Dermatology,* which proceeded to reach a sales level almost twice the prediction and which continued to sell even five years after publication. The subsidy was never mentioned again, because it was neither needed nor desired. The editor's faith in the author was more than amply confirmed.

Also culminating in 1981 were several other major projects of long standing. Chief among these was the "International Textbook of Medicine." In the beginning an innovative publishing venture with far-reaching potential, the International Textbook was altered by world political events and by other factors into something at once greater and less than its concept had promised.

When the Shah still ruled Iran his government laid plans to bring the nation's health care fully up to the high technological standards of the industrialized countries. Leader of the program was the American-trained minister of health, Dr. A.H. Samiy, and the element of the plan that involved the Saunders Company was the development of a new medical textbook.

In Iran as in most developing countries even the best doctors had available, if they had any books at all, little more than an anatomy textbook and perhaps a pathology. The whole sweep of pathophysiologic explication so characteristic of post-1950 medical science in the developed world was closed to these physicians. Furthermore a large part of medical practice in the "third world" was concerned with diseases of infectious origin. Accordingly the "International Textbook" was to comprise three volumes: one on pathophysiology, one on infectious disease, and one on "all the rest" of medicine, which it was thought might most easily be prepared by condensation of an existing major textbook such as "Cecil."

The government of Iran was prepared to underwrite the production cost of the new books and, later, to somehow arrange that the books were made available in developing nations at very low prices. Any medical publisher would have been interested. The opportunity to disseminate the best of contemporary American medicine into parts of the world where even pirated editions were expensive was inherently attractive.

Abridging the "Cecil" textbook was not a new idea. A modest-sized textbook of medicine had long been on the Saunders want list. After Paul Beeson and Walsh McDermott had struggled valiantly and managed to cut practically nothing out of some representative chapters, an altogether new work by authors not involved with "Cecil" was put under contract. It proceeded as far as a comprehensive outline and some sample manuscript before drifting and sadly running aground.

The practical realities of the situation in the late 1970s, with the editorial responsibility for "Cecil" shifting to Holly Smith and Jim Wyngaarden, required that the third volume of the "International Textbook" be in fact the full-blown unabridged Sixteenth Edition of "Cecil," published a year behind the other two volumes but in a similar binding style and identified as part of the "International Textbook" by agreement with Dr. Samiy, who in the meantime had escaped from his native country in advance of the upheaval that deposed the Shah.

Meantime the pathophysiology volume was undertaken by Holly Smith and Samuel O. Thier, then chairman of medicine at Yale, with a relatively small group of distinguished physician-scientists as chapter authors. In execution it was a magnificent single-volume treatment of an extraordinarily complex subject. Filled with illuminating diagrams and buttressed by selected and annotated references, *Pathophysiology* was moreover written in a remarkably short time and was thoroughly up to date when it was published. But a reference work for the third world it was not. It found great favor among American medical residents, whose numbers were hardly sufficient to justify the project, and among academic physicians, too many of whom wished for complimentary copies. Medical students in the main were daunted by its size and price, for in spite of the imperial subvention *Pathophysiology* was a substantial and expensive book. Most unfortunately it ran almost head-on into an existing successful Saunders book—*Pathologic Physiology*, first published in 1950, originally edited by William A. Sodeman of Jefferson Medical College and taken over in later years by his sons William Jr. and Thomas. What had been a sizable market for a single book was now split in two.

Medical Microbiology and Infectious Disease, volume 2 of the "International Textbook," was ably headed up by Abraham I. Braude of San Diego, a scientist of international stature who, by attracting talented contributors from all over the world and by including infectious diseases not commonly seen in developed countries, came closest to realizing the early objectives that had been set for the three-volume work. Sales of this volume were satisfactory if not spectacular, there being two strong competitors for it, but certainly the book filled a long-felt gap in the Saunders list.

In the end there was virtually no combined sale of all three volumes of the "International Textbook," and shipments of the volumes outside the United States were far from uniform in quantity. Each book was promoted on its own, to its own audience, and even the common binding has not been maintained in subsequent editions.

The "International Textbook of Medicine" was not the only sizable project brought to completion in 1981, for in that year as well Saunders published four new clinical reference works as sets of two or more volumes. Especially when several of them are in production at once, such works place unusual burdens on the dedicated Saunders people who labor to accomplish the magical transition from manuscript to book. Manuscript editors, illustration coordinators, typesetters, proofreaders, and production managers struggle every day with incomplete and out-of-sequence manuscript, far-flung and sometimes unreachable contributors, indifferent illustrations and so many more details. In the end only the results of their labors are visible to the reader; but the labor itself is essential to the making of a book.

1982

Once upon a time, when general practitioners and general internists were regarded as more enthusiastic book buyers than they are now, the Saunders commissioned sales force could be relied upon to complain that there simply were not enough titles for these physicians. The sales representatives knew perhaps before the medical schools did that expanding medical knowledge coupled with the inevitable concentration of medical education upon the problems of hospitalized patients left new physicians less than adequately prepared to cope with the continuing care of their ambulatory patients.

Sometimes the salesmen are right. Sometimes they may be right too when they suggest that sales of a book can be spoiled by giving it "a bad title" (or "the wrong title"). Seldom was a title so tediously debated and so frequently changed as in the case of the book that Saunders published in 1982 to address the typical problems presented to office-based internists. In fact, in the first printing of the book, its cover bore one title, its copyright page another—and the catalog data sent to the Library of Congress and printed in the book used yet another title.

Few institutions have been as closely identified with contemporary scientific advances in medicine as the Harvard Medical School and its affiliated hospitals, particularly the Peter Bent Brigham Hospital (now the Brigham and Women's Hospital as a result of consolidation with other nearby institutions). It may seem ironic that a book dedicated to meeting the special needs of the "primary care internist" should emanate from within the walls of the Brigham; but even when the idea for the work first took shape, the provision of an educational foundation for general internal medicine already had a solid history at that hospital. Application of the best of modern medical science to the care of ambulatory patients was being actively studied and taught. What remained was to codify the essentials in book form.

Office Practice of Medicine was edited by William T. Branch, director from its inception in 1973 of the primary care track within the internal medicine residency program at the Brigham, which was started in 1973. Most of the contributors were teachers involved in that program. The book was an expression of their belief "that within a limited number of chapters the vast majority of clinical problems encountered by generalists could be discussed in sufficient depth to be valuable."

That often maligned customer, the general internist, responded enthusiastically, and the commissioned sales force in particular experienced early and continued success with the book. Yet despite that, and considering that such a work might be expected to sell better outside the United States than many more sophisticated and specialized books, the foreign sale was less than 10 per cent of the total. Perhaps the title was wrong. Fortunately the domestic shipments more than made up for the foreign shortfall.

What a range of interesting new titles graced the Saunders list in 1983! This is not a book of lists; but here is a list:

1983

> Bennington *Saunders Dictionary and Encyclopedia of Laboratory Medicine and Technology*
> Bluestone and Stool *Pediatric Otolaryngology*
> Haddad and Winchester *Clinical Management of Poisoning and Drug Overdose*
> Levine, Carey, Crocker and Gross *Developmental-Behavioral Pediatrics*
> Paré and Fraser *Synopsis of Diseases of the Chest*
> Partain *Nuclear Magnetic Resonance (NMR) Imaging*
> Schepens *Retinal Detachment and Allied Diseases*
> Tachdjian *The Child's Foot*
> Tietz *Clinical Guide to Laboratory Tests*

To say a little about each would be to diminish all, so personal preference will be used to pick one that was a more than usually intriguing project. Saunders was not alone among medical publishers in expanding its radiology list as new methods of imaging were developed and introduced. For several years there had been at least as many publishers exhibiting books at the annual meeting of the Radiological Society of North America as at any other specialty meeting. That exhibit hall was equally impressive in the number and scope of equipment displays, even after entangling bureaucratic red tape had begun to restrict the hospitals' ability to go on buying ever more sophisticated tools.

Still there were those in publishing who believed that the radiologic boom had to come to an end, and who were aware that rapid technologic change could work against books essentially technical in nature. Early books on computed tomography, for instance, rapidly became obsolete as later generations of CT scanners replaced the original machines. At the same time medical books in general had come to have shorter lives. Was it possible to develop and publish books even as new imaging modes were just being introduced, with the expectation that such works would not last long but could be justified by the extreme interest in learning about what was new?

C. Leon Partain and his colleagues at Vanderbilt University argued persuasively that radiologists would indeed respond promptly and in considerable numbers to a book intended to explain the physical principles and explore the future possibilities of what was then called "nuclear magnetic resonance" or NMR imaging. When their book was proposed and accepted by Saunders there was not yet a single NMR imaging system set up and functioning anywhere in the United States, though experimental installations existed and equipment manufacturers were gearing up to go into production.

Nuclear Magnetic Resonance (NMR) Imaging was far from a typical clinical reference book. Heavy on physics and light on diagnostic applications, it was quickly though to be sure not carelessly written and just as rapidly published. The sales estimate was cautiously low and the price high. Surely its sales life would not exceed 18 months, so that conservative assumptions were called for.

The 18-month period turned out to be just about right, 90 per cent of the work's ultimate sale being achieved in that time. As for the actual number, it was 50 per cent greater than even the most optimistic projection, serving to demonstrate that at least for a technologically aware group such as radiologists it is possible to publish books right at the cutting edge of advancing medical progress.

1984   For a hundred years or more the great public hospitals of America's large cities were vital elements in the medical care of the indigent population and in medical education. Many of medicine's famed scientists and teachers worked and taught in these public institutions during the late nineteenth and early twentieth centuries. Even after the rise of university-affiliated medical centers the municipal and county hospitals were important in medical education because of the volume and variety of their patients. Only when reduced public funding and increased health insurance coverage (public and private) combined in the years after World War II to diminish the patient populations did the public hospitals begin to decline.

William C. Shoemaker arrived at the Cook County Hospital, Chicago, from a research fellowship at Harvard in 1959, the year in which Saunders published the landmark *Metabolic Care of the Surgical Patient* by Francis D. Moore. Dr. Shoemaker's research interests were centered on the pathophysiology of shock syndromes. The Cook County Hospital was a logical place in which to advance this work, for it not only took care of most of the trauma patients in the midwestern metropolis but also had a history rich in surgical research.

256

Before long Dr. Shoemaker had to confront a serious obstruction to both patient care and research, namely a shortage of qualified nurses at Cook County. The solution to the practical problem of maintaining and improving medical care in spite of the staff shortage was found in an application of a concept already well established in wartime military medicine. Grouping patients according to the severity of their illness made efficient use of a reduced nursing staff, but more than that it suggested to Dr. Shoemaker the possibility of defining and establishing a new field of medical specialization.

During the 1960s the concept of "critical care medicine" was espoused in talks and papers by Dr. Shoemaker and his colleagues in surgery, medicine, pediatrics and anesthesiology. For related reasons other kinds of specialized care units were appearing: trauma units, coronary care units and neonatal intensive care units concentrated clinical expertise on particular categories of seriously ill patients. The "critical care unit" would similarly focus on those who suffered from multiple medical and surgical problems. As a discipline critical care would transcend the boundaries of existing specialties and, in Dr. Shoemaker's words, would be "committed to objective evaluation of physiologic mechanisms that underlie vital organ failures and [to] the development of therapeutic programs and life-support systems for life-threatening problems."

The Society of Critical Care Medicine was founded in 1970 by 26 individuals and had 2,000 members by the end of the decade. To the customary trappings of contemporary specialty societies—a journal, an annual meeting, a periodic self-assessment examination—Critical Care Medicine added an annual state-of-the-art review. Upon approval of subspecialty status, the Society of Critical Care Medicine formulated plans for a comprehensive textbook, which Saunders published in 1984. *The Society of Critical Care Medicine: Textbook of Critical Care*, to use its full and formal title, was edited by Dr. Shoemaker with W. Leigh Thompson and Peter R. Holbrook, and it had contributions from 149 authorities representing fields as diverse as nursing and neurosurgery.

That the textbook should be one of the most widely sold new medical books published by Saunders in the 1980s is not surprising, for its appeal quite naturally cut across traditional specialty lines. The objectives of critical care medicine were impressive too in their far-reaching implications for the future, and they deserve quotation here:

> To define the body of knowledge of critical care;
> To organize and standardize health care professionals' responsibility and authority;
> To define educational objectives and training programs to meet these professional needs;
> To define clinical standards of care for specific diseases and life-threatening conditions;
> To define physiologic criteria and protocols for therapy of critical illnesses based on objective evaluation that can be tested prospectively;
> To develop and test new monitoring devices, automated systems, and other medical instrumentation for use at the bedside;
> To develop and improve life-support systems;

To develop programs for evaluation of cost-effectiveness of specific therapeutic approaches; and

To stimulate research projects and programs to meet specific life-threatening problems.

Only the passage of time will tell whether the *Textbook of Critical Care* was an early signpost on the uncertain road to the hospital of the twenty-first century, a hospital in which continuous automatic biochemical and physiologic measurements provide objective data on the severity of illness and are linked directly to therapy. So vastly different from the public hospitals of fifty years ago where much of medicine was learned and taught, the hospitals of fifty years hence must also be the source of continuing scientific and clinical advances.

1985 New publications were overshadowed by revisions of major works in the Saunders medical list during 1985. Two of the revisions had new authors, as J. Edward Berk led a team of editors in the Fourth Edition of the *Bockus Gastroenterology*, now in seven volumes, and Jean D. Wilson and Daniel W. Foster succeeded Robert H. Williams in the *Textbook of Endocrinology*. Textbooks of medicine, surgery, rheumatology and dermatology also appeared in revised editions during that year.

Five new Blue Books were published in 1985, as were the initial volumes of new paperback textbook series in physiology, medicine and clinical pharmacology. On the clinical side radiology, pathology and surgery were emphasized.

Atlases of surgical procedures were increasingly in demand, and a unique answer to the need was offered among the new books of 1985. Paul D. Kiernan and John P. Hubert, Jr., both former chief residents in surgery at the Mayo Clinic, conceived the idea of gathering into one sourcebook the techniques preferred by Oliver H. Beahrs. Long identified with the general surgery service at the Clinic's affiliated hospitals and widely known as a master of technique, Dr. Beahrs had just retired from the active staff. His younger associates envisioned an atlas as a kind of memorial to his teaching and operating skills; in the end Dr. Beahrs became senior author of the work and contributed much of the focused and detailed commentary on the procedures that brings the illustrations to life.

Among the many categories of medical publishing ventures, surgical atlases are ranked high in two respects. Often they achieve a sale that is not only wide but extends over time—only, to be sure, if they have been well conceived and carefully executed. But they are often difficult to do. Provision of artwork that is anatomically correct and effectively illuminates the surgeon-author's precepts demands extensive skill and experience on the part of the illustrator. Happy combinations of surgeon and artist seldom occur by chance. Even the most auspicious beginnings do not always produce the anticipated results; and preparation of the artwork always takes longer than anyone expected.

Saunders has been fortunate to serve as publisher of many atlases of surgical technique. Introducing each one to the world brings to the Saunders editor a sense of pride in accomplishment somehow different in kind from that which accompanies publication of even the most ambitious of multi-authored clinical references. An atlas is one of the rare books in contemporary medicine that can still depict how one person's experience and considered judgment can turn knowledge into wisdom.

Surgery is an art in which a practical end is sought, so that the interest of a conscientious surgeon in discussion of results and in vivid illustration of effective technique is boundless. Every good surgical meeting and every good surgical book is devoted to the question of how best to attain in both thought and act a desired result.

Acquisition of the Saunders Company by CBS in 1968 was one of many such events happening at about that time as major U.S. corporations sought security in diversity. With the passage of years, and decades, corporate thought turned in other directions. Today the trend is away from diversification, even though the pace of merging and acquiring is, if anything, faster than ever, with deals of breathtaking scope being made almost daily. **1986**

In publishing the mood of the moment is the formation of very large scale organizations, many of them with strong international components. The notion is that markets are better served thereby.

Once again it became the Saunders Company's turn to change owners when CBS arranged to sell all of its book publishing businesses to Harcourt Brace Jovanovich Inc. Announced in October, the transaction was made final at the end of the year. School and college publishing were also involved, and these were areas in which HBJ was already a major force.

The CBS trade publishing operation had already been sold separately, and under its new owners had resumed the old Henry Holt imprint. HBJ in fact had begun back in 1919 when Alfred Harcourt and Donald Brace had left Henry Holt & Sons to go into business on their own.

Prior to the sale to HBJ, CBS had closed the Saunders printing plant, having taken the view that printing and publishing were two different businesses. Long-term contracts were signed with outside printers, who had already taken on much of the company's work. Books with long press runs had been more economically printed outside anyway, especially since new investment in the printing plant had essentially ceased with the loss of the college publishing business several years earlier.

Also in process during 1986 was integration of many Saunders functions into CBS facilities in New York and elsewhere. Order processing and shipping, the customer service office, and almost all back-office operations such as accounting were being consolidated. HBJ moved promptly to replace these plans with new ones that combined Saunders and CBS work into existing HBJ departments in Orlando.

All of these changes, as they evolved, tended to overshadow even the significant publishing during the year. There were 57 new books and 42 new editions with 1986 copyrights, plus 12 imports or translations. Outstanding among the new titles:

- In medical student texts: Andreoli, Carpenter, Plum and Smith: *Cecil Essentials of Medicine*; Hacker and Moore: *Essentials of Obstetrics and Gynecology*; Lookingbill and Marks: *Principles of Dermatology*; Taylor: *How to Choose a Medical Specialty*.
- In clinical medicine: Asbury, McKhann and McDonald: *Diseases of the Nervous System*; Calkins: *The Practice of Geriatrics*; Kokko and Tannen: *Fluids and Electrolytes*; Weber and Janicki: *Cardiopulmonary Exercise Testing*.
- In radiology: Kadir: *Diagnostic Angiography*; Vogler, Helms and Callen: *Normal Variants and Pitfalls in Imaging*; Weissman and Sledge: *Orthopaedic Radiology*.
- In veterinary medicine: Harrison and Harrison: *Clinical Avian Medicine and Surgery*.
- In dentistry: Levine: *Current Treatment in Dental Practice*.
- In nursing: Iyer et al.: *Nursing Process and Nursing Diagnosis*; Knuppel and Drukker: *High Risk Pregnancy*; Ulrich et al.: *Nursing Care Planning Guides*.

There were also far-reaching changes in personnel. Lewis Reines, President of the J. B. Lippincott Company, became the new Saunders president; and Thomas E. Mackey, Jr., President of Grune & Stratton, Inc. (a division of HBJ), became the new Saunders editor in chief with plans to incorporate the Grune & Stratton book list and its strong line of journals into Saunders' operations.

Across many fronts the effort continues: to secure the best authors, to apply the highest production standards and to promote as effectively as we know how. These principles have guided the W. B. Saunders Company through its first 100 years and will guide it as well in the future.

As the writing of this book was being completed the announcement was made that Saunders would celebrate its centenary in new quarters, ending 75 years on West Washington Square. For Saunders as for any publishing house the assets of the business are not the buildings but the people. On their ideas and on their dedicated efforts the first hundred years have been built.

POSTLOGUE

Now that the weary pen is laid down, the jigsaw pieces of leftover manuscript cleared from the kitchen table and the light dimmed, perhaps the author of this memorandum may speak for himself.

I have enjoyed writing this little book, for it is a remembrance of things past—a recollection in tranquility of wonderful association with strong, dedicated, profoundly knowledgeable and sometimes demanding authors. Two things about them might not be suspected by those outside the circle of their work. However authoritative in their decisions, they are surprisingly humble men, for constant preoccupation with disease and death enforces humility.

Nor would one guess from the innumerable self-help style manuals addressed to doctors that the physician-writer is usually a skillful writer. The art of thinking and the art of writing are one, and coherent medicine demands close reasoning. It was a pleasure to read our authors and a pleasure to work with my colleagues at Saunders who respected the good writing of good physicians.

It was an enterprise difficult but enjoyable. An associate of mine once said to a mutual friend, "What a life John leads. Every day he makes decisions, decisions, decisions of far-reaching importance. And you know something? Every once in a while he's right."

Even this small book has required decisions, and I shall be content if a few of them were well-taken. Somehow I recall a decision I once reached after lengthy correspondence with a potential author. After this had gone on for quite a while he wrote, "Dear John: What a beautiful and eloquent letter. So just in its appreciation of my work, so reflective of the rich world of publishing. It was only upon its fourth reading that I realized you were declining to publish my book."

I shall conclude by adapting to myself St. Augustine's famous words: "O Lord, give me chastity and continency, but do not give it yet." I shall say, "O Lord, take from me the burden of my writer's cramp and my writer's itch—but not just yet."

J.L.D.

INDEX OF NAMES

Note: Page numbers in *italics* refer to photographic portraits.

Abian, A., 229
Abt, I.A., 20, 87, 192, *192*, 198, 220
Adams, R., 69, 81
Addison, T., 3
Adler, F.H., 200, *200*
Adrian, E.D., 105
Adriani, J., 192
Aegerter, E., 218
Alan, W., 128
Albee, F.H., 29
Albert, D.M., 200, 233
Albright, F., 59, 75, 80
Alger, H., 43
Allee, W.C., 95, 208
Allen, E.V., 90, 206, *206*
Alvarado, J.A., 234
Alvarez, W., 90, 91, 210, *210*
Amberson, J.B., 193
Andreoli, T., 260
Angell, M., 146
Anson, B.J., 170, 171, 209, *209*
Arey, L.B., 87, 162, 187, *188*, 220, 237
Arny, H.V., 184
Artz, C.P., 221, *221*
Asbury, A.K., 260
Ash, J.E., 205
Aswell, E., 139
Augustine, St., 261
Austrian, C., 106
Avery, M.E., 227, *227*

Bacon, F., 124
Bailey, W., 163
Baker, R.D., 204
Balinsky, B.I., 221
Banks, S.W., 211, *212*
Barcroft, J., 105
Barker, N.W., 90, 206
Barondess, J., 106
Barr, D., 60
Barsky, A.J., 200
Bates, D., 145, 227, *228*
Bateson, W., 76
Bauer, W., 75, 80
Beach, F., 135
Beadle, G.W., 200, *201*
Beahrs, O.H., 258
Bearn, A., 69
Beaverbrook, W., 13, 14
Beckman, H., 113, 120, 196, *196*, 203, 220
Beerman, H., 194

Beeson, P.B., 64–68, 73, 75, 77, 225, 226, *226*, 250, 253
Behnke, J., 95, 208
Behrman, R.E., 111, 250
Bell, J., 95
Bennington, J.L., 234, 255
Bensley, R.R., 53, 54
Bentham, J., 5
Berk, J.E., 204, 258
Bernard, C., 17
Bernhardt, S., 3
Berry, E.W., 80, 101
Best, C.H., 145
Bevan, A., 30, 44
Bickham, W.S., 42, 103, 104, 181, 193, *193*, 214, 220
Bishop of Ravenna, 8
Bistner, S.I., 233
Blackmun, H., 90
Blixen, K., 57
Bloom, M., 52, 54
Bloom, W., 21, 52–55, 162, 196, *196*, 220
Bluestone, C.D., 255
Bockus, H.L., 23, 24, 159, 169, 204, *204*
Bondy, P.K., 69, 232, *233*
Bordley, J., 103, 105, 106, 107, 175, 215, 244
Botsford, T.W., 94, 212, *212*
Boyd, W., 22, 23, 83, 145, 169, 193, *194*
Braasch, J., 93
Braasch, W., 90, 94, 187, *188*
Brace, D., 259
Branch, W.T., 255
Brauckman, G., 171, 213, 232
Braude, A.I., 80, 253
Braun, W., 213
Braunwald, E., 81, 104, 142, 143, 159, 250, 251
Braverman, I.M., 233
Brenner, B.M., 245, 246
Broedel, M., 44, 101, 102, 103, 188, *189*, 192
Brown, J., 167, 168, 172, 207
Buchenau, T., 95, 207, 208, 210
Buchwald, A., 136
Buckstein, J., 201
Burrows, W., 88, 183, *183*
Burt, J., 154
Burton, A.P., 92, 94, 119, 159, 171, *171*, 217
Buschke, F., 200

Cabot, R.C., 106, 185
Calkins, E., 260
Callander, C.L., 104

Callaway, J.L., 204
Callen, P.W., 260
Campbell, M., 94, 159, 199, *199*, 213
Cann, C., 86
Cantarow, A., 197, *197*
Carey, Lewis S., 229
Carey, William B., 255
Carpenter, C., 260
Carter, W., 168, 172, 207, 233
Cattell, R.B., 94, 212, *212*
Cecil, R.L., 59–64, 74, 79, 109, *194*, 195, 210
Cerf, B., 7
Chabner, Davi-Ellen, 244
Chase, R.A., 236, *236*
Cherniack, L., 145, 223
Cherniack, R.M., 145, 223
Child, C.G., 223
Christensen, George C., 224, 229
Christensen, Halvor N., 226
Christie, R.V., 145, 227
Christopher, F., 84, 195, *195*, 199, 216
Christy, N., 69
Church, A., 180
Clark, S.L., 87, 191
Cleveland, G., 20
Clohecy, R.J., 230
Codding, M., 96, 212
Colaiace, W.M., 233
Colcock, B., 93
Cole, W., 92
Collins, W., 49
Compton-Burnett, I., 12
Comroe, J., 80
Conant, N., 204
Conn, Howard, 25, 113–120, 159, 201, 209, *209*, 230, 236
Conn, Rex B., 230
Converse, J.M., 228, *228*
Cooley, D., 84
Cormack, D., 58
Corner, T., 101, 103
Cornwall, J., 163
Cotton, F.J., 184, 185
Cousins, N., 200
Cowdry, E.V., 57, 58, 214, *214*
Craig, E.E., 136
Crile, G.W., 191, *191*
Crocker, A.C., 255
Cruickshank, A.H., 234
Cullen, M.G., 24
Cullen, T., 20, 24, 102, 103, 184, 188, *188*
Curtis, A.H., 196, *196*, 197, 198, 209
Cushing, H., 83, 85, 102, 103, 189, *189*
Custer, R.P., *208*, 209
Cutler, C.W., 203
Cutler, M., 200, *201*

DaCosta, J.C., 20, 170, 176, 177, *177*
Dale, H., 105
Dammin, G., 14
Daniels, L., 206
Dante, 100
Davidsohn, I., 49, 50, 224, 232
Davis, Edith, 85
Davis, Loyal, 30, 84–86, 92, 216, *216*
Davis, Nathan S., 207

Davis, Richard, 83, 85
DeBakey, M.E., 84
De la Vaga, J., 165
DeLee, J.B., 87, 186, *186*, 220
DePalma, A., 219
DeSchweinitz, G.E., 20, 176, *176*
De Voto, B., 80
Dickens, C., 31
Dietz, H., 115–117, 120, 134, 152, 155, 229, 238
Dinesen, I., 57
Dorland, W.A.N., 21, 179, 220
Doyle, A.C., 95
Dripps, R.D., 218
Drukker, J., 260
Dubos, R.J., 225
Duncan, G., 203, *204*
Dunphy, J.E., 80, 94, 145, 212, *212*
Dusseau, J., 69, *171*, 213, 237
Dyck, P.J., 238, *238*

Eckenhoff, J.E., 218
Eckert, W.G., 246
Eckman, J., 91
Edwards, J.E., 90, 223, *223*, 229
Einhorn, M., 191
Eisenberg, M.S., 249
Eisenhower, D., 67
Eliot, T.S., 173
Ellison, E.H., 218
Elwood, P.M., 229
Emerson, A.E., 208
Emmett, J.L., 90, 94, 159, 187, *188*, 227
Engel, G.L., 224
English, O.S., 204
Ettinger, S.J., 224, 238
Evans, Herbert, 44
Evans, Howard E., 224, *228*, 229
Evans, R.W., 234
Ewing, J., 190, *190*, 220

Fawcett, Don W., 55–57, 223, 229, *229*
Fawcett, Dorothy, 56
Federman, Daniel H., 81, 230
Feldman, W., 197, *197*
Felson, B., 223, *223*, 226
Feullian, W., 164
Finland, M., 98, 229
Finney, J., 103
Fischelis, R.P., 184
Fishbein, M., 207, *207*
Fleming, D., 9
Fletcher, S., 154
Florey, H., 214
Fomon, S.J., 230
Fordtran, J.S., 24
Foster, D.W., 258
Francone, C.A., 229
Fraser, R.G., 145, 233, 255
Frederickson, D., 76
Freeman, R.A., 88, 183
Freud, S., 180
Friedberg, C.K., 141, 142, 143, 209, *209*, 251
Friedenwald, J., 211
Friedman, E.A., 87, 186
Friel, J., 155

Friesen, S.R., 218
Frobisher, M., 193, *193*
Frye, W.W., 205
Fulton, J., 186, 206, *206*, 215, 221
Furness, H.H., 203

Gardner, Ernest, 222, *222*
Gardner, L., 233
Garland, L.H., 216
Garrison, F.H., 107, 175, 186, 220
Garrod, A., 76, 77
Gebhard, P.H., 25, 132
Gellis, S., 228, *228*, 234
Gerard, R.W., 54
Gest, J.M., 19
Gibbon, E., 3
Gibbon, John H., 224, *224*
Gifford, S.R., 200, *200*
Gilman, A., 23, 196
Gilman, D., 106
Gleason, E.B., 176
Glickman, I., 212
Glickman, Robert M., 81, 82
Goodman, L.S., 23, 196
Gorman, W., 167, 168
Goss, C.M., 170
Gould, A.P., 180
Gould, George M., 177
Gould, R.P., 56
Graber, T.M., 223
Graham, E., 92, 193, 196, *196*
Gramling, J., 163, *164*
Grant, J.C.B., 145, 171, 209, 248, 249
Gray, Donald J., 222, *222*
Gray, Henry, 12, 147, 170
Graybiel, A., 202
Green, W., 99
Greene, A.M., 110, 126, 203
Greene, Ryland, 7, 21–24, *22*, *25*, 39, 55, 87, 89,
    103, 110, 198, 202, 203, 236
  and advertising policy, 219
  and creation of medical dictionary, 21, 152, 179
  as manager of London office, 167, 180
  as senior editor, 182
  dealings with Loyal Davis, 83, 84
Greenhill, J.P., 87, 186, *186*
Gregg, A., 124, 139
Griffith, J.P.C., 109, 110, 190, *190*
Grimes, A., 27
Gross, Robert E., 93, 94, 100, 202, 212
Gross, Ruth T., 255
Guyton, Arthur C., 147–149, 162, 216, *216*, 219
Guyton, Ruth, 147, 149

Haagensen, C.D., 216, *216*, 226
Hacker, N., 260
Haddad, L.M., 255
Haeckel, E., 208
Haines, W.S., 181
Ham, A., 57, 58
Hamburger, J., 14, 245
Hamburger, V., 95, 215
Hamman, L., 106
Hanley, J., 77, 237
Harcourt, A., 259

Hardy, J.D., 221, *221*, 230, 234
Hare, H.A., 19, 175
Harris, E.D., 77
Harrison, Greg J., 260
Harrison, J.H., 159, 213, *214*
Harrison, Linda R., 260
Harrison, T., 69
Hartman, J., 207
Harvey, A.M., 81, 103, 105, 106, 175, 215, *215*, 244
Harvey, W., 10, 218
Hassall, R., 126, 163, 205
Hassin, G., 54
Hauff, G., 172
Haymaker, W., 205
Hebb, D.O., 218
Heller, L.B., 137
Helms, C.A., 260
Henry, J.B., 50, 232, *232*
Henselman, C., 222
Herrick, C.J., 54, 88, 187, *187*
Hertz, H., 17
Hess, O.T., 54
Hewitt, R., 90
Hill, A.V., 105
Hill, George J., 236, *237*
Hine, M.K., 218
Hines, E.A., 90, 206
Hinshaw, H.C., 216
Hogan, M.J., 211, *211*, 234
Hoguet, E., 119, 128, 232
Holbrook, P.R., 257
Holland, J., 109
Holt, Henry, 259
Holt, L. E., 109
Holzworth, J., 100
Hood, A., 136
Hoover, H., 74
Hotchkiss, D., 21, 119, 201
Howell, W.H., 20, 162, 178, *178*, 206, 214
Huber, C., 20
Hubert, J.P., 258
Huffman, J.W., 197, 209, 224
Hughes, J., 145, 146, 162
Hume, D., 58
Hunter, George W., 205
Hunter, John, 11
Hurley, H., 93, 194, 217
Hurwitz, S., 251, 252
Huxley, T., 91, 121
Hyman, H.T., 141, 159, 206, *207*

Ingelfinger, F., 97, 98, 229
Ingraham, N.R., 194
Isselbacher, K.J., 81
Iyer, P.W., 260

Jackson, Chevalier, 20, 176, 177, 192, *192*
Jackson, Michael, 233
Jacob, S.W., 229
James, W., 99
Janicki, J.S., 260
Jiasi, Hwang, 68
Johns, R., 81, 105
Johnson, Samuel, 11, 155, 156, 165
Johnson, Thomas W., 236

Jones, F.A., 204
Jones, Tom, 31, 44, 45
Jordan, E.O., 87, 183, 220

Kadir, S., 260
Kagan, B.M., 228
Kalckar, H.M., 225
Kanavel, A., 83, 84
Kanehara, H., 164, *164*
Keane, C.B., 152, 154–156, 235, *236*
Keefer, C., 71, 82, 100
Keen, W.W., 20, 176, 186
Keith, A., 193
Keller, W., 76
Kelley, W.N., 75, 77
Kelly, H.A., 20, 103, 182, *182*, 184
Kennedy, R.H., 229
Kerley, P., 168
Kiernan, P.D., 258
King, B.G., 183
Kinsey, A.C., 25, 119, 123–139, *124*, 149, 208, 213
Kirk, R.W., 224, 233
Kirkpatrick, J.A., 218, *218*
Klebs, A.C., 102
Klein, J.O., 245
Kligman, A.M., 93, 194, 216
Knopf, A., 7
Knopf, B., 7
Knuppel, R.A., 260
Kokko, J.P., 260
Kolb, L., 198, *198*
Kottke, F.J., 229
Krebs, H., 65, 80
Krumbhaar, E., 189
Krusen, F., 90, 202, *203*, 229

Labat, G., 191, *191*, 192, 220
Ladd, W.E., 94, 202
Lafayette, M., 22
Lahey, F., 89, *202*
Lambert, E.H., 238
Langman, J., 247, 248, 249
Laufman, H., 211, *212*
Laurie, G., 232
Lea, V.A., 23
Lee, E.W., 27
Leeson, C.R., 145, 229, *230*
Leeson, T.S., 145, 229, *230*
Leonard, A.E., 167
Leonard, Ellis P., 221, 224
Lester, R.G., 229
Levine, Melvin D., 255
Levine, Norman S., 260
Levine, Samuel A., 143, 199, *199*
Levy, B.M., 218
Lichtenberg, G.C., 151
Lightfoot, J., 4, 5
Lilienthal, H., 193, *194*
Lindner, A.E., 234
Linton, R.R., 236, *236*, 246
Livingood, C.S., 26, 204
Loeb, Jacques, 62
Loeb, Robert F., 62–65, 74, 78, 79, 210, *210*, 225
Longcope, W.T., 106
Lookingbill, D.P., 260

Luckmann, J., 152, 238
Ludwig, K., 17
Lundy, J., 90, 203, *204*
Lutz, J., 118, 119, 125, 129, 130, 157–159, 213, 232
Lyons, W.R., 209

MacCallum, W.G., 23, 189, *189*
MacFarland, W., 48, 49
Machiavelli, N., 124
Mackey, T.E., 260
Mackie, T., 205
Macklem, P.T., 145
Macmillan, W., 169
Major, R.H., 199, *200*
Majors, J.A., 159, *160*, 161
Mallory, F.B., 178, *178*, 187
Maloney, M., 31
Marks, J.G., 260
Marlow, D., 152, 223, *223*
Marsden, P., 69
Marshak, R.H., 234, *234*
Marshall, E.K., 105
Marshall, Wayne, 23
Martin, Clyde E., 25, 127, 132, 208
Martin, Joseph B., 81
Masserman, J.H., 88, 206, 214
Masterton, W.L., 230
Maximow, A., 21, 52–55, 162, 196, 198, 220
Mayo, W., 89
McArthur, L.L., 30
McCarty, M., 239
McClendon, J., 159
McConnell, J., 212
McCullough, K., 155
McCusick, V.A., 81
McDermott, W., 64, 66, 69–74, 77, 168, 216, 226, *226*, 250, 253
McDonald, W.I., 260
McGilvery, R.W., 233, *233*
McIntosh, R., 109
McKay, J., 111
McKhann, G.M., 260
McLester, J., 195, *195*
McMillen, C., 123
McMurrich, J.P., 183
Mead, M., 135
Meier, A., 175, 237
Mencken, H.L., 102, 192
Mendel, G., 76
Meschan, I., 161, 211, *211*, 243
Millard, N.D., 183
Miller, Benjamin F., 152–156, 235, *235*
Miller, Malcolm E., 224, 229
Miller, Zelma, 154
Mink, S., 231, 232
Mitchell, A.G., 109, 110, 204
Modell, W., 231, *231*
Moe, H.A., 225
Monsen, H., 171
Moore, Carl, 69
Moore, Francis D., 95, 96, 100, 219, *219*, 230, 256
Moore, J. George, 260
Moore, Joseph, 71
Moore, Keith L., 145, 237, *237*
Morgagni, G.B., 10, 15
Morison, R.S., 124, 225

Moschella, S., 93, 194, 217
Most, H., 91, 119, 136, 138, *164*, 167, 168, *171*, 215, 235
Moynihan, B., 20, 29, 167, 181, 183
Mudd, E., 124
Mudd, S., 124
Mulholland, J.H., 218, *218*
Mumford, L.Q., 7, 41
Munro, D., 117, 118
Murphy, John B., 20, 24, 27–40, *28*, 44, 84, 90, 185
Murphy, Michael, 27
Murray, J., 69, 80
Muschenheim, C., 216
Musser, J.H., 20
Myers, G.H., 159

Nachman, R., 69
Nadas, A.S., 218
Nathan, D.G., 237, *237*
Nelson, M., 110
Nelson, Waldo E., 109–111, 203, 204, *205*
Neufeld, H.N., 229
Newton, I., 10
Nikanov, F., 52, 54
Noller, C.R., 210
Norris, G.W., 189, *189*
Nothnagel, H., 20, 180
Novak, E., 202
Noyes, A.P., 198, *198*

Ochsner, A., 30, 84
Ogle, K.S., 90, 209
O'Rahilly, R., 222, *222*
Oski, F.A., 237, *237*
Osler, W., 14, 106, 180
Owens, A.H., 81

Page, H.J., 167
Paley, W., 26
Paré, Ambroise, 11
Paré, J.A.P., 145, 233, 255
Park, O., 208
Park, T., 208
Parsons, L., 94, 212, *213*, 224
Partain, C.L., 255, 256
Pearl, R., 192, *192*
Pepper, W., 20, 177
Perkins, Maxwell, 7
Perkins, Sherman E., 100, 171, *171*, 220, 221
Pernkopf, E., 170, 171
Petersdorf, R., 65, 66, 81
Peterson, F., 180, 181
Petry, L., 153
Pfister, K., 168
Pierce, W.A., 167, 172
Piette, E., 54
Pillsbury, D.M., 26, 93, 194, 204, 216, *217*
Plum, F., 69, 260
Pollock, L., 83
Pomeroy, W., 25, 127, 132, 208
Poppen, J.L., 93, 221, *221*
Potter, L., 13, 104, 113–120, 126, 141, 203
Prentiss, C.W., 87, 187
Price, A.L., 153

Procter, W.C., 109
Prosser, C.L., 95, 210

Rakel, R.E., 236, *236*
Randall, H.T., 230
Ranson, S.W., 87, 191, *191*, 220
Ravdin, I.S., 92
Reagan, R., 86
Rector, F.C., 245
Reed, S., 92
Reichard, P., 79
Reid, D.E., 95, 224, *225*
Reines, L., 260
Relman, A., 98, 229
Remington, J.S., 245
Resnick, W., 69
Rich, A., 23, 106
Ripol, E., 165
Ripol, M., 165
Robbins, E., 147
Robbins, S.L., 145–147, 162, 218, *218*
Roberts, H.J., 218
Robinson, Judith, 24
Robinson, Roscoe, 69
Robson, A.W.M., 181
Rogers, D., 72
Rolleston, H.D., 182
Romer, A.S., 95, 209
Roosevelt, T., 29, 30
Rosenberg, L.E., 232
Ross, Harold, 7
Ross, J., 149, 162
Ross, Richard S., 81
Rossetti, D.G., 8
Rothman, R.E., 238, *239*
Rowan, R., 86, 95, 97, 118, 120, 135, 159, 171, 213
Rozhestvensky, Z.P., 51, 52
Rubenstein, E., 81
Ruch, T.C., 221, *222*
Ruddy, S., 77
Rutherford, Ernest, 10
Rutherford, Robert B., 246, 247

Sabin, F., 53
Sabiston, D., 86, 224, *224*, 235
Safar, P., 249
Samiy, A.H., 252, 253
Sanford, A., 48, 49, 195, *195*
Saunders, Dorothy, 25, 124
Saunders, Lawrence, 21, *25*, 45, 89, 101, 103, 167, 171, *171*, 215, 231
  and agreement on JAMA advertising policy, 158, 159
  and creation of Art Department, 43
  and international publishing, 168
  and Johns Hopkins Art Fellowship, 26, 226, 227
  and marketing of Conn *Current Therapy*, 118, 119
  and publication of Kinsey report, 124, 125, 127, 128, 132, 135
  as company president, 25, 198–199
Saunders, Louise, 17, 21
Saunders, Walter Burns, 17–21, *18*, 24, 25, 41, 89, 157, 167, 175, 179, 182, 220
Schaffer, A.J., 221, 222, 227

Scheie, H.G., 200, *201*, 233
Schepartz, B., 197, *197*
Schepens, C.L., 255
Schmidt, A., 118
Schmidt, Karl P., 208
Schwartz, G., 249
Scott, J., 172
Scudder, C.L., 20, 180
Sellew, G., 223
Semmelweis, I., 9
Senn, N., 20
Shackelford, R.T., 45, 103–105, 214, *214*, 231
Shafer, W.G., 218
Shakespeare, W. (*King Henry V*), 149
Shambaugh, G.E., 219, *219*
Shanks, S.C., 168
Shaw, Alice C., 44
Shaw, G.B., 9
Shelley, D., 235
Shelley, Walter B., 93, 194, 216, *217*, 235
Shepard, W.C., *41*, 43–45, 118, 205
Shoemaker, W.C., 256, 257
Showers, M.J., 183
Shryock, R.H., 1
Sigerist, H.E., 15
Simeone, F.A., 238, *239*
Skinner, B., 226
Skinner, Eugene W., 199, *199*
Sledge, C.B., 77, 260
Sleisenger, M., 24, 69, 79, 245
Sloane, S.B., 236
Slowinski, E., 230
Smith, Austen, 158, 159
Smith, David T., 204
Smith, Frank, 79
Smith, LeRoy, *25*
Smith, Lloyd H., 70, 73, 74, 77, 79, 80, 81, 253, 260
Snell, A.M., 202, *202*
Sobotta, J., 183
Sodeman, Thomas, 253
Sodeman, William A., *209*, 210, 253
Sollmann, T., 180, *181*, 220
Solomon, S., 31
Sommers, S.C., 224
Sorensen, K., 152, 238
Soskice, F., 137
Spalding, L., 184
Spector, W.S., 217
Spencer, Frank C., 86, 224, *224*
Spencer, William H., 211
Spitz, Harold B., 226
Spitz, Sophie, 205
Squire, L., 233, *234*
Stanbury, J., 75, 76
Starzl, T.E., 227, *228*
Stead, E., 65, 76
Stein, J.H., 81
Stelwagon, H.W., 20
Stengel, A., 180
Stetten, DeWitt, 75, 79
Stevenson, A., 7
Stevenson, R., 229
Stewart, H., 114
Stilwell, D., 236
Stokes, J.H., 93, 194, *194*
Stone, J., 249

Stool, S., 255
Storey, P., 249
Strickland, G.T., 205
Strutynsky, N., 233
Sturtevant, A.H., 200
Sulzberger, M.B., 26, 204
Swartzwelder, J.C., 205

Taber, C.W., 153, 154, 155
Tachdjian, M., 100, 235, 255
Tannen, R.I., 260
Taylor, Anita, 260
Taylor, E., 155
Taylor, N.B., 145
Tedeschi, Cesare, 246
Tedeschi, Luke, 246
Thier, S.O., 80, 253
Thoma, K.H., 199, *199*
Thomas, Clayton L., 153
Thomas, Lewis, 4
Thomas, R.K., 238
Thompson, J.S., 145, 229
Thompson, M.W., 145, 229
Thompson, W.L., 257
Thorn, G., 69, 114
Tietz, N.W., 50, 234, *234*, 255
Todd, J.C., 47–50, 184, 195
Togo, H., 51, 52
Trumper, M., 197, *197*
Tuft, L., 199, *200*

Ulfelder, H., 94, 212, 213, *213*
Ulrich, S., 260
Urban, M., 170
Utz, D.C., 159

Vandam, L.D., 218
vanden Beemt, T., 171, *171*, 235
van der Rohe, M., 13
Vaughan, V., 111
Vesalius, A., 10
Villee, C., 95, 210, *210*
Virchow, R., 17
Vogler, J.B., 260
Voltaire, F., 123
Vondeling, J., 230

Wagner, David, 249
Wagner, Henry N., 231, *231*
Wallace, A., 69
Waller, E., 103
Walsh, A., 14
Walters, H., 101, 102, 103
Walters, W., *201*, 202
Wangensteen, O., 92
Warbasse, J.P., 190, *190*
Warren, John C., 20, 180
Warren, Kenneth W., 94, 212
Warren, R., 99, 226
Warwick, R., 169
Watson, W.D., 19, 21, *25*, 118, 119, 126, 159, 182, 198, 205, 219, 232, 238
Weber, K.T., 260

Webster, J.C., 184, *184*
Webster, Ralph W., 181
Wechsberg, J., 10
Wechsler, I.S., 195, *195*
Weddell, J.E., 234
Weinstein, A.S., 226
Weiss, E., 204, *204*
Weiss, Leon, 56
Weiss, Paul A., 95, 215
Weissman, B.N.W., 260
Welch, W.H., 9, 107
Wells, Benjamin B., 49, 50
Wells, H. Gideon, 88, 183, *183*
Welty, C.J., 224
Wheeler, C., 126, 152
White, E.B., 14
White, J.W., 20, 176
White, Paul D., 141, 202
Wilder, R., 202, *202*
Williams, Hibbard, 79
Williams, Marian, 206
Williams, Peter L., 169
Williams, Robert H., 79, 98, 99, 210, *210*, 258
Willier, B.H., 95, 215
Wilson, J.D., 81, 258

Winchester, J., 255
Windle, W., 202
Wintrobe, M., 69
Witten, D.M., 159
Wodehouse, P.G., 7
Woerdeman, M.W., 247, 249
Wood, Barry, 69
Wood, Paul, 143
Woodhall, B., 205, 209
Worth, C.B., 205
Worthingham, C., 206, *206*
Wright, Almroth, 10
Wright, James H., 178
Wright, Robert E., 152–155, 218, 238
Wyngaarden, J.B., 70, 73–78, 80, 81, 250, 253

Xiancai, Wang, 68

Youmans, J.R., 236

Zuelzer, W., 237
Zuidema, G., 104, 105

This limited edition of *An Informal History of W. B. Saunders Company* was produced by the employees of Saunders and selected suppliers. Carolyn Naylor was the Production Manager. The text was copy-edited by Elizabeth J. Taylor and Evelyn Weiman. Lorraine B. Kilmer designed the text and cover. Patricia Morrison with the assistance of Walter Verbitski handled the illustration processing. Composition and illustration reproduction were provided by the Saunders Typesetting staff.

Text typeface is Palatino and display typography is Palatino and Helvetica. Text paper is 60-pound Smooth Antique Offset by Glatfelter and the end papers are 80-pound Rainbow Parchment by Ecological Fibers. Cover material is Roxite C cloth by Holliston Mills. The cover dies were made by Progressive Brass Die Company. The book was printed and bound at Maple Press.